Outpatient Gynecologic Surgery

Outpatient Gynecologic Surgery

A. JEFFERSON PENFIELD, MD, FACOG
Associate Professor
Department of Obstetrics and Gynecology
Health Science Center
State University of New York
Syracuse, New York

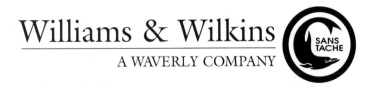

A WAVERLY COMPANY

BALTIMORE • PHILADELPHIA • LONDON • PARIS • BANGKOK
BUENOS AIRES • HONG KONG • MUNICH • SYDNEY • TOKYO • WROCLAW

Editor: Charles W. Mitchell
Managing Editor: Grace E. Miller
Production Coordinator: Raymond E. Reter
Copy Editor: Pamela Goehrig Thomson
Designer: Dan Pfisterer
Illustration Planner: Ray Lowman
Cover Designer: Dan Pfisterer
Typesetter: University Graphics Inc., Atlantic Highlands, New Jersey
Printer & Binder: R. R. Donnelley & Sons, Crawfordsville, Indiana
Digitized Illustrations: University Graphics Inc., Atlantic Highlands, New Jersey

Copyright © 1997 Williams & Wilkins

351 West Camden Street
Baltimore, Maryland 21201-2436 USA

Rose Tree Corporate Center
1400 North Providence Road
Building II, Suite 5025
Media, Pennsylvania 19063-2043 USA

All rights reserved. This book is protected by copyright. No part of this book may be reproduced in any form or by any means, including photocopying, or utilized by any information storage and retrieval system without written permission from the copyright owner.

Accurate indications, adverse reactions and dosage schedules for drugs are provided in this book, but it is possible that they may change. The reader is urged to review the package information data of the manufacturers of the medications mentioned.

Printed in the United States of America

Library of Congress Cataloging-in-Publication Data
Penfield, A. Jefferson (Amos Jefferson), 1927–
    Outpatient gynecologic surgery / A. Jefferson Penfield, with
  contributions by Paul Allen, Ilan Timor-Tritsch, Morris Wortman.
        p. cm.
    Includes bibliographical references and index.
    ISBN 0-683-30176-4
    1. Generative organs, Female—Surgery. 2. Ambulatory surgery.
  I. Title.
    [DNLM: 1. Genital Diseases, Female—surgery. 2. Ambulatory
  Surgery. WP 660 P398o 1997]
  RG104.P3874 1997
  618.1'45—dc21
  DNLM/DLC
  for Library of Congress   96-49541
                                                            CIP

The publishers have made every effort to trace the copyright holders for borrowed material. If they have inadvertently overlooked any, they will be pleased to make the necessary arrangements at the first opportunity.

To purchase additional copies of this book, call our customer service department at **(800) 638-0672** or fax orders to **(800) 447-8438**. For other book services, including chapter reprints and large quantity sales, ask for the Special Sales department.

Canadian customers should call **(800) 665-1148**, or fax **(800) 665-0103**. For all other calls originating outside of the United States, please call **(410) 528-4223** or fax us at **(410) 528-8550**.

Visit Williams & Wilkins on the Internet: http://www.wwilkins.com or contact our customer service department at **custserv@wwilkins.com**. Williams & Wilkins customer service representatives are available from 8:30 am to 6:00 pm, EST, Monday through Friday, for telephone access.

97 98 99 00 01
1 2 3 4 5 6 7 8 9 10

About the Author

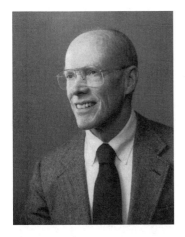

A. Jefferson Penfield has been in private obstetrics-gynecology practice for 33 years. He received his BA degree from Princeton in 1949 and his MD from Johns Hopkins in 1953. After an internship and general practice at the Rochester General Hospital, he served 2 years in the U.S. Army. After an ob-gyn residency at New York Hospital, he established a solo practice in Syracuse and joined the clinical faculty at the Health Science Center.

For the past 30 years, Dr. Penfield has had a special interest in surgical fertility control. He designed his own office surgery for laparoscopy, minilaparotomy, dilation and curettage, loop electrical excision procedure, first trimester abortion, and other procedures, all under local anesthesia. He also initiated similar services at the Syracuse Planned Parenthood Center while serving as medical director from 1966 to 1976. From 1978 to 1985, he traveled abroad under the sponsorship of the Association for Voluntary Surgical Contraception and the Johns Hopkins Program for International Education in Gynecology and Obstetrics to assist with laparoscopy and minilaparotomy programs in Afghanistan, Bangladesh, the Philippines, Indonesia, Mexico, and Jamaica. In 1980, he visited China with an American Association of Gynecological Laparoscopists team under the leadership of Jordan Phillips. He also served as a consultant for laparotomy sterilization and minilaparotomy programs in Baltimore, New York, Boston, Cleveland, Detroit, San Francisco, Los Angeles, and San Diego.

Dr. Penfield has authored two books pertaining to outpatient surgery, namely *Female Sterilization by Minilaparotomy or Open Laparoscopy* (1980) and *Gynecologic Surgery Under Local Anesthesia* (1986).

Preface

The time has arrived for a new and exciting development in gynecologic surgery: the emergence and increasing credibility of outpatient surgical units, free-standing surgery centers, and office surgeries for the performance of laparoscopy, minilaparotomy, hysteroscopy, and other invasive procedures formerly performed only in hospital operating rooms.

What has spurred this new development? Two factors are responsible: the high degree of safety convincingly demonstrated during the past 26 years by individual surgeons in outpatient facilities, particularly when operating primarily under local anesthesia, and the need to curb the cost of surgical care, responding to the demands of third-party insurers.

The immediate catalyst for *Outpatient Gynecologic Surgery* was provided by the First Masters' Course in Outpatient Laparoscopy under Local Anesthesia (OLULA) in Tuskegee, Alabama on May 3–5, 1996. This conference was organized by Beverly Love, MD, and Roosevelt McCorvey, MD, Montgomery, Alabama. For the first time, outpatient laparoscopic surgery was the focus of an International Conference open to all interested practitioners. The list of invited participants at this conference included the following individuals, some of whom have led the way in outpatient laparoscopy for the past 26 years: Paul M. Allen, MD; James Daniell, MD; Larry Demco, MD; James Dingfelder, MD; Joseph Feste, MD; John Fishburne, MD; Ernst Friedrich, MD; Jaroslav Hulka, MD; Gary Lipscomb, MD; Beverly Love, MD; Dan Martin, MD; Roosevelt McCorvey MD; A.J. Penfield, MD; Alfred Poindexter, MD; Fred Schnepper, MD; and Morris Wortman, MD.

In this book I expand the concept of outpatient gynecologic surgery under local anesthesia. I bring together and describe several of the most frequently performed operations in gynecology. My personal experience during the past 23 years, with more than 14,000 patients operated on in free-standing facilities, demonstrates that these operations may be performed *safely* under local anesthesia. Patients appreciate the high degree of pain relief, the absence of side effects, and the rapid postoperative recovery.

The basics of outpatient gynecologic surgery are emphasized to provide a solid background on which the individual gynecologist can introduce his or her favorite instruments and techniques. During the past 10 years, an explosive increase in surgical instrument technology has occurred. A number of innovative operations, including microlaparoscopic procedures, can be safely transferred into the outpatient setting, provided the basic safeguards described in this book are followed. As promising as some of the newer operations appear to be, insufficient time has elapsed since their introduction to determine their value in the future.

Most operations described in this text are well established and time tested in all developed nations. The information and recommendations concerning analgesia and anesthesia, planning of outpatient facilities, patient education and counseling, and surgical safeguards are equally applicable to modern innovative surgical procedures.

The first chapter deals with local versus general anesthesia. The second covers the pharmacology, toxicology, and clinical use of local anesthetic agents. Chapter 3 reviews outpatient facilities. Chapters 4 through 12 are devoted to specific operations, including four by guest contributors. Chapter 6 contains a discussion of hysteroscopic surgery, including endomyometrial excision, by Morris Wortman, MD. Chapter 11, by Ilan E. Timor-Tritsch, MD, and Ana Monteagudo, MD, and Chapter 12 by Drs. Monteagudo, Timor-Tritsch, and Jodi P. Lerner, MD, cover transvaginal ultrasound as it relates to improved diagnosis and puncture procedures. Chapter 13, contributed by Paul M. Allen, MD, deals with risk management, accreditation, and reimbursement.

Repeatedly within the text I stress the importance of sensitive preliminary counseling, supportive conversation with the patient during surgery, the absolute necessity of gentleness in the handling of tissues by the surgeon, and the next day follow-up of the patient by members of the staff.

Outpatient Gynecologic Surgery is offered to gynecologists who wish to operate safely under local anesthesia. In addition, much of the material may interest counselors, nurses, anesthesiologists, and administrators of outpatient surgical clinics.

Contributors

PAUL M. ALLEN, MD, MHA
Chief Executive Officer and Medical Director
Women's Center for Health Care
Pascagoula, Mississippi

JODI P. LERNER, MD
Assistant Professor
Clinical Obstetrics and Gynecology
Columbia Presbyterian Medical Center
New York, New York

WILLIAM E. LINDEMAN, AIA
WEL Designs
Tucson, Arizona

ANA MONTEAGUDO, MD
Associate Professor of Obstetrics and Gynecology
Maternal-Fetal Medicine Specialist
Columbia Presbyterian Medical Center
New York, New York

A. JEFFERSON PENFIELD, MD, FACOG
Associate Professor
Department of Obstetrics and Gynecology
Health Science Center
State University of New York
Syracuse, New York

ILAN E. TIMOR-TRITSCH, MD
Professor of Obstetrics and Gynecology
Director of Obstetric/Gynecologic Ultrasound
Columbia Presbyterian Medical Center
New York, New York

MORRIS WORTMAN, MD, FACOG
Clinical Associate Professor of Gynecology
University of Rochester School of Medicine
Director, The Center for Menstrual Disorders and Reproductive Choice
Rochester, New York

Contents

About the Author / v
Preface / vii
Contributors / ix

1. Local Anesthesia Versus General Anesthesia / 1
2. Local Anesthetic Agents / 9
3. Outpatient Facilities for Operations Under Local Anesthesia / 21
4. Dilatation and Curettage / 29
5. First Trimester Abortion / 41
6. Diagnostic and Operative Hysteroscopy / 65
7. Laparoscopy for Diagnosis or Sterilization / 131
8. Suprapubic Minilaparotomy / 155
9. Outpatient Female Sterilization / 173
10. Additional Gynecologic Operations Under Local Anesthesia / 187
11. Office Ultrasound / 197
12. Transvaginal Sonographic Puncture Procedures / 229
13. Accreditation, Risk Management, and Reimbursement / 245
14. Conclusion / 299

Index / 301

1. Local Anesthesia Versus General Anesthesia

A. JEFFERSON PENFIELD

The choice of anesthetic technique is determined by the personal preferences of the surgeon, the anesthesiologist, and the patient and by the extent of surgery, the patient's medical history, the location of the operating room, and the facilities available.

SUITABILITY FOR A GIVEN OPERATION

For a specific operation to be a relatively painless exercise, it is necessary to select the type of anesthesia that will best fulfill three criteria: safety, minimal disturbance of physiology, and rapid recovery. Thus, these are the three most important factors to consider.

These factors are thoroughly explored by Fishburne (1, 2), who describes indication, techniques, and complications of different types of anesthesia for individual gynecologic operations. Until the early 1970s, most surgical procedures in gynecology and obstetrics in North America were performed under general, spinal, or epidural anesthesia in the hospital operating and delivery rooms. Local or nerve block anesthesia was largely reserved for such minor procedures as episiotomy repair, spontaneous deliveries, or removal of small skin tumors. Occasionally, cesarean sections in severely compromised patients, such as pre-eclamptics, would call for local abdominal wall infiltration. With growing concern regarding safety and economy, a new flood of elective abortions, and the acceptance of sterilizations, however, increasing numbers of gynecologists decided to perform a variety of operations in outpatient or free-standing facilities.

For example, epidural anesthesia for laparoscopy and minilaparotomy, although safe and highly effective if administered by skilled personnel, requires "preloading" with intravenous fluids and proved to be cumbersome and time-consuming in many busy operating schedules. Spinal anesthesia for these operations could be administered more rapidly but was frequently followed by urinary retention or headaches.

Additionally, evidence was accumulating that both first trimester abortion procedures and dilatation and evacuation operations between 13 and 24 weeks' gestation were associated with fewer critical complications when performed under local rather than general anesthesia. Peterson et al. (3) found that the risk of death from first trimester abortion was two to four times higher under general than under local anesthesia, mostly because of a greater likelihood of hemorrhage and perforation. Hemorrhage from uterine relaxation was found to occur most often under halothane and enflurane anesthesia and very infrequently under paracervical block (4). More recently, because of the increasing use of local anesthesia and improved surgical techniques, mortality rates from first trimester abortion have declined. For example, in 1985, only six deaths occurred in the United States, or one death for every 200,000 legal abortions (5). Data on second trimester dilatation and evacuation were presented by Mackay et al. (6). This study shows that hemorrhage requiring transfusion occurred more than four times more often under general anesthesia, although retained products, postoperative hemorrhage, and repeat curettage were more likely if the initial procedure was performed under local anesthesia.

It also became apparent that there was no justification for putting most patients to sleep for diagnostic curettage. The choice of general anesthesia for more major procedures was also questioned. Before 1970, few gynecologists would consider entering the abdominal cavity under local anesthesia except in emergency situations. In the past 26 years, however, worldwide experience has demonstrated the advantages of minilaparotomy and laparoscopy performed under local anesthetic infiltration of the abdominal wall preceded by intravenous analgesic premedication.

As soon as these safer alternatives were demonstrated, concern about risks and complications of general anesthesia increased. When performing laparoscopy, for example, Fishburne (1) described complications of general anesthesia that, although uncommon, continue to occur even in skilled hands, including hypoxia, hypercarbia, pneumothorax, hypotension, hypertension, gas embolism, cardiac arrhythmia, regurgitation, and gastric dilatation. Serious consequences may arise from any of these complications.

Complications of local anesthesia, on the other hand, are far less numerous and only rarely critical, including excessive drug-induced sedation and narcosis and toxicity due to overdosage of local anesthetic drugs (1, 2) (see Chapter 2). If patients are managed prudently, these complications should be rare.

Local anesthesia has gained worldwide acceptance because it is predictably effective and provides a high level of safety, minimal physiologic disturbance, and rapid recovery. In addition, unlike hypnosis or acupuncture, local anesthesia is effective in all patients and requires far less time for counseling and preparation. Clearly, for most major abdominal or vaginal operations, general or conduction anesthesia is required. On the other hand, for such operations as dilatation and curettage (D&C), pregnancy termination, laparoscopy, minilaparotomy, and hysteroscopy, local anesthesia fulfills the above three criteria better than general anesthesia, unless it is contraindicated by medical, surgical, or personal considerations. Unfortunately, in most hospitals today, extraneous factors, mostly personal in nature, usually are responsible for the rejection of local anesthesia.

First, the surgeon is more comfortable if the patient is asleep. The doctor is not distracted by talking with the patient during surgery and can express him or herself freely to nurses or to other physicians without worrying that the patient will be alarmed or upset by what she hears. The surgeon's attention will not be diverted by explaining complications to the patient during surgery. Second, many surgeons object to local anesthesia because they find it cumbersome or because it takes a few minutes of their time.

Third, anesthesiologists feel more useful if their services are fully used. Many gynecologists have told me that they agree reluctantly to the use of general anesthesia because they need the cooperation of their anesthesiologist for their major cases. Operating-room protocol in the United States is frequently dominated by the anesthesiologist, who likes to be in control and can process more cases in a given time period if general or conduction anesthesia is used routinely, particularly if one patient is anesthetized in a connecting room while the previously scheduled patient's operation is being completed.

Finally, some surgeons and anesthesiologists proceed on the basis of the patient's preferences of being asleep or awake during the procedure. Especially if the doctor has not already stated his or her preference, the patient may be influenced exclusively by her fear of pain and say, "I want to be put out." The patient's fears and desires should be respectfully addressed, but I believe that most rational patients will accept the best judgment of their doctor concerning the safest and most appropriate form of anesthesia, once clearly explained.

In a hospital operating room, or in a large surgery center where there is dispersal of responsibility, the pragmatic surgeon is likely to be governed by such extraneous factors as those noted above. The surgeon learns to compromise to operate in a friendly and cooperative environment. On the other hand, a surgeon who has established his or her own office-surgery unit or free-standing center is less likely to be governed by extraneous factors and may choose to operate exclusively under local anesthesia and thus eliminate the need for general anesthesia personnel and equipment.

Let me emphasize that I am referring to the most frequently performed operations in gynecology, namely excisional biopsy, D&C, loop electrical excision procedure, pregnancy termination, and laparoscopy, as well as to less frequently performed procedures, such as minilaparotomy, hysteroscopy, Bartholin cyst marsupialization, and deep cervical conization. If the surgeon is precise and gentle, these operations can be performed under local anesthesia with maximum safety, minimum physiologic disturbance, and optimal postoperative recovery. On the other hand, if extensive manipulations are required, general or conduction anesthesia is indicated. For example, surgeons who perform multiple laparoscopic biopsies, tubal surgery, extensive lysis of adhesions, or laser surgery with two or more abdominal incisions require general or epidural anesthesia in most cases.

PATIENT SELECTION

During the past 22 years, particularly with reference to patients for laparoscopy or minilaparotomy, one question asked by visiting gynecologists is, "How do you screen your patients for local anesthesia?"

The implication of this question is that local anesthesia may not provide sufficient pain relief and there must be a high percentage of patients who are not suitable candidates. On the contrary, in my own practice, only about 0.3% of patients required general or conduction anesthesia for laparoscopy, minilaparotomy, or abortion. The laparoscopies were single incision, most often for purposes of sterilization, but occasionally for diagnosis of obscure pelvic masses, investigation of pelvic pain, or documentation of endometriosis.

Which patients do require general or conduction anesthesia for these operations? Those who cannot relax or cooperate enough for office examination need general anesthesia. They may include (*a*) patients with irreducible anxiety who become rigid at the very prospect of a pelvic examination; (*b*) patients with profound mental retardation who cannot lie still either for examination or surgery (although some retarded patients are remarkably trusting and cooperative and therefore easy to examine); (*c*) adolescents with immature vaginas who cannot relax sufficiently; (*d*) postmenopausal women with vaginal atrophy who cannot tolerate either pelvic examination or surgery while awake; (*e*) patients with a language barrier or severe hearing loss; and (*f*) patients with extreme obesity, physical deformities, or anomalies who require maximal relaxation. However, most patients who can communicate, relax, and cooperate sufficiently for a satisfactory pelvic examination will receive adequate pain relief from local anesthesia.

SURGEON SELECTION

Surgeon selection for local anesthesia is just as critical as patient selection. Many surgeons, because of their own training and experience, are uncomfortable or inept when operating under local anesthesia.

To succeed with local anesthesia for the various operations described in this book, the gynecologist must be sensitive to the patient's needs and apprehension, consistently gentle and confident, and, along with the nurse or counselor, should be ready to talk with the patient during surgery. Many gynecologists prefer to walk into the operating "theater," perform surgically, and walk out. They wish to avoid the distraction of communicating with the patient. If they are training residents or demonstrating procedures, they find it much easier to do so if the patient is asleep. Many are also reluctant to submit the patient even to mild discomfort. These surgeons have chosen to disqualify themselves from the use of local anesthesia. The basic reason why many gynecologists do not attempt surgery under local anesthesia, however, is that they did not learn this procedure during their residency. Fortunately, others did learn the necessary skills after going into practice.

It is hoped that residency directors will follow the lead of individuals such as Jaroslav Hulka and John Fishburne, who pioneered a prototype outpatient laparoscopic sterilization service at the University of North Carolina at Chapel Hill. In that program, residents continue to be taught the indications, limitations, and techniques of local anesthesia in gynecologic surgery.

Other leaders who have taken the responsibility of instructing their residents in laparoscopy under local anesthesia are Ernst Friedrich (7), who pioneered the technique of volonelgesia (vocal reassurance, local anesthesia, and neuroleptanalgesia), and Gary Lipscomb (8), who supervised his resident staff in a comparative study of general versus local anesthesia, with emphasis on cost savings.

A critical warning to the occasionally unwise selection of local anesthesia was expressed to me by David Stark, MD, former chairman of the Department of Anesthesia, Crouse-Memorial Hospital, Syracuse, New York. He states, "Quite often the very sick patient is chosen for surgery under local. Impossibilities are often attempted with consequent loss of confidence in local techniques. Having to 'rescue' a failed local in midoperation is a difficult and dangerous task" (Stark, personal communication).

STAFF SELECTION

Operations performed under local anesthesia require smooth teamwork and minimal turnover in staff personnel. Nurses must become very familiar with techniques, instruments, and surgeons with whom they will work. Each member of the team should be kind and reassuring in communicating with the patient but not overly solicitous. The staff should be skilled in working under local anesthesia and positive in their support.

COUNSELING

Two essential goals in counseling patients about local anesthesia are to win the confidence of the patient and to inform and prepare her so that she will not experience unpleasant surprises or unexpected pain during the operation. If possible, the counseling should be done during the initial visit by the nurse or counselor who will be present in the room for surgery. The physician also interviews and examines the patient during the initial visit and should supplement the counseling as needed.

The advantages of local anesthesia should be stressed, particularly the features of safety and rapid recovery. The patient should be told that she will feel some discomfort (e.g., "pinches when the anesthetic is being injected" or "mild uterine cramps when the tenaculum-sound is being introduced"). The contribution of the patient to the success of the operation when local anesthesia is used should be explained. For example, when a woman is being counseled before a proposed diagnostic laparoscopy under local anesthesia for the investigation of pelvic pain, she should be told that she can provide important information to the surgeon during the operation by telling him or her that the manipulation of certain pelvic structures does or does not reproduce or intensify the pain. Thus, one unique advantage of local anesthesia is that the patient can help the surgeon locate the exact source of her pain (see Chapter 7, under Pain Mapping).

PREOPERATIVE WORKUP, INSTRUCTIONS, AND SCHEDULING

A hematology profile or blood count is unnecessary unless indicated for other reasons, such as a history of chronic menorrhagia or unexplained weakness or pallor. Before abdominal procedures such as minilaparotomy, the patient should have a bowel movement and an enema, if necessary, within the preceding 24 hours. In the case of minilaparotomy, if the patient gives a history of marked bloating or weight gain during the premenstrual phase of her cycle, the operation should be scheduled at some time other than premenstrually. This is because swollen loops of bowel may protrude into the incisional gap and hide the uterine corpus. As a result, it will be difficult for the surgeon to retract the bowel and expose the fallopian tubes without causing pain.

An important advantage of local anesthesia is that it does not predispose the patient to vomiting and aspiration of stomach contents during surgery. Indeed, it is a good idea to instruct the patient to have a light breakfast 1 to 2 hours before coming in for her operation. We usually suggest juice and coffee. Thus, she will avoid hypoglycemia, hunger, and headache.

The patient who is to have her surgery under local anesthesia should be informed at her initial visit that she should be ready to return home with a companion within 1 to 2 hours after her operation. She may experience dizziness or nausea postoperatively either as the result of the surgery or perioperative medications; therefore, she must not expect to drive herself home or walk home alone.

BENEFITS AND RISKS

Aubert et al. (9) and Peterson (10) showed that the principal causes of morbidity and mortality from minilaparotomy, laparoscopy, and abortion are related to general anesthesia. Thus, local anesthesia should be substituted whenever possible. A full discussion of these subjects is found in Chapter 2.

In addition to a higher degree of safety, local anesthesia provides psychological benefits. Many times I have heard patients say something like this: "Thank you, Doctor, for letting me be awake, aware, and in control of myself during the operation." The patient emerges from the experience with an improved self-image and satisfaction that she has been a full participant in the procedure. Postoperatively, she will unlikely feel that she has been taken advantage of or that she has been operated on against her will. On the contrary, she will be pleased to have been a willing partner in her surgical care.

Some patients will not respond favorably to the initial proposal for local anesthesia. These women require more time, more consideration, more supportive counseling, and sometimes more preoperative medications. In an unhurried and reassuring fashion, these individuals can be helped through an otherwise frightening and upsetting experience. Allowances must be made for differences in pain thresholds. "However, no patient should be 'talked into' or persuaded to accept a particular technique against her better judgment" (Stark, personal communication).

PREMEDICATIONS

Before administering a local anesthetic, particular attention must be given to the relief of anxiety. Almost all patients are anxious, and some who are superficially calm have merely disguised their apprehension. Those who are withdrawn frequently require more premedication (and, in addition, more supportive counseling) than those who are openly expressive.

Antianxiety agents not only lessen apprehension but also reduce the dosage of analgesic agent required. Some surgeons instruct patients to take an oral tranquilizer 1 hour before scheduled surgery but most rely on intravenous medication. A widely used agent for the prevention or relief of anxiety is diazepam (Valium, Roche), 10 mg, which may be given orally 1 hour preoperatively or intravenously a few minutes before surgery. A second dose may be given during the procedure if necessary. A word of caution is necessary with respect to intravenous diazepam. Like all other medications delivered directly into the vein, about one quarter of the intended dose should be injected first and at least 1 minute should elapse before slow administration of the remainder of the medication to detect the rare hypersensitivity or idiosyncracy. Intravenous diazepam, for example, particularly in conjunction with a narcotic agent, may produce a hypotensive or syncopal reaction (11). Unfortunately, the importance of a test dose of any intravenous medication is seldom translated into actual practice.

Additional advantages of diazepam, when judiciously administered, include its anticonvulsive effects, its amnesic effects, and its property of raising the toxic threshold of local anesthetic agents (see Chapter 2). However, the outstanding tranquilizing and anticonvulsive properties of intravenous diazepam must be weighed against its occasional side effect of reducing inhibitions and causing some patients to become restless and uncooperative. For this reason I have substituted promethazine hydrochloride (Phenergan, Wyeth), 15 mg, which has sedative, antihistaminic, and anticholinergic properties and seldom causes trouble by reducing inhibitions. It has a potentiating effect on analgesic agents and may be safely mixed in the same syringe with meperidine hydrochloride (Demerol, Winthrop), fentanyl citrate (Sublimaze, Janssen), or butorphanol tartrate (Stadol, Bristol). Promethazine hydrochloride has no significant tranquilizing or anticonvulsant properties and therefore should be replaced by diazepam or midazolam (Versed, Roche) when such effects are desired. Midazolam, because of its rapidity of action, its formulation in aqueous solution (unlike diazepam), and its superior amnesic effects, has become for many clinicians the preoperative tranquilizer of choice.

Whenever Valium or Versed are injected intravenously, the benzodiazepine antagonist flumazenil (Mazicon or Reversed) should be available on the emergency tray for treatment of the rare occurrence of profound hypotension or syncope.

Another advantage of midazolam over diazepam is that it is water soluble. Therefore, it is less likely to cause venous irritation and resultant phlebitis, which is a recognized possibility after intravenous administration of diazepam. Midazolam is twice as potent as diazepam and more consistent in producing amnesia. Antegrade amnesia lasting 20 to 40 minutes has been reported in 90 to 96% of patients after 5 mg of intravenous midazolam. It is important to note that this amnesia may be very distressing to some patients who wish to remain aware and "in control" during the surgery. Therefore, during preoperative counseling, the patient should be informed about the possibility of amnesia so that she may reject either midazolam or diazepam as premedication (12).

RECOVERY

After the use of local anesthesia, recovery is more rapid and discomfort is lessened. There is minimal risk of vomiting and aspiration, diminished likelihood of nausea, and no throat irritation from anesthetic gases or intubation. On the average, 1 hour after surgery, patients are able to sit up, dress themselves, and leave for home.

Gynecologists who use surgery centers will find more available time slots for their local anesthesia cases because afternoon hours are more suitable for the scheduling of patients who can expect rapid recovery and early discharge. Additional afternoon cases, furthermore, will assist in bringing down overhead expenses for the surgery centers. Most surgery centers that operate on an 8:00 A.M. to 5:00 P.M. basis do not schedule cases for general anesthesia after 2:00 P.M.

PRACTICE GUIDELINES FOR NONANESTHESIOLOGISTS

The American Society of Anesthesiologists (13) published a comprehensive set of guidelines for sedation and analgesia compiled by a task force of more than 60 consultants. Among the recommendations are the following:

1. Pulse oximetry with appropriate alarms is valuable but cannot replace the dedicated monitoring of ventilatory function by a properly trained individual who fulfills this primary responsibility throughout the surgical procedure.
2. Electrocardiographic monitoring should be used in patients with significant cardiovascular disease as well as during procedures in which dysrhythmias are anticipated.
3. An individual with advanced life-support skills (should) be immediately available.
4. A defibrillator should be immediately available when sedation is administered to patients with significant cardiovascular disease.
5. Continuous intravenous access is recommended, and, whenever possible, each medication component should be given individually, ideally in small incremental doses.
6. The antagonist naloxone is recommended for opioids and flumazenil for benzodiazepines.

PERSONNEL

Although most surgery centers are prepared to give all forms of anesthesia and therefore employ anesthesiologists and nurse-anesthetists, these individuals need not be present in those centers or office surgeries where only local anesthesia is used. In these locations, of course, no operation should be performed that will subject the patient to even the slightest possibility of major emergency laparotomy. For example, closed laparoscopy that requires the initial introduction of an insufflating needle and sharp trocar involves the risk of major vessel or bowel lacerations. For this operation, general anesthesia backup must be immediately available. Open laparoscopy, on the other hand, carries a negligible risk of major vessel injury. If injury to bowel should occur, either immediate repair with standard instruments can be carried out or the patient can be transferred to a backup hospital operating room for laparotomy in a prompt but unhurried manner (see Chapter 7). Thus, personnel and equipment needs are far less extensive and overhead costs are markedly reduced in centers where local anesthesia alone is used.

RESUSCITATION BACKUP

I recommend the surgeon and all nursing personnel to be certified in cardiopulmonary resuscitation (CPR). This is a sensible precaution, indeed, in any medical or surgical facility.

In surgery centers in which all operations are under local anesthesia, the surgeon observes proper precautions, and patients with serious cardiovascular disorders are excluded, such resuscitation devices as endotracheal tubes and defibrillators are, in my opinion, unnecessary. Those who use these devices rarely should not use them at all, because their safe and effective use requires regular and frequent practice.

Vasovagal episodes or syncopal convulsions will usually terminate spontaneously in 30 to 60 seconds. Oxygen, intravenous atropine sulfate, diazepam or midazolam, and naloxone hydrochloride (Narcan, Dupont) should all be instantly available.

If cardiac or respiratory arrest should occur, standard CPR techniques, skillfully applied, will maintain cardiac output and a functioning airway until the arrival of ambulance personnel.

CONCLUSION

For the operations described in this book, given the proper motivation, knowledge, and experience on the part of the surgeon and staff, local anesthesia is effective, convenient, and safer than general anesthesia.

REFERENCES

1. Fishburne JI. Anesthesia for the outpatient: sterilization and other procedures. In: Symonds EM, Zuspan FP, eds. Clinical and diagnostic procedures in obstetrics and gynecology, Part B: gynecology. New York: Marcel Dekker, 1984.
2. Fishburne JI. Anesthesia for OLULA (office laparoscopy under local anesthesia). Presented at the First Annual Master's Course of the American Association of Office Endoscopy, Tuskegee, Alabama, 1996.
3. Peterson HB, Grimes DA, Cates W, Rubin G. Comparative risk of death from induced abortion at 12 weeks' gestation performed with local versus general anesthesia. Am J Obstet Gynecol 1981;141:763–779.
4. Cullen BF, Margolis AJ, Eger WI. The effects of anesthesia and pulmonary ventilation on blood loss during elective therapeutic abortion. Anesthesiology 1970;32:108.
5. Koonin L, Atrash H, Smith J, Ramick M. Abortion surveillance, 1986–1987. MMWR-CDC Surveillance Summaries. 1990;39(No. SS-2):23–56.
6. Mackay HT, Schulz KF, Grimes DA. Safety of local versus general anesthesia for second-trimester dilatation and evacuation abortion. Obstet Gynecol 1985;66:661–665.
7. Friedrich E. Outpatient laparoscopy under local anesthesia (OLULA) in a procedure room. Presented at the First Annual Master's Course of the American Association of Office Endoscopy, Tuskegee, Alabama, 1996.
8. Lipscomb G. A comparison of the cost of local versus general anesthesia for laparoscopic sterilization in an operating room setting. J AAGL 1996;3:277–281.
9. Aubert JM, Lubell I, Schima M. Mortality risk associated with female sterilization. Int J Gynaecol Obstet 1980;18:406–410.
10. Peterson HB, DeStefano F, Rubin GL, Greenspan J, Lee N, Ory H. Deaths attributable to tubal sterilization in the United States 1977–1981. Am J Obstet Gynecol 1983;146:131–136.
11. Physicians' Desk Reference. Oradell, NJ: Medical Economics Co., 1995.
12. Philip B. Local anesthesia and sedation techniques. In: White P, ed. Outpatient anesthesia. New York: Churchill Livingstone, 1996.
13. Practice guidelines for sedation and analgesia by non-anesthesiologists. Anesthesiology 1996;84:459–471.

2. Local Anesthetic Agents

A. JEFFERSON PENFIELD

The reader will note that most references in this chapter are from the 1970s and 1980s. This is because the landmark studies published during those 10 years have not been superseded by more recent reports. The cited chapter by Dr. Philip (1) indicates general agreement with the classic studies and adds a few recommendations based on her experience in ambulatory surgical settings.

The use of local anesthesia for pain prevention during surgery began 112 years ago in 1884, when Koller, a Viennese ophthalmologist, described the properties of cocaine, an ester of para-amino-benzoic acid (PABA), in the production of corneal anesthesia (2). One year later, in 1885, Halsted of Johns Hopkins Hospital in Baltimore reported on more than 1,000 cases given cocaine infiltration anesthesia (3). It was observed previously that the natives of Peru, who enjoyed chewing the leaves of the plant erythroxylon coca for its mood-elevating effects, also experienced circumoral numbness. In the years that followed, the toxic and addicting properties of cocaine became well known, and the present day use of this agent is largely limited to the production of topical anesthesia, vasoconstriction, and decongestion of the oropharyngeal mucous membranes.

The first injectable anesthetic of value was another ester of PABA, procaine, which was synthesized by Einhorn in 1904. This agent proved to be nonaddictive and far less toxic than cocaine. Other esters have been synthesized, including benzocaine, dibucaine, tetracaine, and chloroprocaine, and these have also demonstrated little toxicity and no addictive potential. Amino esters, however, have shown occasional sensitizing properties, and allergic reactions manifested by urticaria or edema have been reported after their use. These reactions to the esters are due to the metabolite PABA, 90% of which is eventually excreted unchanged by the kidneys. However, if multiple-dose vials of any local anesthetic are used, allergic reactions are most often due to the preservative methyl-paraben.

An important milestone in the development of new anesthetics occurred in 1948 when the Swedish chemist, Lofgren, synthesized lidocaine. This compound is an amide derivative of diethyl-amino-acetic acid. It has superior spreading capabilities, and allergic reactions are extremely rare. Mepivacaine, prilocaine, bupivacaine, and etidocaine are other synthesized amino amides. These are equally free of sensitizing properties. Furthermore, no examples of cross-sensitivity between amino esters and amino amides have been reported Table 2.1).

Amino esters (e.g., procaine) are metabolized by the plasma enzyme pseudocholinesterase, whereas amino amides (e.g., lidocaine) are metabolized mainly by hepatic microsomal enzymes. Therefore, patients with liver disease may show reduced tolerance to the amide-type local anesthetic drugs (4).

PHARMACODYNAMICS OF LOCAL ANESTHESIA

Covino and Vassallo (4) defined local anesthesia as follows: "A loss of sensation in a circumscribed area of the body due to a depression of excitation in nerve endings or an inhibition of the conduction process in peripheral nervous tissue." Such loss of sensation

Table 2.1
Representative Local Anesthetic Agents in Common Clinical Use

Generic[a] and Common Proprietary Name	Chemical Structure	Approximate Year of Initial Clinical Use	Main Anesthetic Utility	Representative Commercial Preparation
Cocaine		1884	Topical	Bulk powder
Benzocaine Americaine[a]		1900	Topical	20% ointment 20% aerosol
Procaine Novocain[a]		1905	Infiltration Spinal	10 and 20 mg/mL solutions 100 mg/mL solution
Dibucaine Nupercaine[a]		1929	Spinal	0.6, 7, 2.5, and 5 mg/mL solutions
Tetracaine Pontocaine[a]		1930	Spinal	Niphanoid crystals—20 mg/mL 10 mg/mL solutions
Lidocaine Xylocaine[a]		1944	Infiltration Peripheral Nerve Blockade Epidural Spinal Topical Topical	5 and 10 mg/mL solutions 10, 15, and 20 mg/mL solutions 10, 15, and 20 mg/mL solutions 50 mg/mL solution 2.0% jelly, viscous 2.5%, 5.0% ointment
Chloroprocaine Nesacaine[a]		1955	Infiltration Peripheral Nerve Blockade Epidural	10 mg/mL solution 10 and 20 mg/mL solutions 20 and 30 mg/mL solutions
Mepivacaine Carbocaine[a]		1957	Infiltration Peripheral Nerve Blockade Epidural	10 mg/mL solution 10 and 20 mg/mL solutions 10, 15 and 20 mg/mL solutions
Prilocaine Citanest[a]		1960	Infiltration Peripheral Nerve Blockade Epidural	10 and 20 mg/mL solutions 10, 20 and 30 mg/mL solutions 10, 20, and 30 mg/mL solutions
Bupivacaine Marcaine[a]		1963	Infiltration Peripheral Nerve Blockade Epidural	2.5 mg/mL solutions 2.5 and 5 mg/mL solutions 2.5, 5, and 7.5 mg/mL solutions
Etidocaine Duranest[a]		1972	Infiltration Peripheral Nerve Blockade Epidural	2.5 and 5 mg/mL solutions 5 and 10 mg/mL solutions 5 and 10 mg/mL solutions

[a]USP nomenclature

From Covino B. *Local anesthetics mechanisms of action and clinical use.* New York: Grune and Stratton, 1976.

may be permanent, such as after surgical interruption of nerves or cauterization with phenol. Local anesthetics, according to de Jong (3), "are drugs that halt the neural traffic along an axon in a predictable and reversible manner, leaving the nerve none the worse for its brief period of rest."

Nerve membranes are composed of lipids and proteins. Differences in rapidity of onset and duration of effect of different agents are principally due to differences in lipid solubility and protein-binding capacity, respectively. Bupivacaine and etidocaine have greater protein-binding capacity and therefore longer duration of action than lidocaine.

The sequence of events in the production of anesthetic block has been broken down by investigators as follows:

1. Displacement of calcium ions from nerve receptor site;
2. Binding of local anesthetic moiety to receptor site;
3. Blockade of sodium channel (reduction of permeability of cell membrane to sodium ions);
4. Decrease of sodium conductance;
5. Depression of rate of electrical depolarization;
6. Failure to achieve threshold potential level;
7. Lack of development of propagated action potential;
8. Conduction blockade (4).

"Local anesthetics inhibit excitation in peripheral nerves by impeding sodium conductance. The site of local anesthetic activity is believed to reside primarily in the sodium channels of the nerve membranes" (5). "The primary electrophysiological effect of local anesthetic agents on the nerve membrane involves a reduction in the rate of the depolarization phase of the action potential" (4). Therefore, several minutes must elapse between the moment of injection of the local agent and the production of complete anesthesia. This is not only because of the time required for diffusion through the tissues, but also because of the additional time taken up by the completion of the above chain reaction, beginning with penetration of the lipid nerve sheath and ending with conduction blockade. This unavoidable delay in attaining satisfactory anesthesia must be borne in mind by the surgeon, who can take good advantage of the 1- to 2-minute waiting period to talk with the patient and check over the instrument tray.

The existence of a waiting period is confirmed by the time schedule adopted by investigators who have recorded the anesthetic potency of various agents. "The intrinsic anesthetic potency of a chemical compound is usually defined as the minimum concentration required to produce *within 5 to 10 minutes* a 50% reduction of the amplitude of the surface action potential recorded from an isolated nerve preparation" (4). Measured in this manner, the comparative intrinsic potency of bupivacaine (Marcaine, Winthrop-Breon) is four times that of lidocaine (Xylocaine, Astra) (4). High intrinsic potency is of value, however, only when the agent must be used in a small volume and confined to a relatively small space, as with spinal or ocular anesthesia.

CLINICAL CONSIDERATIONS

For local infiltration and for paracervical or pudendal nerve block, larger volumes of agents of intermediate intrinsic potency, such as lidocaine or mepivacaine, have been found to be most suitable.

Lidocaine is firmly established worldwide as the standard local anesthetic agent Fig. 2.1). Since its synthesis in 1984 by Lofgren as the first amino amide, it has been studied

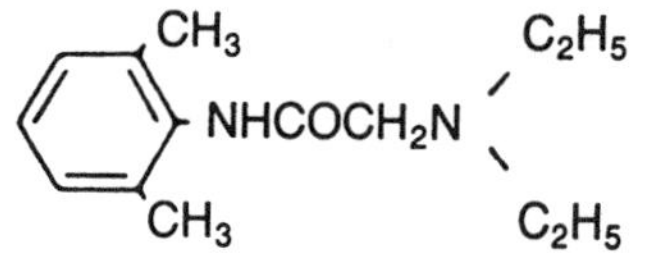

Figure 2.1. Chemical configuration of lidocaine.

and used far more than any other product. Its safety record and effectiveness in clinical practice have not been surpassed by any other agent (Fig. 2.1).

Much clinical research on optimal concentrations of lidocaine and on the usefulness of added epinephrine has been done in the dental field. The effects of infiltration of gingival mucosa by various agents were tested by electrical stimulation of the teeth (6, 7). For example, it was found that adding epinephrine to lidocaine is far more effective in producing a satisfactory degree and duration of analgesia than increasing the concentration of the anesthetic agent. It was found that 1% lidocaine, which was relatively ineffective as a plain solution, was 100% effective when combined with 25 μg/mL epinephrine. Even 4% lidocaine plain (without epinephrine) produced satisfactory analgesia only 80% of the time. It was also found that a much smaller concentration of epinephrine (e.g., 5 μg/mL or 1:200,000) significantly prolonged the duration of anesthesia and retarded systemic absorption of the agent. Vasoconstrictor drugs such as epinephrine not only prevent rapid absorption of the anesthetic agent and prolong its effect, but also produce a relatively bloodless field. Postoperative rebound bleeding when the vasoconstrictive effects have worn off is an uncommon occurrence, provided the surgeon has been careful to clamp and tie all bleeding vessels.

Despite the benefits and safety of the addition of 1:200,000 epinephrine to the anesthetic solution, some patients may experience tachycardia or anxiety from its use. Epinephrine should not be administered to individuals with moderate to severe hypertension.

For the operations described in this book, solutions of 0.5% lidocaine (5 mg/mL), with or without epinephrine 1:200,000 (5 μg/mL), can provide adequate anesthesia. These concentrations are commercially available in the United States in convenient 50-mL multiple dose vials (Xylocaine 0.5% with or without epinephrine 1:200,000, Astra). If only plain lidocaine is available, it may be easily converted to a 1:200,000 epinephrine solution by adding 0.1 mL 1:1,000 epinephrine to each 20 mL.

Epinephrine in 1:400,000 concentration is as effective as 1:200,000 in producing vasoconstriction and hemostasis, according to Beverly Philip, Director of the Day Surgery Unit at the Brigham and Women's Hospital (Boston, MA). In either case, if the patient experiences a significant rise in blood pressure, Dr. Philip recommends an immediate dose of propranolol 0.25 to 0.5 mg (1).

Reasons for the popularity of lidocaine are spelled out by Moore (8), who prefers lidocaine and mepivacaine (Carbocaine, Winthrop) because they are both amides of great stability and low toxicity. They produce sufficiently rapid onset of analgesia in low concentrations. The duration of analgesia is adequate and not unnecessarily prolonged; it is 1.5 hours with the plain solutions and 3 hours with epinephrine added.

Lidocaine has moderate vasodilating properties. Mepivacaine, on the other hand, appears to have its own built-in vasoconstrictive action, so it is unnecessary to add epinephrine to it (8). If epinephrine is added, the duration of effect of mepivacaine is increased by only 15 to 30 minutes. The duration of action of mepivacaine is due to its superior binding power.

Two advantages of lidocaine are that it is commercially available with or without epinephrine and that detoxification is more rapid than with mepivacaine. For any operation described in this book, it would be unwise to use any local agent that produces more than 3 hours of anesthesia, because it is important to be aware of an abnormal degree of persistent or increasing pain in or adjacent to the operative site. Such unexpected pain could be due to an enlarging hematoma, ruptured uterus, or bowel perforation with peritonitis. The early diagnosis of serious complications such as these might be delayed by the use of such longer-acting agents as bupivacaine or etidocaine.

The addition of hyaluronidase to the local anesthetic solution has been recommended by Martin (9) because of the resultant alleged increased rapidity of onset of anesthesia. Hyaluronidase is an enzyme that inactivates hyaluronic acid, which obstructs diffusion of invasive substances in interstitial tissue spaces. Hyaluronidase is nontoxic. It appears to improve the spreading characteristics of the anesthetic agent, thereby speeding the onset of anesthetic block. It also may facilitate the absorption of blood and will occasionally prevent hematoma formation.

A possible disadvantage of hyaluronidase is excessive spread of the anesthetic solution, resulting in an overly extensive block. Analgesia time will be shortened unless epinephrine is added, and toxic reactions to anesthetic or vasoconstrictive drugs are more likely because of accelerated absorption (8).

The recommended dose of hyaluronidase (Wydase, Wyeth) is 150 turbidity reducing units added to 10 or up to 200 mL of anesthetic solution (10). In other words, hyaluronidase is effective even in very high dilutions.

TOXIC, ALLERGIC, AND VASOVAGAL REACTIONS: SAFE DOSAGE LEVELS

Adverse systemic effects of local anesthetic agents should not occur unless blood levels exceed 5 μg/mL. It has been found in the human that a subcutaneous injection of 40 mL 1% lidocaine (400 mg) will result in a peak blood level of 2 μg/mL (11). This level is less than one half the toxic threshold level. Levels slightly higher than 2 μg/mL have been observed after intramuscular injection because of the increased vascularity of muscle tissue, resulting in more rapid systemic absorption. However, 0.5% solutions of lidocaine are equally effective in producing complete local anesthesia and should therefore replace the 1% solutions for most gynecologic procedures.

The maximum safe dose of lidocaine (Xylocaine) with epinephrine for tissue infiltration recommended by the Astra Company and approved by authorities in the field of anesthesia (1, 8) is 100 mL 0.5% or 50 mL 1% (500 mg in either case). Without epinephrine 60 mL 0.5% or 30 mL 1% are recommended as the safe upper limits (10). Peak blood levels from these doses, if absorbed in the expected manner, will approximate 2 μg/mL, which is less than one half the threshold toxic level. However, an unintended intravascular injection of a portion of the solution may result in transient blood levels that approach the toxic threshold. The maximum recommended doses of mepivacaine (Carbocaine) are the same as those for lidocaine (10).

When recommended dosages are followed and the risk of intravascular injection is minimized by repeated attempts to withdraw the barrel of the syringe, toxic levels of anesthetic agents should only rarely occur. Nonetheless, it is important to recognize symptoms and signs of high tissue levels so that no further injections are given and medical treatment can be carried out immediately.

Covino and Vassallo (4) described the following sequence resulting from increasingly toxic levels:

1. Numbness of tongue and circumoral tissues;
2. Lightheadedness and dizziness;
3. Visual and auditory disturbance (e.g., difficulty in focusing and tinnitus);
4. Drowsiness and disorientation;
5. Slurred speech, shivering, and muscle twitching;
6. Tonic-clonic convulsions;
7. Respiratory depression;
8. Respiratory arrest.

Central Nervous System Effects

Initial central nervous system excitation, up to and including convulsions, may occur very early in the sequence of signs and symptoms and is explained by initial inhibitory effects on inhibitory pathways in the cerebral cortex. This inhibition allows facilitatory neurons to function unopposed, leading to increased excitation of the central nervous system. Thus, convulsions may ensue.

In cats, premedication with 0.25 mg/kg diazepam intramuscularly requires a 100% increase in the convulsive dose of lidocaine (12). In the human with a past history of seizure disorder, 10 mg diazepam (Valium, Roche) may be injected slowly intravenously for this purpose and may be safely repeated after a few minutes, should convulsions occur.

Covino's observations that central nervous system excitation may be the first warning of anesthetic agent toxicity is confirmed by the experience of Moore (8), who lists restlessness, tremors, and convulsions as important sign of high blood level reaction. Additional early signs of cortical stimulation noted by Moore include a "metallic taste," dizziness, blurred vision, and "roaring in the ears." If any one or more of the above reactions occur, the patient should receive oxygen immediately. If convulsions occur and persist and if the patient can be safely intubated and mechanically ventilated, succinylcholine (Anectine, Burroughs, Wellcome, or Quelicin, Abbott) 2 mL (40 mg) should be injected intravenously. Succinylcholine is a short-acting depolarizing muscle relaxant that causes transient skeletal muscle paralysis. A repeat dose may be given if needed in 6 to 8 minutes.

Although it is useful to be aware of the most severe possible toxic reactions and their management, such reactions are extremely rare when local anesthetics are administered in the recommended manner.

Cardiovascular Effects

Although the effects of toxic doses of local anesthetic agents on the central nervous system have received the most attention, we must not overlook the critical changes that may be produced in the cardiovascular system, particularly with reference to heart muscle.

In vitro studies of the effect of lidocaine on cardiac muscle reveal an increased efflux of potassium ions from the ventricular muscle cell but not from the atrial muscle cell (13). This is believed to be why intravenous lidocaine, paradoxically, is useful in the treatment of ventricular (but not atrial) arrhythmias. Such treatment should not be carried out without continuous electrocardiographic monitoring. The usual intravenous dose is 50 to 100 mg injected slowly. A second dose may be given after 5 minutes. At these doses, lidocaine does not reduce myocardial contractility or cardiac output. Excessive levels from rapid intravenous administration, however, will reduce contractility and output and may result in circulatory collapse (4).

Unintended intravenous administration of high doses of local anesthetic agents is far more likely to result in cardiac arrest than fibrillation. In either case, the proper immediate treatment is closed-chest resuscitation with mouth-to-mouth breathing if indicated. These maneuvers, skillfully performed, will sustain life until spontaneous recovery occurs. If the patient is in a free-standing facility and normal sinus rhythm does not return within a few minutes, she must be transferred promptly to a hospital emergency room for electrocardiographic monitoring and defibrillation if indicated.

The addition to an anesthetic solution of a vasoconstrictor drug such as epinephrine may cause transient hypertension in a susceptible individual. Such reactions are uncommon in normotensive patients when the concentration of epinephrine is only 1:200,000 and intravenous administration is avoided. In patients already hypertensive, vasoconstrictive solutions must be used with extreme caution, if at all. The adrenolytic drug of choice for a severe hypertensive reaction is chlorpromazine (Thorazine, Smith Kline and French) 12.5 to 15 mg intravenously.

Fatalities from local anesthetic toxicity are exceedingly rare, but these cases should be analyzed carefully to learn how to take the precautions necessary to prevent these catastrophes. For example, Grimes and Cates (14) reported on five women in the United States who died as the result of severe systemic reactions to paracervical anesthetic agents. Lidocaine was the responsible agent in four patients, who received between 200 and 500 mg. Mepivacaine in a 200-mg dosage was the agent in the fifth case. In each case the anesthetic was epinephrine free; thus, undesirable rapid absorption into the bloodstream undoubtedly occurred. Each patient experienced convulsions followed by cardiovascular collapse.

It is not known in any instance whether the physician failed to attempt withdrawal of the plunger of the syringe to minimize the possibility of direct intravenous injection. Neither was it specified whether the physician deposited the anesthetic in several neighboring locations, another technique designed to prevent bolus injection into a large paracervical vessel. However, at least one of five patients experienced an apparent "hypersensitivity" or "intolerance" to the local anesthetic agent. In this case a 20-mL volume of 1% epinephrine-free mepivacaine (200 mg) was injected into the paracervical region. Several seconds later, the patient complained that she did not feel well. She became cold, short of breath, agitated, and pale. Twitching of her face and arms was noted. In a few minutes she suffered cardiovascular collapse and convulsions. Despite intensive resuscitative efforts, she died. This woman had received no more than one half the maximum recommended single dose of 400 mg. Again, it is possible that the injections were made too rapidly, or in too few locations, or directly into a vein because of failure to withdraw the barrel of the syringe before injection. Also, the anesthetic solution, as in the other four cases, was epinephrine free and thus would have been absorbed more rapidly into the systemic circulation. These five exceedingly rare fatalities should serve as a strong reminder to exert maximum caution in the use of local anesthesia. However, no valid statistical conclusions may be drawn from the report regarding the relative safety of lidocaine versus mepivacaine, particularly because, nationwide, lidocaine is by far the most frequently used agent.

Lidocaine and mepivacaine are both amino amides, which are not hydrolyzed but are broken down relatively slowly by hepatic enzymes. Thus, it might be anticipated that toxic reactions from these agents are more likely than from the amino esters such as procaine or chloroprocaine, which are rapidly hydrolyzed by pseudocholinesterase in the bloodstream.

This hypothesis was tested in a bold and ingenious manner by Foldes et al. (15).

Twelve unanesthetized healthy male volunteers 21 to 35 years of age were given intravenous injections of one of three amino esters, procaine, chloroprocaine, or tetracaine, or the amino amide lidocaine. A variable speed pump was used to precisely control the rate of injection.

Physicians trained in cardiopulmonary resuscitation stood by during the experiment. Continuous electroencephalographic and electrocardiographic monitoring was carried out. Although all recognized toxic signs and symptoms up to convulsive activity were observed with each agent, it was demonstrated that the best tolerated anesthetic, volume for volume, was chloroprocaine and the least well tolerated was lidocaine. Furthermore, all signs and symptoms of chloroprocaine toxicity disappeared in an average of 4.7 minutes after the infusion ended, as compared with 18.5 minutes for lidocaine. This apparent advantage of chloroprocaine was reflected by correspondingly lower levels of residual agent in the bloodstream, presumably due to rapid hydrolysis.

As a result of these findings, Foldes et al. (15) recommended chloroprocaine (Nesacaine, Astra) as the preferred agent when large volumes of relatively concentrated solutions are used. This experiment demonstrated in a dramatic fashion the signs of progressive toxicity of each agent when large doses are injected intravenously. Because comparable blood levels cannot occur after tissue infiltration, the experiment cannot serve as a guide to the relative toxicity of these agents in normal clinical use. Large volumes of any agent in greater concentrations than 0.5% should not be used.

Allergic Reactions

"True allergy requires the formation of an antibody to an antigenic substance. To date, no evidence is available that antibodies are formed in response to a challenge by an amide-type local anesthetic drug" (4). This statement by Covino and Vassallo is echoed by most anesthesiologists of my acquaintance, but de Jong, in a search of the literature up to 1967, uncovered three case reports that would appear to support true allergy to preservative-free lidocaine (16–18). In each case, there was a delay of 1 hour or more between injection and the slow development of a pruritic urticarial rash.

Most instances of alleged allergy to lidocaine and other amide anesthetics are in reality vasovagal reactions (to be discussed later), mild epinephrine reactions such as tremors or tachycardia, or exceedingly rare urticarial reactions to methyl- or butyl-paraben in multiple-dose vials (19). A negative local anesthetic skin test in a supposedly allergic individual may be relied on. A positive test, however, is more likely due to the irritancy of the anesthetic agent.

If an allergic reaction occurs, as evidenced by such signs as urticaria, hives, edema, or asthma, 50 mg diphenhydramine (Benadryl, Parke-Davis) may be given by mouth or slowly intravenously. The dose may be repeated every 3 to 4 hours as needed. Also, 0.3 mL of epinephrine 1:1,000 may be given intramuscularly.

Vasovagal Reactions

Vasovagal reactions include a panorama of cardiovascular, autonomic, and central nervous system reactions, such as bradycardia, hypotension, diaphoresis, nausea, and convulsions. A vasovagal reaction may be associated with any surgical procedure in gynecology, from intrauterine device insertion to vacuum curettage to laparoscopic sterilization. The reaction is probably not due to the injection of the anesthetic medication. In fact, skillful administration of local anesthesia will lessen its risk. Rather, a vasovagal reaction may be ushered in as part of a simple anxiety state (i.e., the common fainting spell) or may occur in response to pulling or stretching of tissues, as with cervical dilation or peritoneal traction. In patients without cardiovascular disease, such reactions will terminate spontaneously, usually within a few minutes, without specific therapy.

The preoperative administration of 0.4 mg atropine or a drug such as promethazine hydrochloride (Phenergan, Wyeth), 15 mg, which has an atropine-like effect, reduces the possibility of a vasovagal reaction. An intravenous injection of 0.4 mg atropine may also be given once the reaction has begun, but such treatment is usually unnecessary. Oxygen must always be available in case of prolonged apnea, along with readiness to clear the airway and provide assisted respiration.

CONCLUSION

The surgeon's choice of a local anesthetic agent should be guided by an understanding of features such as safety, potency, duration of action, and side effects. The amino amides are generally preferred over the amino esters because their sensitizing potential as a group is negligible. Most basic research during the past 30 years has focused on lidocaine, which was the first amide to be synthesized. Most gynecologists continue to prefer lidocaine because of its safety record, intermediate potency, and excellent spreading characteristics. Others favor chloroprocaine because of its rapid hydrolysis and extremely low toxic potential [20].

In special situations, more potent longer-acting amides such as bupivacaine (Marcaine) or etidocaine (Duranest, Astra) may be preferred. Lidocaine, however, is the overall favorite for abdominal and perineal tissue infiltration and for uterosacral nerve block. Lidocaine is also most conveniently packaged in the United States in a wide variety of dilutions with or without epinephrine. For example, the 0.5% solution of Xylocaine (Astra) is supplied with or without epinephrine 1:200,000 in multiple-dose 50-mL vials. Various other concentrations and combinations are available in multiple-dose vials, single-dose vials, ampules, and prefilled syringes.

When administering lidocaine for paracervical block, as before dilatation and curettage (D&C), first trimester abortion, or intrauterine device insertion, the addition of epinephrine 1:200,000 not only retards systemic absorption, but also reduces resistance to dilatation of the internal cervical os. This is because of the "catecholamine's beta-adrenergic property of smooth muscle relaxation" [3]. Fortunately, clinical experience has shown that this relaxing effect of epinephrine on the resting tone of smooth muscle does not extend to the myometrium unless it is administered in relatively high doses to a woman in labor at or near term. This is why excessive blood loss from uterine atony associated with pregnancy termination or postabortal curettage is far less likely after paracervical block than with general anesthesia, which puts both the patient and her uterus "to sleep."

During the past 21 years, I have used lidocaine (Xylocaine), with or without epinephrine, for all D&C's, first trimester terminations, minilaparotomies, laparoscopies, skin tumor excisions, and Bartholin cyst marsupializations. During the first 3 years, I used a 1% solution, but in the past 17 years I found that 0.5% lidocaine is equally effective. In 1970, we introduced a first trimester termination service at the free-standing

Syracuse Planned Parenthood Center. One year later, we initiated a vasectomy service, and 2 years later, a laparoscopic sterilization service. These operations were performed under local lidocaine anesthesia.

Except in patients with moderate to severe hypertension, I presently use 0.5% lidocaine with 1;200,000 epinephrine. This epinephrine concentration is effective in reducing absorption and producing a relatively bloodless operating field. A slight rise in pulse or blood pressure may occur.

Among the combined total of over 40,000 patients operated on under local anesthesia between January 1, 1970 and July 1995 at the Planned Parenthood Center and in my office surgery, we have not observed a single toxic or allergic reaction to lidocaine, methylparaben, or epinephrine. Almost all patients, however, have experienced preoperative anxiety of varying intensity. In most cases we are able to lessen this anxiety by preoperative counseling and medications. Once we injected the local anesthetic, we never found it necessary to discontinue the procedure and transfer the patient to the hospital to complete the operation under general anesthesia.

Other gynecologists favor 0.5% etidocaine (Duranest) or 0.25% bupivacaine (Marcaine) because of their rapid onset of action, longer duration of effect (5 to 9 hours), and greater relative intrinsic potency. Darney (21), for example, uses plain bupivacaine with added pitressin for paracervical block before pregnancy terminations and for abdominal wall infiltration before laparoscopic sterilization.

My own continued preference for lidocaine is based on three factors: the enormous body of literature attesting to its unsurpassed safety; its intermediate relative potency, which is adequate; and its 3-hour maximum duration of effect, which is sufficient and less likely to delay the diagnosis of an enlarging hematoma or other painful complication. Etidocaine or bupivacaine, on the other hand, particularly with added epinephrine or pitressin, may produce 6 or more hours of anesthesia, with its attendant masking effect.

In conclusion, successful use of local anesthetics depends on effective patient counseling, judicious premedication, and slow tissue infiltration of minimal effective volumes. Each agent possesses specific advantages and disadvantages with which the competent practitioner should be familiar. A comparison of local versus general anesthesia was presented in Chapter 1. In subsequent chapters, specific details of local anesthetic use for particular operations are outlined.

REFERENCES

1. Philip B. Local anesthesia and sedation techniques. In: White P, ed. Outpatient anesthesia. New York: Churchill Livingstone, 1990.
2. Castiglioni A. The second half of the nineteenth century. Clinical medicine based on the fundamental sciences: growth of the specialties. In: A history of medicine. New York: A. Knopf, 1947.
3. de Jong RH. Local anesthetics. Springfield, IL: Charles C Thomas, 1977.
4. Covino BG, Vassallo HG. Local anesthetics, mechanisms of action and clinical use. New York: Grune and Stratton, 1967.
5. Covino BG. New developments in the field of local anesthesia. Acta Scand 1982;26(3):242–249.
6. Ross NM, Dobbs EC. Mepivacaine HCl (Carbocaine) without vasoconstrictor. J Oral Surg 1963; 21:215–219.
7. Epstein S. Clinical study of prilocaine with varying concentrations of epinephrine. J Am Dent Assoc 1969;78:85–90.
8. Moore DC. Regional block. Springfield, IL: Charles C Thomas, 1973.

9. Martin P. Local anesthesia in the office-based surgical suite. In: Ambulatory gynecologic surgery. Littleton, MA: PSG Publishing Co., Inc., 1979.
10. Physicians' Desk Reference. Oradell, NJ: Medical Economics Co., Inc., 1995.
11. Scott DB, Jebson PJR, Braid DP, Ortengren B, Frisch P. Factors affecting plasma levels of lignocaine and prilocaine. Br J Anaesth 1972;44:1040–1049.
12. de Jong RH, Heavner JE. Diazepam prevents local anesthetic seizures. Anesthesiology 1971;34:523–531.
13. Kabela E. The effects of lidocaine on potassium efflux from various tissues of dog heart. J Pharmacol Exp Ther 1973;184:611–618.
14. Grimes DH, Cates W. Deaths from paracervical anesthesia used for first-trimester abortion, 1972–1975. N Engl J Med 1976;295:1397–1399.
15. Foldes FF, Molloy R, McNall PG, Pearl MB, Koukal L. Comparison of toxicity of intravenously given local anesthetic agents in man. JAMA 1960;172:1493–1498.
16. Eyre J, Nally FF. Nasal test for hypersensitivity, including a positive reaction to lignocaine. Lancet 1971;1(693):264–265.
17. Holti G, Hood FJC. An anaphylactoid reaction to lignocaine. Dent Pract Dent Rec 1965;15:294–295.
18. Rood JP. A case of lignocaine hypersensitivity. Br Dent J 1973;135:411–412.
19. Schorr WF. Paraben allergy. A cause of intractable dermatitis. JAMA 1968;204:859–862.
20. Altman AM, Stubblefield PG, Schlam JF, Loberfeld R, Osathanonh, R. Midtrimester abortion with laminaria and vacuum evacuation on a teaching service. J Reprod Med 1985;30:601–606.
21. Darney P. Ambulatory surgery under local anesthesia: avoiding complications and litigation. Presented at the Round Table, Annual Meeting of American College of Obstetricians and Gynecologists, San Francisco, CA, May 1984.

3. *Outpatient Facilities for Operations Under Local Anesthesia*

A. JEFFERSON PENFIELD

Most practicing gynecologists in the United States perform outpatient surgery in units incorporated in or connected to a hospital in which they have major operating privileges. Others have chosen to use free-standing surgery centers, some of which are administered by anesthesiologists. A prototype facility in the United States is the Phoenix Surgicenter, which has served as a model unit for the past 25 years.

Most conspicuous among free-standing centers for gynecologic surgery have been abortion and sterilization clinics, both public and private, developed in almost all urban areas to meet the increasing demand for fertility control. Administrators and personnel of abortion clinics are particularly gratified to expand their services to include the more "constructive" operations of laparoscopic sterilization, minilaparotomy tubal ligation, and vasectomy. While I was Medical Director of the Syracuse Planned Parenthood Center from 1966 to 1976, I discovered how logical and easy it was to add sterilization to abortion services, particularly because we continued to perform all operations under local anesthesia. We required no additional operating space, the existing operating lights were adequate, our autoclaves could sterilize the additional instruments, and cold-sterilizing solutions were used for laparoscopes and other equipment that could not be autoclaved.

A few examples of the many abortion clinics that have added female sterilization services are The Pre-Term/Planned Parenthood Clinic in Brookline, Massachusetts (open laparoscopy); The Planned Parenthood Clinics in Los Angeles, California and Augusta, Georgia (closed laparoscopy, open laparoscopy, and minilaparotomy); The Women's Clinic in Ft. Lauderdale, Florida (closed laparoscopy); and the Baltimore and Grand Rapids Planned Parenthood Centers, Baltimore, Maryland and Grand Rapids, Michigan (minilaparotomy).

Kaali and Landesman (1) reported on 520 laparoscopic tubal sterilizations with Falope rings performed at the Women's Medical Pavilion in Dobbs Ferry, New York, a free-standing surgical unit that also provides abortion services. A total of 435 patients requested and received general anesthesia with endotracheal intubation and assisted respiration; only 85 procedures were performed under local anesthesia.

This apparent preference for general anesthesia was found to be even more pronounced by Greenspan et al. (2) in their review of ambulatory tubal sterilizations in the United States in 1980. Although admittedly an incomplete survey because many private facilities do not report their cases, information was gathered from 141 free-standing facilities out of 330 potential responders. About 16,500 tubal sterilizations were performed in the reporting facilities in 1980, 97% of them under general anesthesia. A total of 90.9% were laparoscopic. Approximately 70% of the tubal sterilizations were by bipolar coagulation, silastic band, and surgical ligation; 2.1% were by clip; and 5.7% were by "other method."

Although most outpatients in the United States are operated on in hospital-connected or free-standing centers, I believe that the office surgical facility offers unique advantages of safety, convenience, and economy. Safety is promoted by the exclusive use of local anesthesia and minimal turnover of personnel. There is convenience for the patient because of her familiarity with the office setting and for the gynecologist because of control of scheduling. There is greater economy due to lower facility overhead costs and the option to reduce fees for patients in financial distress.

The following recommendations are based on my personal experience during the past 25 years with five separate free-standing surgical units. Three have been private office surgical facilities; one was the Syracuse Planned Parenthood Center and one was the Health Center in Fulton, New York. The operations I performed in these units include the following:

1. Diagnostic or therapeutic dilatation and curettage (D&C);
2. First trimester pregnancy termination (vacuum and standard curettage);
3. Bartholin duct marsupialization;
4. Minilaparotomy tubal ligation;
5. Open laparoscopy for diagnosis of pelvic pain, obscure pelvic masses, suspected endometriosis, tubal patency, and so forth;
6. Open laparoscopy for tubal sterilization, initially by unipolar coagulation, then by the Yoon silastic band, and most recently by the Hulka clip;
7. Removal of skin tumors, vulval biopsies, excision of vaginal septa, and so forth.

Gynecologists who plan to build a private office surgery will have their own list of operations they would like to offer patients. In addition to or in place of any of the above, they might include procedures such as cervical conization, hysteroscopy, and hysteroscopic myomectomy or endometrial ablation (see Chapter 6). Before designing and constructing an office surgery, however, two important prerequisites must be fulfilled. First, the gynecologist must possess the basic skills, enthusiasm, and patience for operating under local anesthesia. Second, there must be a community need for such a facility. The second prerequisite is difficult to analyze in a precise manner, just as is the question of the appropriate number of specialists in a given area. Nonetheless, the evaluation must be made and a positive conclusion reached to justify the considerable cost of constructing, staffing, and equipping a new surgical unit. Where the anticipated needs of the community and the gynecologist are already met by a hospital in-and-out surgery, for example, it would be a needless extravagance to develop an office surgical unit.

Government regulations in certain localities may restrict the performance of surgery in a private office setting, and the individual practitioner should inquire as to whether a certificate of need must be obtained. For example, in New York City at the present time, the Health Department has the authority to regulate certain procedures such as abortion and sterilization in an office surgery. However, some gynecologists in private practice in New York City have taken the viewpoint that what they do in their own private suites is their own business. As a result, large numbers of D&Cs and first trimester abortions are performed in private office units without public health supervision. The Maternal and Child Health Committee of the New York State Department of Health has disapproved the concept of office laparoscopic sterilization because of their concern that poorly qualified physicians will set up their own services (McLean, personal communication).

What about peer review or quality assurance committees to oversee the work done in such facilities? I have been asked this question by practitioners who operate in hospital-based surgical units and who are inclined to regard free-standing facilities as uncontrollable. Risk management in outpatient surgery is discussed by Dr. Paul Allen in Chapter 13. For a general presentation of the concept and practice of ambulatory surgery in the United States, the reader is referred to *Outpatient Surgery* edited by George J. Hill, MD (3).

Office-based surgery has come of age. One of its original exponents was the late Purvis Martin, MD, a Board-certified gynecologist who practiced in San Diego, California. He mobilized leaders in his own and other specialties, including ophthalmology, urology, general surgery, plastic surgery, orthopedic surgery, and otolaryngology, to form the Society for Office-Based Surgery. Dr. Martin published a book that outlines the planning of facilities, the use of local anesthesia, record-keeping recommendations, accreditation mechanisms, and malpractice risks, as well as other important topics (4). He has been a pioneer in establishing the credibility of office-based surgery in the eyes of his colleagues, as well as in the eyes of insurance company executives. His book covers, in detail, safe and high-quality practice patterns and techniques suitable to the office surgery. Most recommendations are also applicable to the ambulatory surgical unit or the hospital operating room. For a full discussion of this important topic, see Chapter 11.

Office surgery may never appeal to most gynecologists who are satisfied with their access to hospitals and surgery centers. For the practitioner who anticipates a sufficient volume of surgery to justify his or her own unit and who appreciates the high degree of safety and control over his or her own scheduling that such a unit would provide, however, an office surgery may be a worthwhile investment.

What about the cost of developing and equipping a free-standing unit? This is the major stumbling block for many practitioners. Among the many factors influencing the cost are

1. Basic construction costs in the community;
2. Increased rental or leasing costs of added operating and recovery-room space;
3. The cost of equipment and instruments;
4. The cost of additional nursing and counseling personnel;
5. The hiring of anesthesia personnel and equipment, should the option of general anesthesia be offered on the premises;
6. The decision concerning formal certification of the office surgery.

Let me present my own experience in building and equipping my current office surgery in 1983. Figure 3.1 shows an architect's final drawing for a solo practitioner's unit on the second floor of an office building in Syracuse, New York, a city of about 250,000. I was fortunate to have the opportunity, with the cooperation of the landlord, to plan the office surgery from the ground up. This model is offered as an arrangement that has permitted private counseling, personal care during surgery, and adequate supervision during the immediate recovery period.

Our unit is designed for a solo-practice gynecologist. The operating rooms (Fig. 3.2) accommodate surgical procedures, most often scheduled during morning hours. These same rooms serve as examining rooms during afternoon hours. Emergency procedures, such as a D&C for uterine hemorrhage or a completion of an incomplete abortion, may be fitted into the morning or afternoon schedule.

A private room is assigned to the nurses for initial patient interviews and counseling, and the recovery room is just large enough for two couch-and-chair combinations with an intervening privacy curtain suspended from a ceiling rack. A collapsible wheelchair is

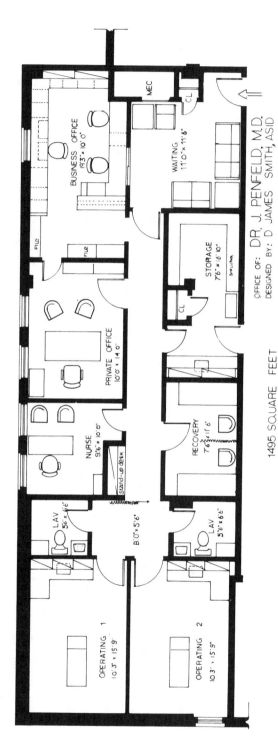

Figure 3.1. Plan for office surgery.

CHAPTER 3 / OUTPATIENT FACILITIES FOR OPERATIONS UNDER LOCAL ANESTHESIA

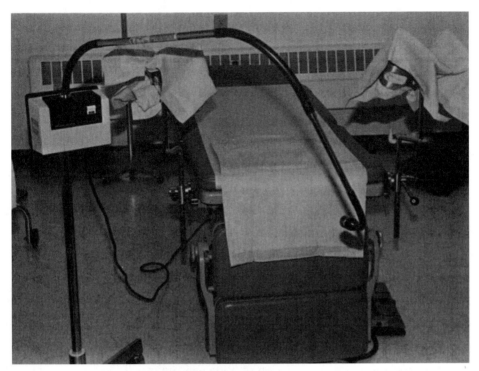

Figure 3.2. Operating room.

stored in the recovery room and is used regularly for the postoperative transport of patients by the nurse to the elevator and out of the building to a waiting car.

The office plans include room dimensions I consider to be close to the minimum for the provision of comfortable uncrowded accommodations. Room shapes and dimensions may be varied to suit the individual floor plan. A group practice would require a far more elaborate arrangement in a much larger overall space.

Accreditation of a free-standing facility will carry with it the added benefit of public assurance of quality care. However, the process of certification and periodic recertification will add substantial expense to the operation of the facility because of rigorous design and equipment requirements. The practitioner will probably attempt to recoup these additional costs by increasing the facility fee for each operation performed.

Facility certification for the purpose of insurance reimbursement is generally considered appropriate and even essential for group practice units that offer the option of general anesthesia, requiring added personnel and safeguards. My own choice as a solo practitioner, however, has been to perform operations in my office surgery exclusively under local anesthesia. I admit to the hospital all patients requiring general anesthesia. Therefore, I have been able to hold down my outpatient surgical fees and have not found it necessary to charge facility fees.

When an office surgery is set up for the performance of operations under local anesthesia, the following basic safeguards are, I believe, essential:

1. An auxiliary light source. In case of power failure, a portable battery-powered lantern may be used to complete the surgery;

2. Certification and annual recertification of the surgeon and assistants in cardiopulmonary resuscitation (CPR);
3. Oxygen and emergency medications, including diazepam (Valium, Roche) or midazolam (Versed, Roche), atropine, and a narcotic antagonist (Figs. 3.3–3.5);
4. Ready availability of an ambulance service;
5. Hospital backup within a few minutes' ambulance drive.

For sterilization of instruments, one autoclave should be placed on the counter near the sink in each operating room (Fig. 3.6). After each surgical procedure, instruments are immediately washed, rinsed, and placed in packets or on trays for repeat autoclaving.

Busy hospital units ordinarily isolate instrument sterilization and hand-washing from the operating room environment. Indeed, health department regulations in certain localities mandate such separations to promote asepsis, even in free-standing units. Nonetheless, for most small office surgeries serving one or two practitioners, where patient scheduling is tightly controlled and daily cleaning routines are immaculate, the construction of separate scrub and sterilization rooms is both unnecessary and prohibitively expensive.

With increasing demand throughout the United States for outpatient, free-standing, and office surgical facilities for procedures under local anesthesia and with the growing realization that even invasive operations, such as minilaparotomy and laparoscopy, can be safely performed in these centers, practice guidelines have been formulated for optimal patient care and to assist insurance companies in providing appropriate reimbursement. These and other related topics are discussed in Chapter 13 by Paul Allen, MD.

The emerging need for accreditation of outpatient units will result inevitably in the introduction of sophisticated and expensive equipment and electronic monitoring devices. There is evidence, for example, that pulse oximetry, a noninvasive monitoring of hemoglobin saturation, will detect hypoxia earlier than is possible by clinical observation alone (5). However, hypoxia does not occur in a patient who is breathing normally and engaged in conversation with her nurse attendant. Even in centers where all operations are under local anesthesia supplemented by minimal analgesia and sedation, there will be demands for on-site defibrillators. Who will trust a gynecologist to operate one of these?

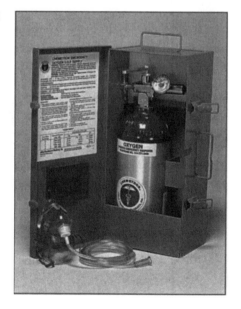

Figure 3.3. Portable oxygen tank. (Photo courtesy of Allied Healthcare Products, 1720 Sublette Avenue, St. Louis, MO 63110.)

CHAPTER 3 / OUTPATIENT FACILITIES FOR OPERATIONS UNDER LOCAL ANESTHESIA 27

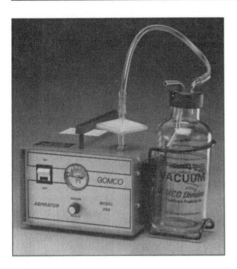

Figure 3.4. Emergency oropharyngeal suction equipment. (Photo courtesy of Allied Healthcare Products, 1720 Sublette Avenue, St. Louis, MO 63110.)

In my opinion, patients will be far better safeguarded if physicians and staff are regularly certified in life support techniques (CPR or Advanced Life Support (ALS)). In the rare event of cardiac arrest, these measures should be promptly applied while awaiting ambulance transfer to a nearby hospital. Obviously, a patient with a history of significant cardiac dysrhythmia who presents for any procedure that may be dangerously stressful should have an anesthesiologist in attendance with the kind of monitoring equipment normally present only in the hospital operating room. It is understood that patients with this disorder or any equally threatening condition are not candidates for office surgery,

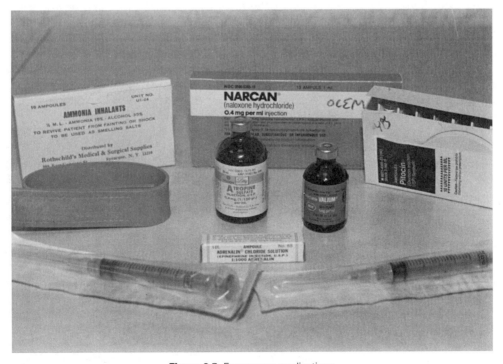

Figure 3.5. Emergency medications.

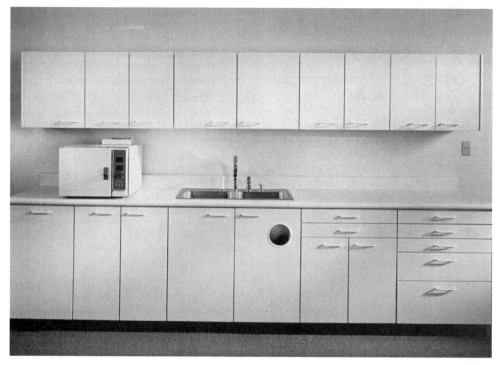

Figure 3.6. Autoclave. (Photo courtesy of Pelton & Crane, P.O. Box 7800, Charlotte, NC 28241-7800.)

but for virtually all other patients, every operation described in this book can be adequately monitored clinically by an alert surgeon and nurse attendant.

The decision to equip a free-standing or office surgical facility with electronic monitoring and resuscitation devices will be based in most instances not so much on a realistic desire to improve safety as on the requirements for accreditation and reimbursement.

Notwithstanding individual variations in monitoring techniques, the modern office surgical facility provides an excellent setting for the performance of outpatient surgery under local anesthesia.

REFERENCES

1. Kaali SG, Landesman R. Tubal sterilization with the Falope ring in an ambulatory-care surgical facility. NY State J Med 1985;85:98–100.
2. Greenspan JR, Phillips JM, Ruber GL, Rhodenhiser EP, Ory HW. Tubal sterilizations performed in free-standing ambulatory-care surgical facilities in the United States in 1980. J Reprod Med 1984; 29:237–241.
3. Hill G, ed. Outpatient surgery. Philadelphia, PA: WB Saunders, 1988.
4. Martin P. Ambulatory gynecologic surgery. Littleton, MA: PSG Publishing Co., 1979.
5. Tremper K, Barker S. Oxygenation and blood gases. In: Staidman L, eds. Monitoring in anesthesia. Boston, MA: Butterworth-Heinemann, 1993:1.

4. Dilatation and Curettage

A. JEFFERSON PENFIELD

Each year in the United States, apart from the estimated 1.5 million abortions, dilatation and curettage (D&C) is the most frequently performed operation in gynecology. However, during the past 10 years, in modern gynecologic practice this procedure as a diagnostic tool has been largely supplanted by hysteroscopically directed biopsies. As surgical therapy for severe chronic dysfunctional uterine bleeding, hysteroscopically controlled endometrial ablation or endomyometrial resection has produced superior results (see Chapter 6). Nonetheless, a skillfully performed D&C is equally effective in controlling most cases of severe acute menorrhagia and is a far simpler and rapid approach to the treatment of the very common problem of incomplete abortion, retained products, or bleeding decidua (1).

The main disadvantage of D&C is that it is a blind procedure that occasionally fails to reveal localized pathology. The main advantage is that it requires minimum instrumentation and can be performed in most cases in an outpatient setting or emergency room under local anesthesia with minimal expense.

This chapter covers the indications, contraindications, counseling, performance, and complications of D&C under local anesthesia. First trimester abortion (voluntary interruption of pregnancy) is covered as a separate subject in Chapter 5.

SENSORY INNERVATION OF THE UTERUS AND RATIONALE FOR UTEROSACRAL BLOCK

"The nerves of the uterus are derived from the hypogastric and ovarian plexuses and from the third and fourth sacral nerves. Afferent (sensory) fibers from the uterus enter the spinal cord solely through the eleventh and twelfth thoracic nerves" (2). Note that afferent pain fibers traveling from the body of the uterus through the ovarian plexuses cannot be interrupted by uterosacral block. Therefore, it is not possible to anesthetize the uterine corpus transvaginally (Fig. 4.1). Neither can the entire inferior hypogastric plexus be blocked. However, accurate placement of anesthetic solution into the uterosacral ligaments blocks most if not all of the nerve fibers supplying the region of the internal cervical os (Fig. 4.2). Thus, it is possible to obliterate most pain sensations from cervical dilatation.

Patients may experience mild to moderate reflex uterine pain during the course of cervical dilatation. Frequently, they will liken this sensation to a "menstrual cramp." It is rare indeed for a patient during cervical dilatation to experience uterine pain even approaching the intensity of labor pain. Her reactions are governed by her basic physiologic threshold for pain, her degree of anxiety, the effectiveness of pre- and intraoperative counseling, the presence or absence of cervical stenosis, and the gynecologist's skill in administering a paracervical block.

Once the cervix has been adequately dilated, little additional uterine pain other than ordinary menstrual cramps will be elicited by gentle, slow, deliberate, and systematic manipulation of the uterine curette to retrieve endocervical and endometrial tissue.

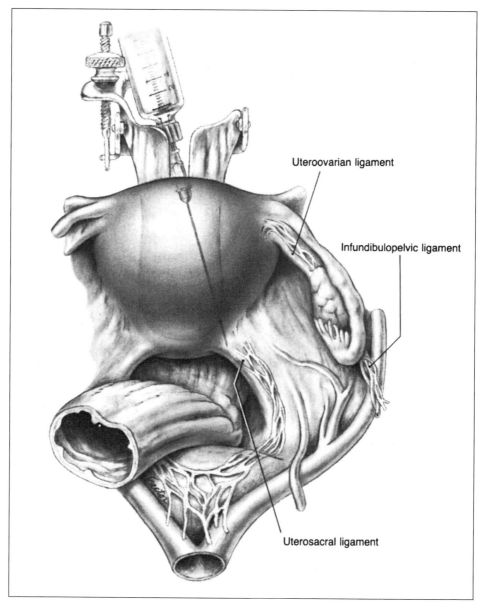

Figure 4.1. Sensory innervation of the uterus and uterosacral block.

INDICATIONS

Abnormal uterine bleeding is the primary indication for D&C (Table 4.1). It is important to note that certain systemic diseases, such as thyroid or other endocrine disorders, leukemia, or bleeding diatheses, may cause abnormal uterine bleeding and must first be ruled out. Iatrogenic causes such as estrogen-progestin therapy must also be diagnosed and managed before any consideration is given to curettage.

Most cases of abnormal uterine bleeding call for preoperative transvaginal sonography (see Chapter 11). An abnormally thick endometrium, for example, may suggest hyper-

CHAPTER 4 / DILATATION AND CURETTAGE

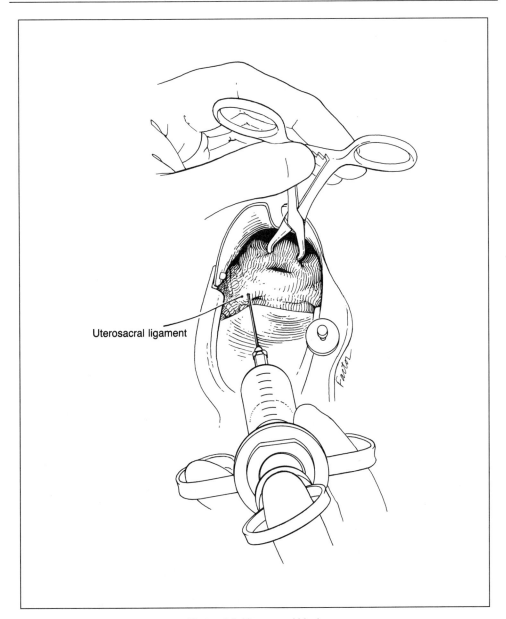

Figure 4.2. Uterosacral block.

plasia; polyps and submucous myomata can be diagnosed preoperatively and may be managed preferably hysteroscopically (see Chapter 6).

Apparent "dysfunctional" menometrorrhagia that has proven to be refractory to progestogen or other hormonal therapy is an indication either for D&C or for hysteroscopically directed sampling, ranging from directed biopsies to endomyometrial resection (see Chapter 6.) When D&C is selected, it should accomplish three goals: obtain a maximal sampling of endometrium for microscopic examination, rule out carcinoma, and provide hemostasis, both immediate and long term.

On four occasions during the past 24 years, patients have arrived in my office surgery

Table 4.1
Indications for Dilatation and Curettage

Abnormal uterine bleeding
    Refractory dysfunctional bleeding
    Endometrial or endocervical polyps
    Adenomyosis or myomata: if submucous, hysteroscopy preferable
    Grand multiparity
    Incomplete abortion
    Retained products, postabortal or postpartum
    Subinvolution, endometritis, or hydatid mole
    Suspected endometrial carcinoma
Refractory dysmenorrhea
Hematometra or pyometra

hemorrhaging from the uterine cavity with hypotension and tachycardia. Two women were miscarrying and two were experiencing severe "dysfunctional" menorrhagia. Because we always have trays of sterile instruments ready, I was able to start intravenous fluids and perform a curettage under paracervical block on each patient within 5 minutes of their arrival. Thus, there was a prompt normalization of pulse and blood pressure in each case.

Unfortunately, protocol in most hospitals in the United States requires that all such patients be started on an intravenous infusion and be typed, cross-matched, and frequently transfused before anesthesia personnel are permitted or willing to take responsibility for the patient in the operating room. To overcome these dangerous delays, an emergency operating room or office surgery, in which the gynecologist is fully responsible for giving local anesthesia, can provide a superior setting for the prompt management of life-threatening uterine hemorrhage.

Incomplete abortion, or persistent postabortal bleeding suggesting the possibility of retained products, subinvolution, endometritis, or hydatid mole, is an indication for D&C. In the United States during the past 30 years, as hospital costs have skyrocketed, increasing numbers of gynecologists have discovered the convenience of a private office surgery or a small outpatient operating room, possibly adjacent to the hospital emergency room, where prompt uterine evacuations for incomplete abortions may be carried out. Local anesthesia, possibly supplemented by an intravenous analgesic, is adequate for these cases. General anesthesia is frequently contraindicated because the patients may have eaten recently.

Puerperal bleeding due to retained secundines, subinvolution, endometritis, or retained molar tissue and postmenopausal bleeding are indications for D&C. If a postmenopausal woman on cyclic estrogen-progestogen therapy is having withdrawal periods that are gradually diminishing in volume and duration, curettage is not indicated. Otherwise, with rare exceptions, any episode of uterine bleeding unassociated with typical premenstrual symptoms that occurs more than 6 months after the menopause calls for curettage. Most postmenopausal bleeders can be curetted without difficulty under local anesthesia, but some patients, because of vaginal atrophy, require general anesthesia for muscle relaxation and pain relief and to permit a satisfactory pelvic examination.

Refractory dysmenorrhea, possibly secondary to stenosis of the internal os of the cervix, is an indication for D&C. On the other hand, primary dysmenorrhea is most often due to incoordinate uterine activity that should be treated first with antiprostaglandins, oral contraceptives, or by other conservative measures. Dysmenorrhea secondary to endometriosis may require lupron, danazol, or high-dose progestogen therapy. Cervical dilatation with or without uterine curettage is seldom justified as initial therapy for dysmenorrhea. Even when performed after all conservative measures have failed, a D&C will probably not prevent symptoms for more than 6 months. The rare case of congenital stenosis of the internal cervical os, on the other hand, does require cervical dilatation.

Hematometra or pyometra secondary to cervical stenosis, obstruction, radiation fibrosis, or postmenopausal atrophy is an indication for D&C.

COUNSELING

Especially for the patient who presents with specific complaints, it is important for the gynecologist or counselor to stress that the proposed D&C has therapeutic and diagnostic purposes. Not only is full disclosure consistent with good medical care, but I found that patients are inclined to be more relaxed and cooperative for a procedure under local anesthesia when they are well informed beforehand.

If a patient is constipated, she should take an enema the evening before the surgery, both for her own comfort and to facilitate pelvic examination. On the morning of surgery, she may have a clear liquid breakfast. If possible, a companion should take her home after surgery.

When describing the paracervical block to a patient, it is important to tell her that this is a form of anesthesia. Several years ago a 45-year-old woman with menometrorrhagia returned to the referring physician after her preoperative visit in my office. She was upset because I had recommended a D&C without anesthesia! What I had actually told her was that she would feel some "pinches" as I injected the local anesthetic around her cervix. The word "anesthetic" had escaped her attention; therefore, I had failed in my effort to communicate. Some physicians will supplement their counseling with written information or videotape.

The patient should understand that in addition to the "pinches," she will feel some uterine cramps during the cervical dilatation. Pain fibers from the internal os can be blocked, but the uterine corpus cannot be anesthetized through the vagina. I have occasionally injected 5 mL 1% lidocaine transcervically into the endometrial cavity, but in my hands the technique has not been uniformly successful in preventing uterine pain. It helps the patient to relate to something familiar by explaining that she is likely to experience menstrual cramps. She should be told that the procedure will be completed in 10 to 15 minutes and the cramps will subside postoperatively, allowing her to go home within 30 to 60 minutes. We usually ask her to return for a visit at 6 weeks, at which time I will re-examine her if necessary and review the pathology findings and follow-up instructions.

We prefer to discuss all above details with the patient at the first preoperative visit. Such a policy is not only consistent with good medical care but is also reassuring to the patient, who realizes that we regard the D&C as a part of her ongoing care.

Whenever appropriate, while counseling the patient, the advantages of local anesthesia—safety, convenience in the outpatient setting, and rapid easy recovery—should be emphasized.

TECHNIQUE

Most patients for diagnostic or therapeutic curettage do not require any preoperative medication. However, an unusually anxious patient may benefit from 10 mg oral diazepam (Valium) 1 hour before surgery. If necessary, 10 mg diazepam or 5 mg midazolam (Versed) may be injected intravenously immediately before the operation. If a patient has a history of "easy fainting" or previous vasovagal episodes, she should be given 0.4 mg atropine sulfate intravenously as soon as she is on the operating table. If there is any reason to suspect that she may have an unusually low pain threshold, a dose of meperidine, fentanyl, or butorphanol may be given intravenously.

I then examine the patient to confirm the original findings and to rule out intercurrent developments such as early pregnancy. When in doubt, a urine pregnancy test is done. The vagina and vulva are prepped with full-strength povidone-iodine solution. I put on sterile gloves and position a fenestrated drape to frame the vaginal opening. A medium or large bivalve speculum is introduced and opened sufficiently to expose the cervix and bring into view the posterior fornix and cervicovaginal junction.

I fill a 10-mL Luer-Lok syringe with a solution of 0.5% lidocaine with 1:200,000 epinephrine, attach a 2.5-inch 22-gauge needle, and inject 1 to 2 mL barely beneath the cervicovaginal mucosa at 4, 8, 10, and 2 o'clock. If these injections are made with great care, most patients feel no pain. However, I precede each puncture with the spoken word "pinch" so that no patient will be startled. Then, with a comment that she may feel a mild cramp, I attach a tenaculum to the anterior lip of the cervix.

At this point I am ready to perform the paracervical block. Having already achieved superficial anesthesia, the introduction of the needle into each uterosacral ligament is less likely to cause any pain. Nonetheless, I always caution the patient that she may feel a pinch. To avoid contributing to the patient's anxiety, the word "pain" should not be used when describing the sensation the patient is likely to experience. A properly performed injection into the uterosacral ligament should result in no more than mild to moderate transient discomfort; 3 to 4 mL of the anesthetic solution in each ligament is adequate. The injection should be made slowly and interrupted at least once with an attempted withdrawal of the piston of the syringe to avoid an intravascular administration.

The speculum nut should now be loosened to allow the blades to come together so as to give the patient at least a minute to relax and regain her composure as the anesthetic is taking hold. During this brief interval, I arrange my instruments and gauze sponges and reassure the patient that the procedure will be completed in 10 to 15 minutes. I also caution her to expect some mild menstrual cramps. Success with local anesthesia requires this kind of reassuring communication and gentle deliberate maneuvers.

Occasionally, despite our best efforts, a patient has called out in pain or broken down with uncontrollable crying. My remedy for these situations is to discontinue the procedure, take the patient's legs down, and sit beside her to talk in a reassuring manner while she regains her equanimity. Additional tranquilizers or analgesics administered intravenously may be helpful. In each such case during the past 24 years, we were able to complete the procedure without further difficulty. I can recall no more than two or three out of several thousand surgical cases under local anesthesia in which it was necessary to discontinue and resume the operation in this manner. In no case have we transferred the patient to the hospital or surgery center for general anesthesia.

Gentle traction should now be placed on the tenaculum to partially straighten the cervicouterine angle. The curved uterine sound should be held lightly between the thumb and first or second finger as the tip is "dropped" into the cervical canal (Fig 4.3). Resistance is usually encountered at the internal os, but with a careful search for the proper angle of passage, it is normally possible to negotiate the canal with only a very slight increase in pressure.

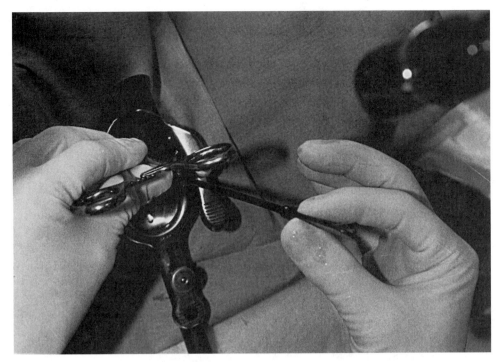

Figure 4.3. Gentle sounding of internal cervical os.

If true stenosis of the internal os is encountered, a fine hemostat may be used to effect entry into the uterine cavity. Rarely, it may be necessary to administer oral or vaginal estrogen for 3 to 4 weeks to bring about sufficient softening of the cervix to permit passage of the sound. This measure has proven effective in two of my patients whose cervices were not otherwise safely negotiable.

Having determined the exact cervicouterine angle with the aid of the sound, the 5-mm and larger dilators are introduced in exactly the same direction, as downward traction is applied to the cervical tenaculum. Dilators should be grasped in the same manner as the sound, that is, between the thumb and index finger. As dilators with 0.5-mm incremental diameters are introduced, increasing resistance is likely to be encountered at the internal os. It may be necessary to replace the single-tooth with a double-tooth tenaculum (Jacobs) for a firmer grasp of the cervix. As internal os resistance increases, so does the risk of uterine perforation. Therefore, it may be necessary for the operator to return to smaller dilators and patiently work his or her way back up to the larger ones. This situation is most often encountered in the postmenopausal patient with an atrophic uterus.

The cervix should not be dilated any further than necessary for the indicated procedure. In the postmenopausal patient, for example, dilatation to 7 mm is adequate, permitting passage of the small sharp curette.

One important advantage of paracervical block before cervical dilatation is that the local anesthetic relaxes the internal os, particularly if epinephrine is incorporated into the solution. I saw a dramatic demonstration of this phenomenon under general anesthesia in the surgery center. The patient was asleep and the uterine corpus was relaxed, but the internal os remained firm and nonnegotiable until local anesthetic solution was injected into the uterosacral ligaments.

After the cervix is sufficiently dilated, a small sharp curette may be introduced and a systematic curettage of the cavity carried out. The patient should again be cautioned that she will feel some cramps during this portion of the operation. The curette should be introduced gently and repeatedly to the fundal wall, and whatever endometrial tissue is dislodged should be brought out at the end of each downward stroke and deposited on a gauze or Telfa sponge. Systematic longitudinal strokes should be taken with the curette in a clockwise or counterclockwise fashion (Fig. 4.4). I know of no justification for the "egg-beater" technique favored by some surgeons, who practice a vigorous mixing maneuver that merely churns up the endometrium and increases uterine cramping.

The entire procedure is unlikely to take more than 15 to 20 minutes, including the time required to produce satisfactory local anesthesia. General anesthesia is unnecessary unless the patient cannot be adequately examined while awake.

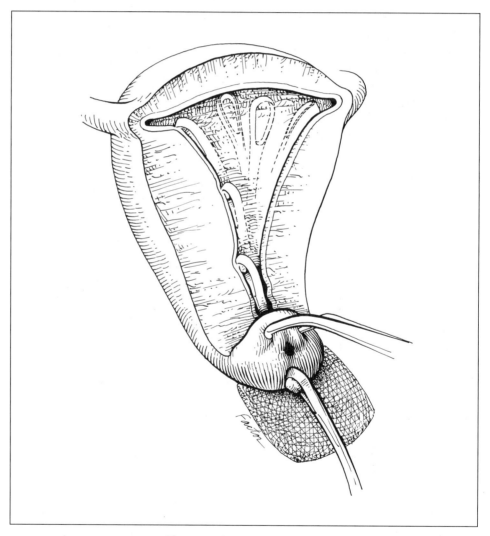

Figure 4.4. Systematic curettage.

COMPLICATIONS

Uterine Perforation

This accident may occur when the sound is introduced with too great a force in the wrong direction (Fig. 4.5). It is most likely to occur in the postmenopausal patient with a firm fibrotic cervix, a stenotic internal os, and an atrophic corpus. Uterine perforation is not completely preventable, because there are occasions when the surgeon's attempt to overcome the usual internal os resistance allows the tip of the uterine sound to perforate the wall, usually at the cervicouterine junction. The accident rarely results in serious consequences, provided it is promptly recognized and the procedure is discontinued. Most perforations occur near the midline of the uterus, which is relatively avascular, both anteriorly and posteriorly, and most will heal spontaneously. One advantage of local

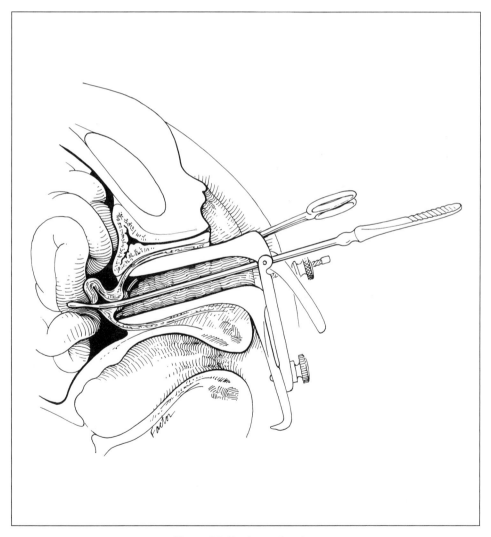

Figure 4.5. Uterine perforation.

anesthesia is that if a perforation does occur, the patient is likely to complain of a steady dull pain, unlike the pain of a menstrual cramp. The patient then assists in making the surgeon aware of the complication sooner than if she were under general anesthesia.

If the perforation is not recognized until the cervix has already been at least partially dilated, the cautious meticulous surgeon should be able to safely introduce a small curette and obtain enough endometrial tissue to establish a diagnosis. Such a patient should be monitored with vital signs for at least 1 hour postoperatively. Continued pain or signs of peritoneal irritation may call for hospitalization and possible laparoscopy.

Cervical Laceration

Occasionally, a cervix at or near the internal os will give way or split, either because of overly forceful dilatation or because of a thinned-out scar of the cervix that allows it to lacerate easily. It is not always possible for the surgeon to predict which cervix is particularly subject to laceration. Certainly, a pale fibrotic cervix or one with a deep longitudinal scar extending into the lower uterine segment calls for extreme caution. If during dilatation the cervix splits laterally across the uterine vessels, serious hemorrhage may result, requiring immediate transfer to a major hospital operating room, laparotomy for control of bleeding, evacuation of hematoma, or even hysterectomy. This should be an exceedingly rare accident.

Should the patient at risk for cervical laceration be given general anesthesia to provide better relaxation? The answer is no. As pointed out earlier, the internal os relaxes far better under a paracervical block, particularly if epinephrine 1:200,000 is included in the anesthetic solution. Furthermore, a laceration or a perforation is more promptly recognized in the awake patient, who usually complains of an unexpected dull steady pain immediately after the injury occurs.

Vasovagal Reactions

These occur commonly during or after a wide variety of surgical procedures in the awake patient. The vasovagal syndrome, its prevention, description, and treatment, are covered at length in Chapter 2. Briefly, bradycardia or even convulsions and syncope may be experienced by the patient during the introduction of a paracervical block or during cervical dilatation. The reaction is less likely if she has already received 0.4 mg intravenous or intramuscular atropine sulfate prophylactically. Even without this medication, spontaneous prompt recovery from a vasovagal reaction should be expected in any patient who does not suffer from serious cardiovascular disease. The procedure need only be discontinued long enough for full recovery to occur, usually within 3 minutes. In my experience, serious reactions are so unusual with a D&C that routine preoperative atropine sulfate or other anticholinergic drugs are unnecessary.

Although I have never seen a vasovagal reaction or a cardiac dysrhythmia severe enough to require aggressive intervention, I continue to believe that the surgical staff must be trained in basic cardiopulmonary resuscitation and oxygen therapy. Oxygen and assisted ventilation should be administered immediately for apnea, cyanosis, or dysrhythmia.

CONCLUSION

In the interests of safety, convenience, and economy, I recommend that most D&Cs, excluding those that immediately precede major surgery, should be performed in outpatient settings under paracervical block. General anesthesia simply increases the risk, postoperative discomfort, and expense and should be reserved for those patients who must be asleep for adequate examination.

REFERENCES

1. Grimes DA. Diagnostic dilatation and curettage: a reappraisal. Am J Obstet Gynecol 1982;142:1–6.
2. Gray H. Anatomy of the human body. 30th ed. Philadelphia, PA: Lea and Febiger, 1985.

5. First Trimester Abortion

A. JEFFERSON PENFIELD

RU 486: A COMMENTARY

There has been wide media coverage recently about the conditional approval by the Food and Drug Administration (FDA) for the oral administration of RU 486 (mifepristone) to terminate pregnancies before the ninth week. RU 486, developed in 1980 by Roussel-Uclaf in Paris, France, is a steroid that has been studied and marketed in France, Britain, and China for several years. Mifepristone blocks the effects of progesterone and disrupts the process of decidual maturation. It may also initiate endogenous prostaglandin synthesis (1).

To complete the abortion, most patients require, in addition, a prostaglandin analogue (misoprostol) administered either vaginally or by mouth 48 hours later. Thus, continuous medical supervision is necessary for at least several days.

RU 486 has already been used by 250,000 women in Europe and China to terminate their pregnancies. A multicenter European study of 16,173 patients who received RU 486-prostaglandin combination showed an overall success rate of 95.3% (2). The mean duration of bleeding was 8 days, and 0.8% of patients required a follow-up vacuum curettage or a dilatation and curettage. A blood transfusion was necessary in 0.1% of women (11 patients).

A Chinese study of 1,572 women who received mifepristone followed by misoprostol reported somewhat less satisfactory results. Complete abortion occurred in 91.2%, incomplete abortion in 4.8%, and continued pregnancy in 3.9%. Nausea and vomiting was reported by 22.3% of women, prolonged abdominal pain by 10.2%, headache and dizziness by 4.1%, and diarrhea by 2.8% (3).

The conditional U.S. FDA approval of mifepristone/misoprostol for medical abortion followed a New Drug Application presented in March 1996 by the Population Council in New York at the conclusion of a 2-year multicenter trial across the United States. The findings of this trial did not vary significantly from those reported from Europe and China.

To quote from the Population Council Report, "The most frequent adverse effects experienced in the U.S. clinical trial were painful uterine contractions and gastrointestinal effects (nausea, diarrhea, and vomiting). Most of these events (65%) took place immediately after taking the misoprostol at the second visit" (4). Full FDA approval awaits the selection and certification by the FDA of a U.S. distributor.

Despite the drawbacks cited by European, Chinese and U.S. studies, RU 486 will be very appealing to many women seeking abortion before the ninth week of pregnancy. They will welcome any method that offers some assurance of privacy and is less frightening to contemplate than surgical abortion.

However, judging from the study findings cited above, I will add my commentary. Many women will find that medical abortion is accompanied by prolonged uterine contractions and more nausea, vomiting, and/or diarrhea than surgical abortion. Regarding the privacy issue, either method of pregnancy termination requires two or more visits to an office or a clinic. Medical abortion, after all, will be supervised by a physician who is qualified to determine the duration of pregnancy, rule out ectopic pregnancy, and provide backup emergency care including surgical abortion or evacuation of retained products if necessary.

In conclusion, there will continue to be a need for skilled sensitive surgical abortion throughout the first trimester. Under local anesthesia, it is a 10- to 15-minute procedure that should cause only moderate transient uterine cramps and should allow the patient to return promptly to her normal activities.

The reader is referred to Chapter 4, on dilatation and curettage, for a review of counseling, technique, and complications. The material in those sections relates exactly to early pregnancy termination. This chapter emphasizes important features of first trimester abortion counseling, technique, and complications. For a more detailed description of operative abortion, both first and second trimester, the reader is referred to *Protocols for Office Gynecologic Surgery* by Darney et al. (5) or *Abortion Practice* by Hern (6). My own experience with induced abortion during the past 24 years is largely limited to operative termination of pregnancy up to 10 weeks from conception or 12 weeks from the first day of the last menstrual period.

COUNSELING

Most patients who present for abortion are upset and frightened. Unplanned pregnancies are disturbing, at least initially, even to those women who within a few weeks accept the pregnancy and look forward to delivery.

But what about the women who refuse to accept the result of failed contraception or no contraception and decide to terminate their pregnancies? Ever since the demonstration of the effectiveness of vacuum curettage by the Japanese, who faced an intolerable population explosion after World War II, safe elective abortion has become an option for millions of women around the world, provided they can surmount religious and political barriers and then locate and afford the necessary surgical services.

In the United States, a Supreme Court ruling in 1973 (Roe *v* Wade 410 US 113) upheld the right of a woman to terminate an unwanted first or second trimester pregnancy. The public debate continues, however, in religious and political circles about the rights of the embryo versus the rights of the pregnant woman. Thus, it should be no surprise that many women presenting for abortion are troubled by a sense of guilt and shame because of social and religious disapproval. A substantial segment of society is telling these women that they are contemplating a selfish and destructive act.

Many intelligent and thoughtful women, however, particularly those whose partners are loving and supportive, are rapidly able to recognize operative abortion as a responsible solution to their contraceptive failure or lack of contraceptive use. If a woman's husband or partner has shared in the decision for abortion, she will approach the event with greater equanimity.

The effective abortion counselor must be sensitive to the enormous variety of human responses to unplanned pregnancy. When a patient first telephones us for an appointment, we often suggest that she obtain a urine pregnancy test unless she has already received confirmation by pelvic or laboratory examination. If she does not know her blood type, we order this also. (All Rh-negative patients receive anti-D immunoglobulin [Micrhogam Ortho] on the day of the procedure.)

The patient is instructed to have clear liquids only (e.g., juice and coffee) in the morning before surgery. She is invited to bring her partner or companion into the counseling session if she wishes. The counselor, preferably a mature compassionate woman, should be, first and foremost, a perceptive listener and competent history taker. All options, including continuation of pregnancy to term and placing the child for adoption, must be introduced and discussed. The counselor must be as certain as possible that the decision for abortion is the patient's own decision and that she is not being coerced by her husband, partner, family, or friends.

Discussion with the counselor serves to inform and reassure the patient and provides the basis for the ready acceptance of vacuum curettage under local anesthesia. It is particularly comforting to a woman to know that her counselor will be with her during the procedure. Under exceptional circumstances, if the patient's husband or partner is supportive and well prepared, it may be helpful for him to be present at the operation also.

We found that a 15- to 30-minute counseling session on the day of the operation is adequate to provide peace of mind for the patient. Frequently, we offer the unusually agitated patient a tranquilizer such as diazepam, 5 mg by mouth, as soon as she registers with the receptionist.

In a private practice setting, the fee for the procedure must be discussed at the time of the initial inquiry. Although payment at the time of service may be requested, it is unconscionable to endanger the patient's health by refusing or postponing the procedure because of her inability to pay in advance. Because affordability is a major source of anxiety to many patients, at least in the United States, I believe that the physician should be ready to adjust fees or immediately assist the patient in making alternative arrangements. The woman whose anxieties, financial and otherwise, are resolved is in a much more relaxed frame of mind to cooperate during an operation under local anesthesia that requires her complete trust and confidence.

Just as with a planned dilatation and curettage for any procedure, the counselor should describe the proposed paracervical block, cervical dilatation, and vacuum curettage in a nonthreatening manner. The word "pain" should be avoided if possible, and words such as "pinches" as the anesthetic is being given and "menstrual cramps" as the cervix is being dilated should be used instead. The word "vacuum" has fewer unpleasant connotations than "suction."

In my opinion, graphic color illustrations of the abortion procedure are more likely to alarm than inform. Few patients, indeed, are eager to learn every specific detail of the operation. I frequently emphasize after the initial counseling session that I will make no attempt to identify an embryo during the procedure and that I will simply empty the uterus gently and safely and dispose of the tissue promptly. (Tissue is sent to the laboratory only if it appears in any way abnormal [i.e., with vesical formation] or if very little tissue is obtained.)

We tell the patient that the operation will take no more than 5 to 10 minutes after the anesthetic has been injected. The manner of the counselor should be sensitive, warm, and "laid-back." At the same time, the counselor must be firm and confident. During the procedure, the counselor must not be overly solicitous or protective; these are attitudes that can only increase the patient's anxiety.

Each patient should be told that the procedure is safe, particularly under local anesthesia, and that the risks of hemorrhage or uterine perforation are remote. If either of these events occurs, it is comforting for her to know that the skills and facilities are immediately available for effective management. A good deal of tact and discretion must be exercised in discussing these matters. The operative consent form must make reference to them in general terms. The consent form must be signed by the patient and also by a parent or other adult of her choice if she is under 16 years of age.

PREOPERATIVE EXAMINATION

There is no situation in gynecology more fraught with possible confusion and error than a pelvic examination before an intended operative termination of pregnancy. Even those patients who are relaxed and easy to examine, not obese, and with clearly identifiable pelvic structures may lull the gynecologist into a false sense of security. In dealing with abortion under local anesthesia in women who are no more than 10 weeks from conception, it is essential for the operator first to determine the position of the uterus and to outline its dimensions as exactly as possible. With the corpus in an anterior position, estimation of size is not difficult unless the patient is tense or obese. Tension may be relieved by counseling, premedication, and gentleness, but obesity may force the examiner to rely principally on vaginal findings.

A markedly retroverted uterus requires a rectovaginal examination for better delineation and for a gentle attempt at manual repositioning to facilitate the procedure. The additional congestion resulting from chronic retroversion will enlarge the uterus at least 2 weeks beyond the gestational size of a corpus in midposition or anteversion. A unicornuate uterus may present a special challenge if the lateral enlargement simulates an adnexal mass. Large uterine myomata will also obscure the true pregnancy dimensions and may present serious operative difficulties if they encroach upon the lower uterine segment.

Adnexal masses are particularly difficult to evaluate because the enlarged uterus may displace them too far laterally to be detectable by bimanual examination. Alternatively, an adnexal mass may present directly behind the uterus, either in the cul-de-sac or behind the corpus. An example of this difficulty was demonstrated in a patient who came to me for a second opinion. Her gynecologist had diagnosed an intrauterine pregnancy 12 weeks from conception; in response to her request for termination, he had scheduled her for a vacuum curettage in the hospital. She came to my office surgery and was interviewed by the nurse-counselor. We asked her to empty her bladder and assisted her onto the examining table. She placed her legs comfortably into the knee stirrups to allow for complete relaxation. Upon bimanual examination, I found that her uterine corpus was enlarged to a pregnancy size no more than 6 weeks from conception, and there was a 8-cm cystic mass directly behind and above the fundus. These findings were confirmed by sonography. A few days later, I terminated her pregnancy by vacuum and standard curettage under paracervical block in my office surgery. As we hoped, the cyst, which was probably a giant corpus luteum cyst of pregnancy, collapsed spontaneously a few days later without causing any problems, and pelvic examination 1 week after abortion revealed a normally involuting uterus and no adnexal mass.

Exactly the reverse anatomic relationship was noted upon my examining a young woman on the occasion of her visit to our gynecology clinic. She had been referred by a physician who concluded from pelvic examination 1 week earlier that she was 3 months pregnant. My examination confirmed the presence of a symmetric, firm, tense, cystic, midline, 12-week-size pelvic mass. However, there was also a 6-week uterine corpus directly behind the mass. I informed her that she had a normal 6 weeks pregnancy and also a rather large ovarian cyst that should be removed if it was still present in another 6 to 8 weeks. Presumably, the utero-ovarian and infundibulopelvic ligaments had elongated sufficiently to allow the cystic ovary to float up anterior to the uterus (Fig. 5.1).

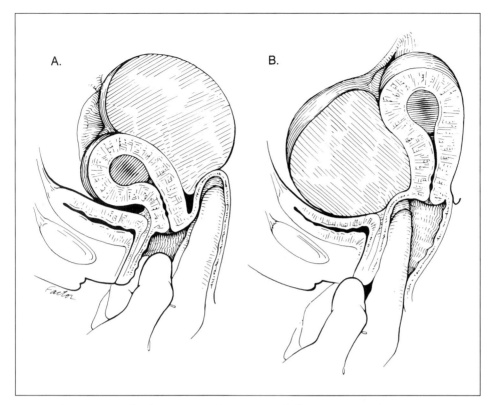

Figure 5.1. (**A**) Ovarian cyst posterior to uterus. (**B**) Ovarian cyst anterior to uterus.

The patient was referred to a private obstetrician who confirmed these findings and proposed a laparotomy for excision of a large ovarian cyst after the completion of her first trimester. It so happened that this cyst also collapsed spontaneously, in the tenth week of her pregnancy, and she progressed normally to term.

In each case, the first examiner mistook the larger of the pelvic masses for a pregnant uterus. One advantage of operating regularly under local anesthesia is that the gynecologist develops the skills necessary to win the patient's confidence and help her relax to outline pelvic structures and uterine size with greater accuracy.

Sonography has taken much of the guesswork out of pelvic examination. The most critical indication for sonography is the suspicion of a possible ectopic pregnancy. Sonographic findings concerning the presence or absence of an intrauterine sac or an adnexal mass may be most helpful in arriving at an accurate diagnosis. Negative adnexal findings, however, cannot be relied on to rule out a tubal pregnancy. Adnexal pain in early pregnancy should immediately alert one to the possibility of an ectopic pregnancy, as should any adnexal mass contiguous to the uterus.

VALUE OF PELVIC SONOGRAPHY

There are four observations, any one of which should trigger suspicion of the presence of an unruptured tubal pregnancy:

1. Unilateral adnexal pain;
2. An adnexal mass, elongated, tender, and contiguous to the uterine cornu;

3. An unexpectedly small volume of aspirated or curetted tissue from the uterine cavity (and a subsequent failure to identify placental villi on microscopic examination);
4. An empty uterine cavity or, at most, a "pseudocyst" within the uterus by pelvic sonography.

The sonogram may demonstrate an adnexal mass consistent with, but not diagnostic of, a pregnancy within the tube. Occasionally, the sonographer will identify an embryo in the tube with evidence of movement and cardiac activity. Rarely, simultaneous ectopic and intrauterine gestations are discovered.

The most likely and helpful sonographic aid to the diagnosis of ectopic pregnancy is the absence of an embryo in the uterine cavity in the presence of a positive pregnancy test (beta-subunit of chorionic gonadotropin). Conversely, the presence of an ultrasound image of an intrauterine embryo will, with rare exceptions, rule out the possibility of a tubal pregnancy.

If the gravid uterus on pelvic examination is "larger than it should be," based on presumed date of conception, then ultrasound will be helpful in confirming the suspicion of multiple pregnancy or hydatid mole. If, on the other hand, the uterus feels "smaller than it should," the sonographer will be able to corroborate the diagnosis of a missed abortion, "blighted ovum," incomplete abortion, or trapped products of conception after attempted uterine evacuation.

A pelvic sonogram is also most useful in determining the duration of pregnancy when the patient is difficult to examine because of obesity or in the presence of uterine myomata.

During the past 10 years, many American gynecologists and clinics have leased or purchased their own sonographic equipment. Transvaginal sonography has revolutionized abortion practice in assessing uterine contents and ruling out ectopic pregnancy (see Chapter 11).

OPERATIVE TECHNIQUE

Essential instruments for first trimester abortion are shown in Figure 5.2. Also shown (Fig. 5.2*B*) and described below are cervical dilators, single- or double-ended, with 17 incremental diameters. When the duration of pregnancy and the position of the uterus have been ascertained and an ectopic pregnancy has been reasonably excluded, I proceed as follows.

Preparation

A medium-sized speculum is inserted to expose the vaginal walls. The vagina and cervix are washed with povidone-iodine solution. The speculum is removed and the perineum is washed with povidone-iodine. The surgeon puts on sterile gloves and places a sterile fenestrated drape over the perineum. No mask is worn. A large sterile bivalve speculum is introduced and opened wide enough to expose the posterior fornix and cervicovaginal junction.

Local Anesthesia

Using a Luer-Lok syringe with frequent attempted withdrawals of the piston, a solution of 0.5% lidocaine with 1:200,000 epinephrine is injected through a 2.5-inch 22-gauge needle; 2 mL are injected barely beneath the cervicovaginal mucosa at 4, 8, 10, and 2 o'clock. Preceding each of these injections, the patient is told that she may feel a pinch. We have found that by anesthetizing superficially at first in this manner and then waiting

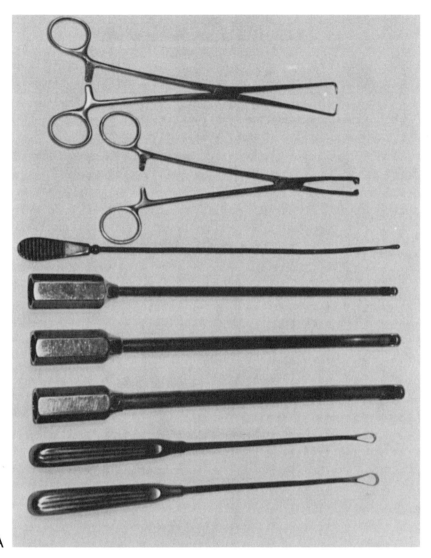

Figure 5.2. (**A**) Essential instruments for first trimester abortion (see text for description of dilators): Top to bottom, single-tooth cervical tenaculum, double-tooth (Jacobs) tenaculum, malleable uterine sound, vacurettes (6, 9, and 11 mm internal diameter), and standard curettes, medium and large. (**B**) Denniston Plastic Cervical Dilators. (Photo courtesy of Berkeley Medevices, Inc., 907 Camelia St., Berkeley, CA 94710.) (**C**) Vacurettes. (Photo courtesy of Berkeley Medevices.) (**D**) Uterine Aspirator. (Photo courtesy of Berkeley Medevices.)

30 to 60 seconds before injecting the uterosacrals, about one-half of our patients feel no pain whatsoever. The others may feel a momentary sharp pain of mild to moderate severity.

A single-tooth tenaculum is attached to the anterior lip of the cervix and upward traction exposes the cul-de-sac and outlines the position of the uterosacral ligaments. Each uterosacral ligament is injected about 0.5 cm from its uterine insertion with 3 to 4 mL of 0.5% lidocaine with 1:200,000 epinephrine. The speculum blades are partially closed and readjusted to reduce the vaginal pressure and give the patient 30 to 60 seconds of rest before sounding the cervix.

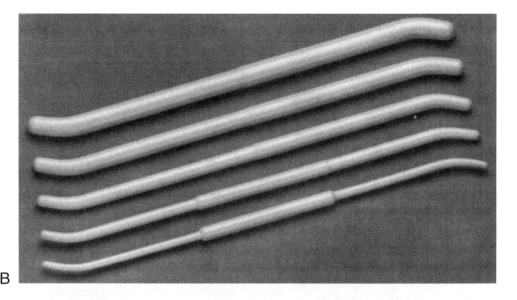

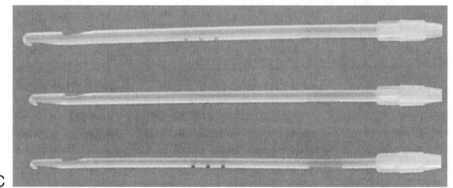

Figure 5.2 (*continued*)

Sounding the Cervix and Uterus

With continued traction on the cervical tenaculum, the uterine sound is gently "dropped" into the cervical canal, being careful to follow the previously noted angle between cervix and corpus. Passing the sound into the uterine cavity may be the most critical step in the performance of abortion. It confirms or reveals the position of the corpus, showing its degree of anteversion, retroversion, or inclination to the left or to the right. A pronounced lateral inclination suggests a unicornuate uterus. One may also find varying degrees of persistence of a lesser horn with the possibility of a double uterine cavity. I have had the experience of sounding two separate cavities and surmising that the larger of the two contained the products of conception. Vacuum curettage did indeed remove the products from the larger cavity. A medium-sized standard curette was then used to ensure that both cavities were empty.

When unusual resistance is encountered by the tip of the sound, the surgeon must assume that he or she has miscalculated the exact location of the internal os. He or she should then be prepared to spend as long as 1 or 2 minutes gently probing for the internal

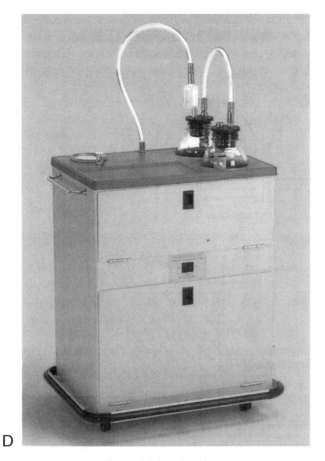

Figure 5.2 (*continued*)

os in all directions. The surgeon must keep in mind that firm traction on the cervical tenaculum may have straightened or even reversed the original angle between the cervix and corpus. Not infrequently, I have introduced the curved sound in an upside down position to accommodate a retroflexed corpus only to find that cervical traction has reversed the angle, thus requiring that I again reverse the curve of the sound and enter the cavity in an anterior direction.

Occasionally, because of excessive tightness of the internal os, the surgeon will be forced to conclude that a laminaria tent should be inserted or the procedure be postponed for a few weeks to allow for additional softening of the cervix. These alternative solutions will be covered in the next section.

Cervical Dilatation

Most practitioners favor the use of tapered dilators (e.g., Pratt's dilators) that require less propulsive force on the part of the operator. The advantage of such dilators was demonstrated by Hulka et al. (7), who devised a technique to compare forces necessary to overcome internal os resistance. However, I have found the parallel-sided relatively blunt Hegar dilators, in 0.5-mm incremental diameters, to be satisfactory and probably slightly less likely to perforate the uterus. As mentioned previously, the required insertional force is significantly diminished not only by the paracervical block but also by the addition of epinephrine to the anesthetic solution deposited into the uterosacral ligaments. All dilators should be copiously lubricated with a sterile, water-soluble lubricant such as K-Y jelly immediately before insertion. It has been my practice to begin with a 6-mm dilator and progress by 0.5-mm gradations to 8 mm for a uterus 6 weeks, 10 mm for 8 weeks, and 12 mm for 10 weeks from conception. (Add 2 weeks if calculating duration from the first day of the last period.)

Each dilator must be introduced at the same angle as the uterine sound, and excessive force must be avoided. It may be necessary to replace the single-tooth tenaculum with a double-tooth Jacobs tenaculum to avoid lacerating the anterior lip of the cervix. It may take 15 to 30 seconds to enter the uterine cavity with a dilator, and with experience the operator learns to recognize when too much resistance is encountered. When this occurs, it is best to back off, reintroduce a dilator 0.5 mm smaller, and leave it in place for 30 to 60 seconds. A second attempt with the larger dilator is then almost always successful.

During the entire process of dilatation, which normally takes no more than 5 minutes, the patient should be quietly reminded that she is likely to experience intermittent menstrual cramps and that, although they may become progressively somewhat stronger, no new or startling sensations will be experienced.

Vacuum Curettage

The external diameter of the vacurette should be the same as, or slightly smaller than, the diameter of the last dilator inserted. Note that many manufacturers label the vacurette with the number in millimeters of its internal, not external, diameter. For example, a cervix dilated up to a number 11 Hegar dilator will accommodate a number 9 stainless steel Gomco vacurette. Sometimes it is necessary to introduce a dilator 0.5 mm larger in diameter so that the vacurette may be inserted and withdrawn easily (e.g., a 11.5-mm dilator for a 9-mm internal diameter vacurette).

The vacuum machine must be one that cannot reverse the flow of air and produce embolization of vessels. The vacurette tip should be fully introduced through the cervical canal, but not to the top of the fundus, before the vacuum is turned on. Initial evacuation of the cavity should allow some contraction and thickening of the wall of the uterus. This will improve the safety of the remainder of the evacuation, because the operator will feel a much firmer resistance as the tip of the vacurette encounters the fundal wall with subsequent insertions.

Just as one would handle the curette during standard curettage (see Chapter 4), the vacurette after initial evacuation should be introduced repeatedly and gently to the top of the fundus and withdrawn slowly and systematically with longitudinal strokes, allowing the vacurette aperture to press against the internal wall of the uterus. As these strokes are taken in a clockwise or counterclockwise direction, it is often possible to sense the site of implantation. If so, several repeated strokes should be taken across that site to accelerate evacuation.

As tissue is evacuated through the transparent tubing into the collection bottle, the surgeon should repeatedly inspect its appearance. With experience it becomes easy to identify amniotic fluid and products of conception. For philosophic reasons that are shared by most patients, I am not interested in confirming the presence of embryonic parts. I am very interested, however, in noting the volume of products and in detecting the presence of vesicles that would suggest a hydatid mole. If an unexpectedly small amount of material is obtained, suggesting the possibility of an ectopic pregnancy, or if any grossly abnormal elements are observed, all tissue retrieved is sent to the pathologist for microscopic examination. If, on the other hand, the expected amount of normal-appearing tissue is obtained, we do not send a sample to the pathology laboratory for tissue confirmation, unless the patient or her referring physician has requested we do so for specific medical or medicolegal reasons.

It is usually possible to detect a uterine contraction against the vacurette when it encounters increasing resistance as the uterus is emptied, and at this point the patient may complain of a strong menstrual cramp.

Standard Curettage

The vacurette is removed and a medium or lange standard sharp curette is used for careful systematic scraping of the endometrial cavity in a circumferential manner. It is important also to scrape horizontally across the top of the fundal cavity. These maneuvers will loosen and deliver most remaining tissue fragments and shave off thickened areas of decidua. As a result, postoperative bleeding will be greatly reduced and rapid uterine involution will be facilitated. It is surprising how often patients will call us 2 or 3 days later, concerned because they have had no bleeding at all since the operation. On the other hand, overly vigorous curettage is not helpful and may indeed result in the later development of uterine synechiae.

MANUAL VACUUM ASPIRATION

An alternative method of surgical first trimester pregnancy termination, particularly appropriate before the eighth week of gestation, is manual vacuum aspiration (MVA). MVA refers to the evacuation of the uterus through a flexible cannula into a valved syringe in which a partial vacuum has been created by withdrawal and locking the barrel. No aspiration pump is required (Fig. 5.3).

MVA has been a remarkably safe and effective procedure where access to abortion services is limited. In the United States, for example, Judy Tyson, MD, has taught the method for the past 20 years to physicians and nurse practitioners for use in Northern New England. During the past 23 years, syringes and cannulas have been distributed to more than 100 countries by International Projects Assistance Services (IPAS). The instruments are inexpensive, portable, and easily adapted to an office surgery or emergency room. The syringe and cannula are equally effective in the management of incomplete abortion.

An outstanding video film describing MVA was produced in 1996 by Jerry Edwards, MD, Medical Director, Planned Parenthood of Houston and Southeast Texas. Inquiries regarding purchase of copies of this video and related information may be made to IPAS, 303 E. Main Street, P.O. Box 999, Carrboro, NC 27510.

POSTOPERATIVE EXAMINATION

The cervical tenaculum and vaginal speculum are removed and a careful bimanual examination is carried out. It is important to be sure that the uterus is contracting down

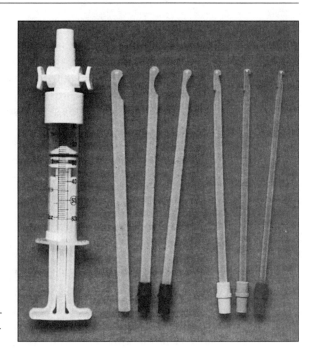

Figure 5.3. IPAS Manual Aspiration Instruments. (Photo courtesy of IPAS, 303 E. Main St., Carrboro, NC 27510.)

well. After late first trimester abortions, particularly in multigravida patients, the corpus may be noted to be somewhat flaccid as the result of inertia. Bleeding is likely to continue until gentle bimanual massage has been carried out. It is possible to accomplish this in the awake patient without causing any significant pain. As the uterus contracts down and becomes smaller, the operator may be able to bring it well forward and examine the adnexal regions carefully. Tubal thickening suggesting a possible ectopic pregnancy, or an ovarian mass, either of which may have been inaccessible to the examining fingers preoperatively, are now readily palpable. The surgeon should bear in mind the remote possibility of simultaneous intrauterine and ectopic pregnancies.

The paracervical and parametrial areas must be palpated carefully to rule out a developing hematoma from an unrecognized uterine perforation or cervical disruption; this is discussed more fully in the section on complications in this chapter.

One advantage of paracervical anesthetic block, particularly for late first trimester abortion, is that it brings about increased uterine muscle tone, in contrast to the marked relaxing effect of general anesthesia. Therefore, under local anesthesia, it is rarely necessary to administer intravenous oxytocics to facilitate uterine contraction. Nonetheless, an intravenous infusion should be immediately available so that 50 units of oxytocin (Pitocin, Parke-Davis) in 500 mL of dextrose in water may be started if postevacuation bimanual massage of the uterine corpus fails to correct uterine atony. In my experience, however, intravenous oxytocin has been indicated in no more than 1% of late first trimester abortions under local anesthesia.

TRANSFER TO RECOVERY ROOM

After resting for 10 minutes and provided the pulse and blood pressure are stable, the patient may sit up and be escorted, walking, to the recovery room, where she should continue to rest, attended by a nurse or companion for at least 30 minutes before returning home. Strong uterine cramps may persist for 5 to 10 minutes, but in 30 minutes the patient is usually asymptomatic and no further analgesics are required.

If the patient is Rh negative, she is given an injection of Micrhogam.

Postoperative counseling and instructions are given (Fig. 5.4), and after a 30- to 60-minute rest, the patient returns home with a companion.

An oral oxytocic, methylergonovine maleate (Methergine, Sandoz, 0.2 mg every day for 3 to 5 days), is prescribed only if uterine atony and excessive bleeding occurred during or immediately after the procedure. Antibiotics are not prescribed unless the patient has a history of pelvic inflammatory disease or demonstrates an obvious purulent cervicitis.

PROBLEMS

Abortion is often referred to as a simple procedure, particularly by those who never perform the operation. However, when the surgeon sets out to work under local anesthesia and to provide a maximum degree of safety for the patient, he or she must be prepared for a large number of variables, complicated by the fact that the procedure is a blind one that depends for its successful completion on the proper functioning of contractile and hemostatic mechanisms over which the surgeon has little control.

Apprehension

There are those who maintain that general anesthesia is the best treatment for unmanageable apprehension. Rarely, this is true, and most particularly in the moderately to severely retarded patient who cannot cooperate even in the absence of apprehension. If the physician and staff maintain a consistent, firm, confident, and kindly manner, however, it should become apparent to most patients, regardless of how frightened they are at the outset, that their welfare will be far better served by being awake and experiencing the few uterine cramps that will occur during the procedure. There is of course enormous variability in pain threshold among patients. This threshold is unique to the individual and applicable to virtually all painful stimuli to which she may be subjected. The pain threshold may be lowered precipitously by fear or anxiety; a large part of the success of the physician in working with local anesthesia will depend on his or her skill and the skill of the staff in helping each patient overcome or diminish her apprehension.

It is unfair to ask the patient at the first visit if she would prefer to be asleep. Many will answer in the affirmative simply out of fear or ignorance. The very question suggests two things to the patient: first, that it must be just as safe as any other technique of anesthesia and, second, that the physician is letting her call the shots. Most women facing abortion desperately want a professional who is skilled, confident, and compassionate. They are greatly relieved to discover that local anesthesia is not only safer but adequate, and most find that the abortion experience in the awake and conscious state reassures them that no one has taken advantage of them. Their self-image has been improved because they have been full and willing participants in the termination of the pregnancy.

Any physician who chooses to belittle these feelings and emotions is insulting patients and will probably fail in helping them to cope with their inevitable apprehension. As a direct consequence, the surgeon will not succeed in the effort to operate under paracervical block and will soon give up and suggest general anesthesia as a better choice.

> *A. Pat Doe, M.D., P.C.*
> *1234 Fifth Street*
> *New York, New York 13201*
> (555) 321-1234
>
> TERMINATION OF UNPLANNED PREGNANCY
>
> Post-operative Instructions:
>
> 1. You must leave the office with a companion.
>
> 2. Rest in bed or on a couch for the remainder of the day.
>
> 3. You may get up for lunch or dinner, or to go to the bathroom.
>
> 4. You may return to work or your normal activities the day after the procedure.
>
> 5. You may have a tub-bath or shower as soon as you wish.
>
> 6. Expect dark menstrual-like flow on and off for several weeks. Some women have very little bleeding while others will have cramps and pass a few large clots at some point between one and ten days after the procedure. Both patterns are normal.
>
> 7. Use external pads for three days, then internal protection if you wish.
>
> 8. Your first period may come any time between two and six weeks. Please contact the office if you have not had a period within six weeks.
>
> 9. No intercourse for at least three weeks following surgery.
>
> 10. You may douche or use vaginal medication after two weeks.
>
> 11. Return to your own physician when your next Pap Smear is due.
>
> 12. Please call us anytime if you have questions. Phone promptly in case of <u>HEMORRHAGE, PAIN, OR FEVER</u>.
>
> A. Pat Doe, M.D.

Figure 5.4. Postoperative instructions.

Tranquilizers, such as diazepam 5 mg by mouth 30 minutes preoperatively or the same dose intravenously immediately before surgery, are helpful in combating apprehension. They are far less important, however, than the demeanor and attitude of each individual in the operating room. One final caution is necessary. Beware the overly solicitous nurse or counselor who hovers over her "suffering victim" practically imploring her to be brave, telling her that she really will be alright if she can just bear with it for a few minutes. On the other hand, a skilled counselor at the head of the table is enormously helpful. She or he should be firm, reassuring, and almost matter of fact to lessen the aura of crisis.

Obesity

In a markedly obese woman, it may be impossible to determine the duration of pregnancy by pelvic examination alone. In such a case, pelvic sonography will reveal gestational age. Furthermore, in the preoperative evaluation of an obese patient, the gynecologist should bear in mind that even postabortally he or she may miss a significant adnexal mass on pelvic examination. Therefore, if any woman, particularly one who is obese, presents for early pregnancy termination and also complains of unilateral pelvic pain, a pelvic sonogram may be indicated to help rule out an ectopic pregnancy.

Obesity may hinder examination of the upper vagina and cervix and interfere with accurate injection of anesthetic solution into the paracervical tissues and uterosacral ligaments. Exposure of the upper vagina in an obese woman may be facilitated by using an extra large speculum.

Uterine Retroversion

A retroverted corpus is almost always somewhat larger than one would expect on the basis of duration of pregnancy. This is because retroversion or, more frequently, retroflexion (corpus on cervix) causes venous obstruction at the cervicouterine junction. This results in chronic engorgement and enlargement of the corpus. Thus, in such a case, a 10-week-from-conception-sized corpus is probably only 8 weeks from fertilization. Careful initial sounding of the retroflexed uterus requires introduction of the sound or small dilator with concave curve facing downward. The cervicouterine angle will become less acute by traction on the cervical tenaculum. Any patient with significant retroflexion should be instructed to rest on her abdomen as long as possible during the first few hours after the abortion to help the uterus "fall forward" and contract down better. Postoperative bleeding will thus be lessened.

Infantile Cervix and Relative Stenosis of Internal Cervical Os

Most often seen in the young primigravida, the infantile cervix is immediately recognizable. It is unusually small, firm, and pink in early pregnancy rather than enlarged, congested, and blue. The external os may be pinpoint. The passage of a sound through the canal of such a cervix may be difficult. Much resistance may be encountered at the internal os, creating a risk of perforation. Even if the sound and the 6-mm dilator are passed without encountering too much resistance, the force needed to introduce larger dilators rises sharply, thus greatly increasing the risk of cervical laceration and perforation at the level of the internal os.

There are two possible solutions to the problem of the nonnegotiable cervix. The first is to discontinue the procedure and ask the patient to return 2 to 3 weeks later, provided that the return visit will not take her beyond 10 weeks from conception. Late in the first trimester, most infantile cervices soften up from the effect of increasing progesterone levels. This development allows greater safety in sounding and dilatation. The second solution is one that I prefer and is the one favored by most gynecologists, some of whom use the following technique in all primigravid patients. A laminaria tent (Laminaria Japonica, Milex Products Inc., Chicago, IL) is inserted into the cervical canal, preferably just beyond the internal os. Ideally, it should be left in place for 12 hours to swell to its maximum dimension, but many practitioners find that a satisfactory degree of dilatation is achieved after 4 to 6 hours. Therefore, they can examine the patient for the first time in the morning, insert the laminaria, and proceed with the termination late in the afternoon (Fig. 5.5).

In my experience, the incidence among primigravidae of an infantile cervix is less than 1 in 100. Stenosis of the internal cervical os is also an unusual finding. Consequently, I have found the need for either postponing the termination or using laminaria to be most uncommon.

Obstructing Myomata

These may be single or multiple. They occupy the lower uterine cavity, thus "displacing" the products of conception further away from the cervical canal. Sonography and occasionally lower segment hysterography may be helpful in determining the degree of obstruction and the duration of pregnancy. I have had occasion to terminate first trimester pregnancies under local anesthesia in several patients in the presence of obstructing myomata, and I was fortunate to experience no particular difficulty in any case. With each patient, the vacurette was felt to push the smooth myoma easily to one side, and the

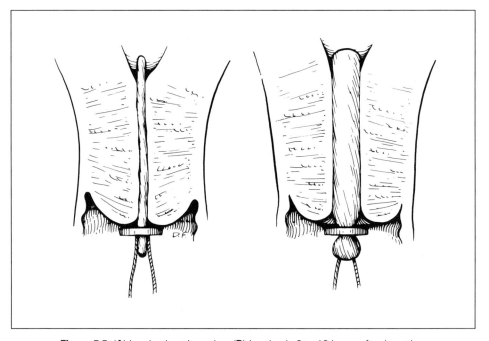

Figure 5.5. (**A**) Laminaria at insertion. (**B**) Laminaria 6 to 12 hours after insertion.

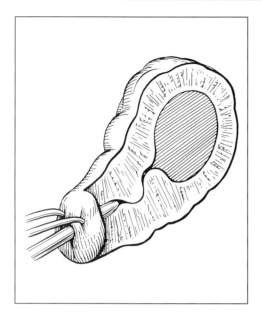

Figure 5.6. Obstructing lower segment myomata.

products of conception were reached and evacuated. I recognized beforehand that the vacurette would need to pass 2 to 3 inches deeper than normal to encounter the top of the fundus. No unusual bleeding followed the procedures. It is well known that these low lying myomata, if encountered in a laboring woman at term, react in a very convenient fashion and usually cause no difficulty (Fig. 5.6).

Nonetheless, one must proceed with extreme caution in such cases. When in doubt, the operator should have blood available for the patient and be prepared to evacuate the uterus under sonographic guidance (see Chapter 11).

Trapped Products

One advantage of paracervical block for first trimester abortion is the fact that the uterine corpus contracts forcibly during the evacuation procedure, thus assisting in the expulsion of the products of conception. As a result, the uterine wall becomes thicker and the risk of perforation is diminished. At least, that is what usually happens. Occasionally, however, the fundus will contract prematurely and trap some of the products of conception before complete evacuation has been accomplished. Usually, after 3 to 5 minutes, the contraction will subside, the upper and lower uterine cavities will communicate with one another, and the procedure may be completed. Before this happens, however, the operator may mistakenly assume that the cavity has shrunk down remarkably rapidly, when in reality the tip of the vacurette is simply "knocking at the door" of the upper uterine cavity. Many a case of delayed bleeding requiring a second curettage for retained products could have been prevented by the operator's waiting for that "door" to open and then completing the vacuum and standard curettage (Fig. 5.7).

In my experience, the patient does not complain of sustained pain during this period of entrapment of products of conception. The operator should reassure the patient that he or she is waiting for the uterus to relax a little so that the procedure can be completed.

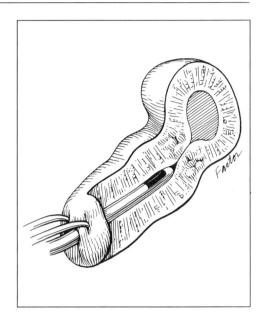

Figure 5.7. Trapped products of conception.

COMPLICATIONS AND THEIR MANAGEMENT

Uterine Atony and Hemorrhage: Prevention and Management

The procedure of uterine curettage that follows vacuum aspiration of the products of conception brings about strong uterine contractions, particularly if the operation is performed under local paracervical block anesthesia that does not interfere with spontaneous contractile mechanisms of the uterus. General anesthesia, on the other hand, puts the uterus and the patient to sleep and thus predisposes to uterine atony and hemorrhage. Thus, curettage under paracervical anesthetic block is highly effective in the prevention and treatment of uterine atony.

Uterine atony is rarely seen after adequate uterine evacuation and curettage under local anesthesia during the first trimester. Immediate uterine blood loss in excess of 300 mL (in the absence of laceration or perforation) is very uncommon in these cases. However, if bleeding after satisfactory curettage appears to be excessive, then vigorous bimanual massage of the corpus should be carried out. This maneuver will usually bring about a firm, sustained uterine contraction, and fresh bleeding will cease. If it does not, then it is my practice to give a rapid infusion of 50 units of oxytocin in 500 mL of 5% dextrose in water. An alternative oxytocic, 0.02 mg of methylergonovine maleate, may also be given intramuscularly, but its effect, if any, will not be noted for at least 3 to 5 minutes, by which time the intravenous oxytocin will have already produced a maximal response.

Although Pitocin and Methergine are highly effective in stimulating uterine contractions in late pregnancy or after delivery, oxytocics in general are rarely beneficial after first trimester abortion because the uterus in early pregnancy is relatively insensitive to these agents. In 1970, I administered 50 units of Pitocin intravenously to 50 consecutive first trimester abortion patients and then performed abortion on the next 50 patients without an oxytocic. All patients were operated on under paracervical block. The blood loss varied from 80 to 150 mL, and we were unable to detect any difference between the two groups.

I believe that first trimester abortion patients should receive oxytocic agents only for persistent bleeding. This opinion is shared by the contemporary British authority, G. M.

Filshie (8). In the definitive American text, *Abortion Practice*, Hern (6) states that he restricts the use of oxytocics to those patients who are bleeding excessively or who may be expected to bleed excessively during late first trimester abortion procedures. This is also the practice recommended by Darney et al. (5).

Methylergonovine maleate taken by mouth after first trimester abortion may bring about an occasional mild uterine cramp but is of no value in reducing bleeding. Therefore, I would challenge the routine administration of one 0.2 Methergine tablet every 6 hours for 2 to 3 days after first trimester abortion. This practice should be discontinued not only because it has no significant effect on the postabortal uterus, but because the occasional patient who has an unexpected sensitivity to the vasospastic properties of ergot alkaloids may experience a stroke or a coronary occlusion directly as the result of its administration. One such case was reported to me (Walden, personal communication). A previously normotensive 40-year-old woman with no history of cardiovascular disease was admitted to a large teaching hospital in New York because of a vasospastic reaction leading to a heart attack and a stroke. After an uncomplicated first trimester abortion, she had taken one Methergine tablet by mouth every 6 hours as instructed. On the second postoperative day, she developed chest pain and was admitted to the hospital in critical condition. Examinations showed that she had suffered an acute coronary occlusion and a cerebrovascular accident with serious neurologic sequelae. This case was presented at a subsequent obstetrics-gynecology department meeting, and the conclusion was reached that oral methylergonovine maleate is contraindicated after first trimester abortion.

After my first 50 patients demonstrated no benefit from intravenous Pitocin, none of the approximately 7,000 abortion patients operated on under local paracervical block in my private office surgery received oxytocics during the procedure. Only three of these patients experienced delayed uterine atony and hemorrhage on the 4th, 10th and 54th days, respectively, after the first vacuum curettage. I performed a prompt secondary curettage under paracervical block on each of these three patients. In each case, sustained uterine contractions occurred without benefit of oxytocics, and the bleeding was controlled.

Rarely, uterine hemorrhage persists or recurs even after secondary curettage and parenteral oxytocics. It may be that in these rare situations spiral arterioles open up and bleed profusely through patches of necrotic decidua. There is no known means of preventing this occurrence. Hysterectomy may be the only rational solution in removing the source of bleeding.

The complication of persistent postabortal uterine atony after secondary curettage is most likely to occur in a multiparous patient who has experienced previous endometrial scarring or fibrosis. The only such patient in my personal series of approximately 7,000 patients was a 32-year-old woman who had three previous term deliveries and three previous first trimester abortions, all without complications. Ten days after an uneventful vacuum and standard curettage under paracervical block at 9 weeks from conception, she hemorrhaged, was admitted to the hospital, and received 3 units of packed cells. While a Pitocin infusion was rapidly administered, a second curettage was carried out under general anesthesia by another gynecologist during my absence from the country. Although the relaxing effects of general anesthesia probably diminished the spontaneous ability of the uterus to contract, the curettage with Pitocin infusion curbed the bleeding. The patient was discharged from the hospital with a prescription for Methergine and iron. The curettings were read by the pathologist as follows: "Necrotic decidual tissue with large blood vessels and blood clot." No products of conception were identified.

The patient continued in good condition at home with only slight spotting. However, 8 days after discharge from the hospital, she experienced an abrupt uterine hemorrhage of over 500 mL while grocery shopping. She was readmitted to the hospital where intravenous Pitocin and intramuscular ergotrate were given. This patient had previously requested a sterilization procedure, and after consultation with her and her husband, a prompt abdominal hysterectomy was carried out by the same gynecologist who had performed the secondary curettage. The uterus was examined by the pathologist who submitted the following report: "The myometrium and endometrium contain numerous enlarged and thick-walled blood vessels. Some of the endometrial surface is necrotic with occasional decidual cells."

The patient's hemoglobin was 8.8 and hematocrit was 25.6 on the day after her hysterectomy, so she received two more units of packed cells. Her hemoglobin rose to 11.1 and hematocrit to 32.8. She was discharged home on iron medication 5 days after her surgery.

The ultimate resort to hysterectomy for management of intractable postabortal hemorrhage will be a rare experience for the competent gynecologist. Postabortal uterine atony and hemorrhage will normally respond to vigorous bimanual massage and, if necessary, to a secondary curettage, preferably under paracervical block anesthesia, which promotes uterine muscle contractility. If, after secondary curettage, the uterine wall remains flaccid and hemorrhage persists, then vigorous bimanual uterine massage should be carried out with concurrent intravenous oxytocin administration. If these measures are not promptly effective, immediate hysterectomy is indicated.

Uterine Perforation

If the sound or the dilator, or even the vacurette or standard curette, passes further than it should, the operator should immediately suspect that he or she has perforated the uterus. If the suspected perforation is detected at the time of the introduction of the sound or one of the smaller dilators, the wisest course of action is to remove the instruments, massage the uterus gently, and immediately discontinue the operation. The patient should be observed for at least an hour to ensure that hemorrhage, as manifested by external bleeding, pelvic pain, or an enlarging parauterine hematoma, does not occur. If she has no pain and her vital signs are normal, she should be sent home on broad-spectrum antibiotic coverage. Follow-up telephone calls should be made daily for at least 3 days, and the patient should return for vacuum and standard curettage in 2 weeks when her perforation site could be expected to have healed over.

If, on the other hand, the perforation is not suspected until the vacuum or standard curettage is under way, then gentle extremely cautious use of the standard curette is indicated to remove remaining products. Under no circumstances should vacuum curettage be resumed because of the obvious risk of aspirating omentum or bowel.

This patient also should be observed for an hour and then allowed to return home. Telephone follow-up would again be important and the patient should take prophylactic antibiotics. After 1 to 2 weeks, the patient should return for evaluation regarding the need for a second curettage to remove remaining products of conception. This need would be influenced by the operator's impression of how completely he or she was able to evacuate the uterus the first time and also by the presence of such findings as subinvolution or an intercurrent history of continuous bleeding or cramping.

Some gynecologists, after diagnosing uterine perforation during the performance of abortion, advocate immediate emergency laparoscopy to evaluate the extent of injury to uterus or bowel, to rule out intra-abdominal hemorrhage, and to assist in the completion of the evacuation procedure under laparoscopic guidance. In my opinion, such a course of action rarely is indicated. Almost all perforations result in self-limited bleeding. On the other hand, if the patient develops signs of intra-abdominal or pelvic hemorrhage, such as pelvic pain, enlarging pelvic-abdominal mass, or shock, she requires immediate transfer to a hospital operating room, blood transfusion, and laparotomy for control of bleeding. When the patient's vital signs are stable, the abortion procedure may then be completed with extreme caution and gentleness by a second surgeon, while the first surgeon observes the uterus through the open abdominal incision. In such a case of obvious internal hemorrhage, a preliminary laparoscopy is superfluous and further endangers the patient by delaying definitive management.

Cervical Disruption

This all-inclusive term refers either to the laceration of an apparently normal cervix by excessive propulsive force of a dilating instrument or to the tearing or giving way of a thin, fibrous, scarred segment of a previously lacerated cervix. This latter accident is one of the most feared complications of abortion, because it can occur even during gentle dilatation. If the operator recognizes such a scar on preoperative examination, the patient may be a good candidate for the preliminary insertion of a laminaria tent. Cervical disruptions should occur rarely, certainly in less than 1% of unselected groups of patients. Unfortunately, when they do occur, a large proportion are found to be lateral, in which case there is a significant risk of associated laceration of uterine vessels. If this occurs, bleeding is more likely to be concealed than external, and a parametrial hematoma may not be suspected until the patient develops increasing pelvic pain from 1 to several hours after the abortion (Fig. 5.8).

This complication calls for immediate hospitalization and laparotomy for an enlarging hematoma. It is hoped that evacuation of the hematoma and deep suturing of the cervix may suffice. If the bleeding cannot be controlled promptly, hypogastric artery ligation or hysterectomy may be indicated.

In my own experience, I have had two patients who experienced a cervical disruption and broad ligament hematoma immediately after an apparently uncomplicated abortion. One did well after laparotomy, hematoma evacuation, and cervical suture. The other developed increasing pelvic pain 1 hour after the patient had returned home. I admitted her to the nearby hospital, diagnosed a left broad ligament hematoma on pelvic examination, and discussed therapeutic options with the patient. We then prepared for transfusion and took her to the operating room. At laparotomy, I found a 500-mL hematoma extending laterally from the internal cervical os on the left side. She was bleeding from a lateral lower uterine laceration. Because the patient had previously requested a tubal sterilization, I evacuated the hematoma and performed a total hysterectomy rather than attempt to control her bleeding by suturing or by ligating the internal iliac artery.

These rare accidents are effective reminders that all patients for abortion should be informed preoperatively of the risks of perforation and hemorrhage.

Antibiotic Prophylaxis for Endometritis

There are wide differences of opinion among experienced clinicians as to the usefulness of prophylactic antibiotics. Hodgson (9) prescribed them routinely and believes she has proven their usefulness in a study of 4,000 cases with control subjects. She argued that

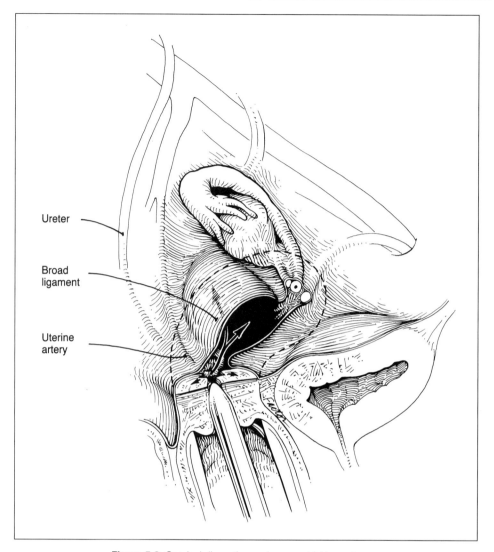

Figure 5.8. Cervical disruption and parametrial hematoma.

in her particular practice with clinic (nonprivate) patients, early warning signs of infection such as fever, pain, or discharge are often not reported. Consequently, Dr. Hodgson believed that all patients should be given antibiotics to benefit the small percentage of patients who might otherwise become infected and delay in seeking treatment.

Hern (6) states that the "prophylactic use of antibiotics following abortion is a controversial issue." In dealing with a large clinic population, where patients are often lost to follow-up, he has adopted the following practice: "As a matter of routine, we provide patients with enough 500 mg tetracycline capsules for 5 days, with instructions to take 1 capsule 4 times a day."

The principle of antibiotic prophylaxis is rejected as a routine by four other current authorities in the practice of abortion. Their objections are expressed in the following quotations. "The routine use of antibiotic prophylaxis is not advised unless there is some justification, such as suspected contamination" (10). "Most clinicians do not routinely use antibiotics after abortion because of the low incidence of infection and the questionable efficacy of prophylactic antibiotics in many medical areas" (11). McGregor (12) has also concluded that prophylactic antibiotics are unjustified for unselected abortion patients. He cites the experience of Stewart (13), who evaluated the use of tetracycline in 2,000 first trimester abortion patients and found no benefit from tetracycline versus placebo in preventing postabortal infection. McGregor goes on to point out that routine antibiotic administration will occasionally lead to complications such as hypersensitivity, photosensitization, and monilial overgrowth. Darney et al. (5) prescribed prophylactic antibiotics for patients "at risk" but not routinely for all patients.

In my own care of over 7,000 private abortion patients during the past 25 years, I have been aware of the occurrence of postoperative infection as indicated by fever, endometritis, or parametritis in less than 1% of cases. Without exception, these few patients, having reported their problem to me promptly, have responded rapidly to doxycycline 100 mg bid or other broad-spectrum agents. Therefore, I have concluded that the routine administration of prophylactic antibiotics to private patients undergoing first trimester abortion is unnecessary and will allow the proliferation of resistant more dangerous bacteria.

Endometritis should be suspected in any postabortal patient who develops increasing uterine and possibly adnexal pain with definite tenderness on palpation. Increasing leukorrhea is generally a late manifestation, and fever may not be present at all. If endometritis is detected early, the patient will almost always respond within 24 hours to any broad-spectrum antibiotic. If, on the other hand, the patient presents with a pelvic infection more than 5 days postabortally, she may be a candidate for an antibiotic such as clindamycin or metronidazole to eradicate anaerobic organisms.

Postoperative Depression

Continued supportive care by the patient's husband or companion is of particular importance in the immediate postoperative period. Guilt feelings may surface postabortally, and the patient should be given, or encouraged to seek, supplemental counseling if persistent depression occurs. Profound depression is rare except in women who already demonstrate a tendency to depressive episodes. Such a patient should receive very close postoperative attention for several weeks, especially if she becomes sullen or morose or if she expresses suicidal thoughts.

Late Complications of Abortion: Uterine Synechiae and Cervical Incompetence

Uterine synechiae and even total amenorrhea after overly vigorous curettage are very rare complications with which I have had no personal experience. After three or more consecutive abortion operations on the same patient, I have noticed on occasion a decided diminution in resistance of the internal cervical os to dilatation. However, I do not personally know of any such patient who has in subsequent pregnancy experienced premature labor on the basis of iatrogenic cervical incompetence. Nonetheless, several European reports (14–16) indicate that women who have undergone multiple operative abortions experience a significant increase in premature labor in later pregnancies. It is hoped that improved surgical skills and the gentle insertion of half-size dilators (and laminaria when indicated) will diminish the possibility of damage to the internal cervical os leading to premature labor.

A study in Boston of 1,235 women who were aborted by optimal techniques and who were followed for as long as 3.5 years showed that induced abortion did not affect subsequent fertility rates nor increase pregnancy complications (17).

REFERENCES

1. Somell C, Olunda A, Carlstrom K, et al. Reproductive hormones during termination of early pregnancy with Mifepristone. Gynecol Obstet Invest 1990;30:224–227.
2. Ulmann A, Silvestre L, Chemama L, et al. Medical termination of early pregnancy with mifepristone (RU 486) followed by a prostaglandin analogue. Study in 15,369 women. Acta Obstet Gynecol Scand 1992;71:278–283.
3. Wu S, Gao J, Wu Y, et al. Clinical trial on termination of early pregnancy with RU 486 in combination with prostaglandin. Contraception 1992;46:203–210.
4. The Population Council. Presented at the Presentation Advisory Committee Hearing to the U.S. Food and Drug Administration on Mifepristone/Misoprostol Medical Abortion, July 19, 1996, New York.
5. Darney P, Horbach N, Korn A. Protocols for office gynecologic surgery. Cambridge, MA: Blackwell Science, 1996:158–219.
6. Hern W. Abortion practice. Philadelphia, PA: J.B. Lippincott, 1984.
7. Hulka JF, Lefler HT Jr, Anglone A, Lachenbruch PA. A new electronic force monitor to measure factors influencing cervical dilation for vacuum curettage. Am J Obstet Gynecol 1947;120:166–173.
8. Filshie GM. First trimester termination of pregnancy. In: Symonds M, Zuspan F, eds. Clinical and diagnostic procedures in obstetrics and gynecology. Part B. Gynecology. New York: Marcel Dekker, 1984.
9. Hodgson JE. Prophylactic use of tetracycline for first trimester abortions. Obstet Gynecol 1978;16:204.
10. Lauersen NH. Spontaneous and therapeutic abortion. In: Schaefer G, Graber E, eds. Complications in obstetric and gynecologic surgery. Hagerstown, MD: Harper & Row, 1981.
11. Margolis A, Goldsmith S. Aspiration abortion in an office setting. In: Glass B, ed. Office gynecology. Baltimore, MD: Williams & Wilkins, 1976.
12. McGregor JA. Prophylactic antibiotics unjustified for unselected abortion patients [letter]. Am J Obstet Gynecol 1985;152:722–723.
13. Stewart GS. Evaluation of tetracycline in first trimester abortion. Presented at the Annual Meeting of Association of Planned Parenthood Professionals, Denver, Colorado, 1981.
14. Pantelakis SM, Papadimitriou GC, Doxiadis SA. Influence of induced and spontaneous abortions on the outcome of subsequent pregnancies. Am J Obstet Gynecol 1973;116:799.
15. Papaevangelou G, Vrettos AS, Papadatoc C, Alexiou D. The effect of spontaneous and induced abortions on prematurity and birthweight. Br J Obstet Gynaecol 1973;80:418.
16. Richardson JA, Dixon G. Effects of legal termination on subsequent pregnancy. Br Med J 1976;1:1303.
17. Stubblefield GG, Monson RR, Schoenbaum SC, Wolfson CE, Cookson DJ, Ryan KJ. Fertility after induced abortion: a prospective follow-up study. Obstet Gynecol 1984;62:186–193.

6. *Diagnostic and Operative Hysteroscopy*

MORRIS WORTMAN

MODERN HYSTEROSCOPY: A HISTORICAL PERSPECTIVE

In the 1960s, hysteroscopy was referred to as "a tool looking for an indication." Almost three decades of technologic development and clinical research have transformed hysteroscopy into an indispensable method of diagnosis and treatment. However, although orthopedic surgeons and urologists would not consider formulating a diagnosis without an endoscopic examination, many gynecologists are content to examine the uterus blindly, using tactile sensations and curettage. An understanding of uterine anatomy may offer an explanation for the delay in the acceptance and full appreciation of hysteroscopy. The uterus does not have a maintained space found in joints and its thick muscular wall cannot be as easily distended as the urinary bladder. Moreover, the tough, thick-walled uterus has lent itself quite well to "scraping," as a method of "finding out what is going on inside." Because of the distinct anatomy of the uterus, the development of instruments and techniques for endoscopic examination has been challenging.

Modern hysteroscopy shares its historical roots with all other forms of endoscopy in medical curiosa that began almost two hundred years ago. When Bozzini, in 1805, used a hollow tube, mirror, and candle to observe the vagina, rectum, urethra, and nose he was censured by the medical faculty of Vienna for his "undue curiosity." In 1853, Desormeaux reported the use of the first cystoscope/urethroscope to the Imperial Academy of Medicine in Paris. His ingeniously designed "light source" burned alcohol and turpentine and had a self-contained "smoke stack." He made some wonderful observations and actually spoke of the possibility of using such a device to explore the inside of the uterine cavity. It was Pantaleoni in 1869 who made the first observation of the uterine cavity using the Desormeaux "scope." In 1886, Pantaleoni reported on finding and destroying an endometrial polyp in a 60-year-old woman suffering from postmenopausal bleeding. He was also the first to describe using laminaria to dilate the cervix before "hysteroscopic examinations."

The next major "advance" in modern endoscopy came in 1879, when Maximillian Nietze, a urologist, closed the viewing tube and added a lens system that provided magnification to his cystoscope. He was also responsible for the addition of a platinum wire loop at the distal end that was energized by an electric current. This "distal illumination" actually came before Edison's incandescent bulb. Although credited as being the father of modern endoscopy, Nietze never made intrauterine observations. He was, after all, a urologist.

A year later, in 1880, Edison invented the incandescent bulb. In 1883, Newman used the Edison lamp as a light source for endoscopic equipment. But it was not until 1885 that Bumm used Nietze's instrument to make the first intrauterine observations. Charles David produced the first instrument to resemble a modern day hysteroscope in 1908. The distal end was sealed to keep blood and debris out of the lens system (located more proximally) and was equipped with an incandescent bulb.

Once adequate illumination for examination of the uterus had been achieved, it became abundantly clear that there could be no precise examination without a method for distending the uterus. In 1914, Heinenberg used a water system to provide cleansing of the telescope's distal end and limited distention of the uterus. Six years later, Rubin replaced water with oxygen for insufflation to assess tubal patency. By 1921 he had replaced oxygen with carbon dioxide. This logically led to attempts to distend the uterus for examination. However forward looking this was, Rubin's technique was not successful. In 1934 Schroeder reported the necessity of distending the uterine cavity to achieve adequate visualization and to control bleeding. He found that an intrauterine pressure of 25–35 mm Hg would distend the uterus. This pressure could be achieved using a column of water originating 65–95 cm above the uterus (the first gravity-fed system).

Consistently good methods of uterine distention were not invented until the 1970s when Lindeman, working with carbon dioxide; Edstron, using Dextran 70; and Normant, experimenting with 5% dextrose in water, published their individual works.

Among the exciting developments in instrumentation that were taking place concurrently with advancements in distention media was the single most important improvement in telescope design, the replacement of the proximal incandescent bulb with the external light source that was transmitted through quartz fibers (1). Because of the remote location of the light source, heat could be controlled, and the use of very bright illumination became possible.

Surgical techniques, using endoscopy in gynecology, began with Schroeder's work (1934) in transcervical sterilization (2). In 1950, Asherman (3) suggested that a hysteroscopic means might one day be used to divide intrauterine adhesions. A lost intrauterine device was retrieved by Hepp and Roll (4). During the late 1970s and early 1980s, the technology for making accurate observations of the uterine cavity was well established as illustrated by Hamou and Taylor (5). However, the technologic leap needed for the development of hysteroscopic surgical instruments and techniques had not occurred. The invention of Inglesias et al. (6) of the continuous flow urologic resectoscope (1975) and Neuwirth and Amin's (7) resection of uterine fibroids, using a standard urologic resectoscope, were at the forefront of wellspring of hysteroscopic instrumentation and techniques that would lay the foundation for advancing a variety of hysteroscopic surgical procedures. The incorporation of a variety of energy sources was soon to follow. Goldrath et al. (8) were the first to report on the use of the Nd:YAG laser to accomplish thermal destruction (ablation) of the endometrium. High-frequency electrosurgical wave forms were used by DeCherney and Polan (9) to perform endometrial resection, and electrosurgical ablation with the roller-ball electrode was introduced by Lin (10). Despite this flurry of activity, gynecologists practicing in the 1970s and 1980s saw hysteroscopy as a diagnostic tool of purely academic value. The question was "Why bother looking into the uterus when the patient would need to have a hysterectomy anyway?" With the Food and Drug Administration (FDA) approval of the continuous flow gynecologic resectoscope in 1989 (Karl Stortz Endoscopy, Culver City, CA), the need to master hysteroscopic skills became obvious because for the first time, an inexpensive minimally invasive alternative to hysterectomy was put into the hands of all gynecologists.

INTRODUCTION TO HYSTEROSCOPY AND HYSTEROSCOPIC SURGERY

Why learn to perform diagnostic hysteroscopy? Why build the skills required for hysteroscopic surgery? As one of the least invasive diagnostic and therapeutic techniques available to the gynecologist today, hysteroscopy offers the physician and patient procedures that have few risks and can be easily accomplished in the medical office or in an outpatient operating setting. Diagnostic hysteroscopy, performed in the physician's office, provides significant savings in time and aggravation for the physician, greater participation for the patient, and a shorter recovery period. Significant savings in cost are also enjoyed by patients and the health care system.

Hysteroscopy, as a diagnostic method, is nontraumatic and has a wide spectrum of indications. Diagnostic hysteroscopy also forms the foundation for an array of therapeutic interventions that are minimally invasive and organ sparing. Among the many success stories of hysteroscopic technology is its striking effectiveness in the diagnosis and treatment of abnormal uterine bleeding. For decades, physicians have attempted to diagnose and treat abnormal uterine bleeding, the most common patient complaint in the gynecologist's office, with dilation and curettage (D&C). D&C is only partially effective as a diagnostic tool and enjoys little respect as a method of treatment for abnormal uterine bleeding. Benign pathology, such as fibroids and polyps, are the cause of abnormal uterine bleeding in 25% of cases. These lesions usually go undetected by the gynecologist's curette. Most studies show that a return to previously established abnormal menstrual patterns reoccurs in two to three cycles after D&C. The final destination for many patients with abnormal uterine bleeding has been hysterectomy. Of the 650,000 hysterectomies performed annually, more than half are done for complaints of excessive bleeding, at a cost of $1.5 billion dollars. In many cases, the pathology found would hardly warrant such dramatic surgical intervention.

Direct visual inspection of the uterus allows the physician to make a definitive diagnosis and to accurately locate pathologic structures. Information collected during the examination is used to formulate the best therapeutic plan for the patient. Hysteroscopic surgery offers the patient a variety of alternatives to the more invasive, expensive, and morbid procedure, hysterectomy.

Physicians know that hysterectomy involves more serious risks to the patient and requires a lengthier hospitalization and recovery period than less invasive hysteroscopic procedures. Additionally, hysterectomy carries with it greater expense to insurers and increased liability risks for physicians. Hysteroscopic surgery, because it targets only dysfunctional tissue (10–20% of the uterus), can safely remove endometrium, polyps, and fibroids without injury to adjacent organs and structures. These techniques can be learned by all gynecologists willing to devote the same amount of time and energy as they spent on learning hysterectomy. With a well-planned training period followed by regular practice, physicians will strengthen diagnostic abilities and also develop the subtle manipulations and techniques necessary for efficient and safe hysteroscopic surgery. Gynecologists who master diagnostic and operative hysteroscopy are keen to offer this precise, minimally invasive, organ-sparing alternative in an office or outpatient surgical unit.

This chapter introduces the physician to diagnostic hysteroscopy and describes endomyometrial resection (EMR) and hysteroscopic myomectomy, two of the most important alternatives to hysterectomy for the treatment of abnormal uterine bleeding.

INTRODUCTION TO OFFICE-BASED DIAGNOSTIC HYSTEROSCOPY

Hysteroscopy has had a profound impact on the management of many common gynecologic problems. No longer is it necessary to wander around the uterine cavity, blindly tapping at its confines with a curette, only guessing at the causes of abnormal uterine bleeding, infertility, recurrent pregnancy loss, and amenorrhea.

This chapter introduces the physician to office-based diagnostic hysteroscopy. In the physician's office, the patient finds a structured and familiar atmosphere that is too frequently absent in today's hospital operating room. The patient is surrounded by well-trained efficient staff members who understand the procedure and the equipment and are prepared for the physician's preferences and routines. The physician and office staff convey, with a single voice, what the patient may expect as she plans for this simple office procedure—preoperatively, intraoperatively, and postoperatively.

A woman who participates in the procedure is rewarded with a firsthand look at her own anatomy and insight into a problem that she can now visualize. This setting allows most women to undergo this relatively quick procedure without a major anesthetic. She may even elect to be accompanied by a support person who can provide additional comfort. Office-based hysteroscopy, performed in a well-coordinated environment, enables the patient to receive a tremendous amount of "real time" information during a carefully choreographed examination that is diagnostic, conversational, and informational. Unimpaired by anesthesia, the office patient has an opportunity to ask questions and to receive immediate answers from the physician.

Physicians also benefit from the office-based setting. They may choose experienced personnel and protocols that can be individualized to the patient. Carefully selected equipment can be properly assembled, disassembled, cleaned, maintained, and stored with a degree of efficiency often absent in the cacophonous and wasteful routines that characterize hospital operating suites. When was the last time you participated in a hospital-based procedure that was suddenly brought to a standstill when you learned that the equipment was "not available" or because the circulating nurse was unfamiliar with it? How often have you worked with a technician who prefaced entrance into the operating room with "Doctor . . . I've never done this before!"? No wonder hospital-based procedures "require" a general anesthetic.

Finally, office-based hysteroscopy provides an excellent opportunity for the physician to hone his or her skills in a more familiar and less stressful setting. By mastering the hand–eye coordination that is essential to a thorough diagnostic examination, the physician may now purposefully place the hysteroscope in every corner and crevice of the uterus. It is precisely the development of these skills that will form the foundation for progressing to more advanced techniques. Mastery of diagnostic hysteroscopy prepares the physician to undertake the deliberate and orchestrated movements required for ablation and resection techniques.

CREDENTIALING IN OFFICE HYSTEROSCOPY

Medical practice is the quintessential learned profession. Physicians undertake a lifelong commitment to continuing their education, sharpening their skills, and keeping abreast of the most current medical science. As members of this profession, doctors, first and foremost, must honestly credential themselves, reaching even beyond the minimal standards set by professional organizations. Although presently no formal credentialing guidelines exist for performing office-based diagnostic hysteroscopy, the American Association of Gynecologic Laparoscopists (AAGL) and American College of Obstetricians and Gynecologists (ACOG) credentialing guidelines for operative endoscopy procedures suggest that a credentialing process should involve three separate and distinct phases. The physician should attend a recognized didactic course that addresses the role of hysteroscopy in gynecology, introduces basic hysteroscopic instrumentation, and teaches hysteroscopic technique. The second phase, observation, requires that the physician watch an accomplished hysteroscopist performing the procedure in a hospital setting. Finally, in a hospital, the trainee should conduct a number of hysteroscopic examinations on anesthetized patients under the close supervision of a recognized expert. Only after the physician has mastered the techniques involved in obtaining consistently successful examinations should he or she perform hysteroscopy in an office environment. Incorporating this procedure into a private medical office is a complex task involving expensive equipment purchases, development of protocols, and education and coordination of the entire office staff. This is discussed at greater length below.

It is of the utmost importance not to confuse the credentialing process for diagnostic hysteroscopy with that for operative hysteroscopy. ACOG, AAGL, and the Accreditation Council on Gynecologic Endoscopy (ACGE) all clearly prescribe the credentialing process for operative hysteroscopy (see Appendix).

ESSENTIALS OF OFFICE-BASED HYSTEROSCOPY

Office hysteroscopy requires the careful assembly of equipment, staff, and thoroughly developed protocols in a suitable environment.

Equipment: Assembling "the Right Stuff"

Examination Tables

The most important consideration when choosing a table for diagnostic hysteroscopy is whether or not it will accommodate a pair of high-quality supportive stirrups. Wide comfortable tables that may be raised and lowered are especially useful when examining a woman with an anteverted uterus. Otherwise, you may find yourself on bended knee straining to peer into the upper recesses of the uterine fundus. Using a video system when performing hysteroscopy will eliminate the need for raising and lowering the table. The need for achieving various degrees of Trendelenburg or reverse Trendelenburg is not a factor when choosing a table.

Stirrups

The stirrups that are built into standard gynecologic examination tables are somewhat limiting. Allen Universal stirrups (Fig. 6.1) (Allen Medical Systems, Bedford Heights, OH) are useful and well tolerated by patients because they support the patient's entire leg. This becomes especially important in situations where intravenous sedation is used. Sedative hypnotic medications will render most patients incapable of the balancing act required for secure positioning in standard gynecologic stirrups. Moreover, patients with a history of knee, ankle, hip, or back surgery require the additional protection that is provided only by a strong supportive stirrup.

Open-Sided Specula

An open-sided speculum, in the smallest size necessary, should be used for locating the cervix. After the tenaculum and diagnostic sheath are in place, the speculum is removed so that enhanced patient comfort and improved maneuverability of the hysteroscope can be achieved. In most cases, an open-sided Pederson speculum is adequate. However, three or four specula of different shapes and sizes should be readily available.

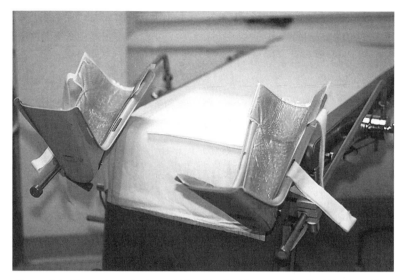

Figure 6.1. Allen universal stirrups (Allen Medical Systems, Bedford Heights, OH).

Tenaculum

A simple single-toothed tenaculum is used to grasp and stabilize the cervix for most rigid hysteroscopic procedures. A tenaculum is usually unnecessary when using a small-caliber flexible scope.

Dilators

An assortment of Hank, Pratt, Denniston, and Hegar dilators, in varying sizes, should be available. Diagnostic hysteroscopic telescopes are available in sizes ranging from 3.0-mm flexible fiber optic scopes to 6.5-mm continuous flow hysteroscopes. Most patients do not require cervical dilatation to accommodate up to a 5.0- or a 5.5-mm hysteroscopic sheath and lens. Dilators are a necessity with the larger continuous flow hysteroscopes. In addition to dilators, cervical "finders" (Fig. 6.2) (Zinnanti Surgical Instruments, Chats-

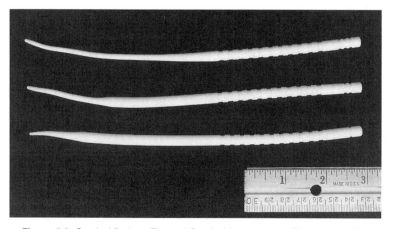

Figure 6.2. Cervical finders (Zinnanti Surgical Instruments, Chatsworth, CA).

CHAPTER 6 / DIAGNOSTIC AND OPERATIVE HYSTEROSCOPY

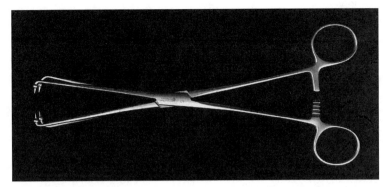

Figure 6.3. Gimpelson tenaculum (Richard Wolf Instrument, Corp., Rosemont, IL).

worth, CA) are very useful in overcoming mild to moderate degrees of cervical stenosis, avoiding "false passages" and resultant uterine perforations.

Cervical Sealing Instruments

A four-pronged tenaculum, a cervical sealing device (Fig. 6.3) designed by Dr. Richard Gimpelson (Richard Wolf Instrument Corp., Rosemont, IL), is very useful in situations that present the physician with the challenging combination of a carbon dioxide distention system and a patulous cervix. Significant carbon dioxide loss from the cervix precludes adequate uterine distention and impairs inspection of the uterine cavity as carbon dioxide bubbles form distal to the hysteroscope and escape in a retrograde fashion. Two single-toothed tenacula in combination may provide similar results, albeit in a more cumbersome fashion.

Telescopes

The diagnostic telescope is the instrument of central importance in the discussion of hysteroscopic equipment. There are a variety of endoscopes (Figs. 6.4–6.6), ranging from the familiar rod-lens systems ($2,500–2,800) to the small diameter semirigid fiber optic hysteroscopes ($4,200) to the sophisticated flexible fiber optic scopes ($7,000–7,500). Before purchasing a scope, a physician should carefully and comprehensively evaluate all options. This evaluation should include telescope lens angle or angle of tilt, angle of view, telescope diameter, flexible versus rigid, rod-lens system optics versus fiber optic image bundle, accommodation for a variety of sheaths, and utility with various distention systems.

All scopes serve two functions. First, they must transmit enough light to the uterine cavity to facilitate panoramic and "macroscopic" observations. Second, they must return a high resolution image to the operator's eye, video camera, or 35-mm camera for documentation.

Angle of Tilt

Telescopes for hysteroscopy come with a variety of lens angles (Fig. 6.7) that allow the physician to inspect the fundus, tubal ostia, and side walls from an optimal perspective.

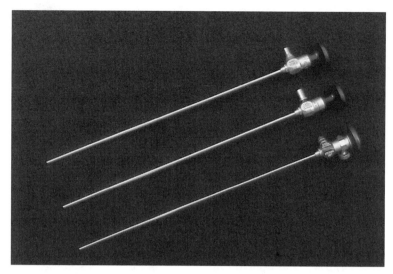

Figure 6.4. Rigid endoscopes (Karl Stortz Endoscopy, Culver City, CA).

Most commercially available hysteroscopes are manufactured with the lens placed at a 0°, 12°, or 30° tilt. For the remainder of this chapter, what the manufacturers refer to as "angle of lens" is referred to as "angle of tilt." A zero degree lens transmits the most intense illumination but only visualizes the objects directly in front of it, not allowing the physician to adequately view the cornua and tubal ostia. Because the visual field is not limited to the space directly in front of the scope, 12° and 30° fore oblique lenses are beneficial for most gynecologic investigations. The greater the angle of tilt, the less effectively light will be transmitted in the scope. For light to pass through the lens placed at a tilt, it must be reflected by prisms, which results in a loss of illumination. The angle of tilt for a particular telescope is readily available from manufacturers and is generally printed on the telescope.

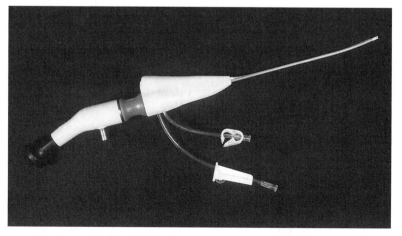

Figure 6.5. Semirigid endoscope (Imagyn, Laguna Niguel, CA).

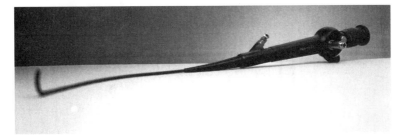

Figure 6.6. Flexible fiber optic endoscope (Karl Stortz Endoscopy, Culver City, CA).

Angle of View

Not to be confused with the telescope's angle of tilt is the angle of view (Fig. 6.8), which in most commercially available hysteroscopes varies from 70° to 120° and corresponds to the lateral field of vision of the scope. Selecting a telescope with a maximum angle of view will prove advantageous to the physician and the patient. Telescopes with a wide angle of view offer a panoramic view and require less manipulation of the hysteroscope, which in turn will ensure a clearer picture. They function much like a wide-angled camera, capturing a large amount of information at relatively close distances. Wide-angled lenses tend to distort the relative size of objects, enlarging those that are within the central portion of the lens and reducing those that lie at the periphery. This is not usually a problem in high quality lens systems with an angle of view of 90° or less. As angle of view increases, magnification decreases. This is not only acceptable but even advantageous to diagnostic procedures.

Telescope Diameter

Telescope manufacturers, understanding the need to obviate cervical dilatation, are developing telescopes with ever decreasing diameters. Smaller diameter telescopes carry less light to the object and may fail to provide adequate light for video documentation. Resolution of the image is also reduced in some smaller scopes. Cervical dilatation, necessary

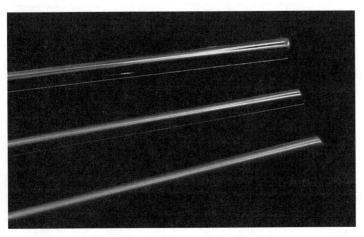

Figure 6.7. Angle of tilt, 0°, 12°, and 30°.

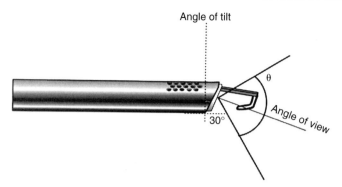

Figure 6.8. Angle of view.

to accommodate the larger diameter scopes, increases the need for analgesia and the risk of intraoperative bleeding. Thus, the physician must seek a balance between patient comfort and image quality.

Conventional Endoscopes: Hopkins Rod-Lens System

In a conventional scope (varying from 2.7 to 4.0 mm in diameter), the relay system consists of a long metal tube fitted with a series of glass rod lenses, 20 mm in length, interspersed with small air spaces. The rod-lens system (Fig. 6.9) is a great improvement over the "traditional" system that used small glass lenses and large air spaces (11). Rod-lens optical systems are superior because they provide illumination and resolution that surpasses even the best fiber optic endoscopes. This increased illumination is a result of the intensifying effect of the high refractive index (2.25–2.72) of the glass rods and the increased clear aperture space in which light may travel. Image contrast and detail rendition are improved because of the precision production of rod-lenses (12).

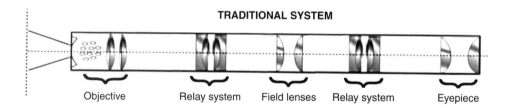

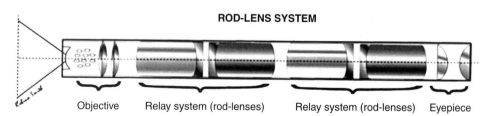

Figure 6.9. Evolution of the Hopkins rod-lens system.

Semirigid Fiber Optic Endoscopes

A semirigid hysteroscope (Fig. 6.5) with a 1.6-mm scope diameter has recently become available at a cost of $4,200 (Imagyn Medical, Inc., Laguna Niguel, CA). Disposable continuous flow sheaths are available for this semirigid hysteroscope. What is unique about this endoscope is that, for the present, at 3.6 mm o.d., it is the smallest continuous flow office hysteroscope available, obviating the need for cervical dilatation in most patients. Smaller scopes, using semirigid fiber optics, convey an optical image through glass fibers composed of a high refractive index glass core surrounded by a low refractive glass cladding. Light travels by repeated reflections between the core and cladding. The fibers are arranged in an ordered (coherent) bundle, that is, each fiber occupies the same relative position at the exit face of the bundle as at the entry face. Each fiber in the image bundle carries a small part of the image. The need for exact ordering is the reason an image bundle is so much more expensive than the incoherent bundles used for light cables. Although semirigid fiber optic scopes have a smaller scope diameter, they offer resolution quality that is somewhat intermediate between that produced by a rod-lens system and flexible fiber optic scope. One clear advantage of the semirigid technology is that these scopes illuminate the endometrial cavity in an unexpectedly superior fashion—not unlike the rod-lens endoscopes of far greater diameter. The semirigid scope's properties are the result of a specially designed cladding material that allows many fiber optic bundles to be concentrated in a small surface area.

Flexible Fiber Optic Endoscopes

Several companies are now producing flexible fiber optic endoscopes for hysteroscopy (Fig. 6.6) similar to those used by surgeons for gastroscopy and sigmoidoscopy. These systems enjoy superior patient comfort and greater maneuverability and require fewer manipulations that exert pressure on the cervix. They also offer excellent views of the uterus laterally, superiorly, inferiorly, and posteriorly. Flexible fiber optic scopes can be threaded along a myoma or a large polyp, revealing its points of attachment. The limitation of the number of fiber bundles that can be accommodated in a telescope with a diameter of 3.0 mm precludes good resolution often resulting in a poorer image than a more conventional rod-lens system. The $7,000 price tag, reduced illumination, and inability to incorporate a continuous flow distention system are disadvantages of the flexible fiber optic scopes.

Accommodation of Sheaths

It is most economical to select a telescope that is compatible with various diagnostic and operative sheaths. My preference is to select an endoscope that will accommodate a non-continuous flow sheath for carbon dioxide distention, a continuous flow sheath for low viscosity fluids (LVFs), and a resectoscope operating element and continuous flow sheath.

Light Cables

Light cables are composed of flexible glass fiber bundles that carry the light produced by halogen, metal halide, or xenon bulbs in the light source. Because the purpose of the cable is only to convey light and not to transmit an image, there is no need for the fibers to be in corresponding order at the two ends (incoherent bundle). Due to a number of factors, including reflective light loss at air–glass interfaces, only 40% of the light from the light source reaches the scope. An additional 20% is lost at the junction between the cable and fiber optic scope due to mismatched fibers (12). Extending the light cable length beyond 2 m will result in additional light loss. Expensive hysteroscopes and light sources frequently do not to live up to their full potential because of old or mistreated light cables. With mishandling, inadvertent dropping, and twisting, fiber bundles "drop out" over a period of time. This can be easily tested for using the so-called "ceiling test." By holding one end of the cable up to a fluorescent light and observing, one can see how many "black spots" (or nonfunctioning fibers) can be visualized at the other end. Optimally, 75–80% of the light bundles should be intact. When in doubt, replace. The usual cost is about $250.

Light Sources

There are a variety of light sources available today. They can be classified by the amount of light they produce (watts), the type of bulb element (xenon, metal halide, or halogen), and whether they are intended for purely "diagnostic" uses or for "video" uses. A high power light source is needed because of light loss in different parts of the illumination system and the small diameter of the endoscopic lens or fiber optic bundle. Illumination using a high intensity xenon arc or metal halide light source is powerful enough and sufficiently white for both still and video photography. A xenon light source, with a color temperature of 5,600 K, mimics daylight and provides greater illumination in the blue-green spectrum. A xenon light source emits the kind of light necessary for diagnosis based on subtle color differences. With a color temperature of 5,600 K, metal halide provides, like xenon, bluer light but suffers from uneven spectral distribution. For color photography, a xenon light source is a must. Halogen light, with an even color temperature of 3,400 K, is more intense toward the red end of the spectrum and can compress color variations in the tissue. A high intensity light source will cost between $3,000 and $4,000. If video documentation is not desired, a standard 150-W halogen system is adequate. Single-bulb systems will cost between $125 and $250, and replacement bulbs can be purchased from any photography store that sells carousel projectors for approximately $25. The cost of these light sources makes them well suited for the novice who has not yet established the role of hysteroscopy in his or her office practice.

The choice of a light source for video documentation is much more complex. It may be advantageous to try several light sources before making a selection. Most companies will allow the use of a light source on a trial basis before the purchase is made. There are some hidden costs to consider, including the bulb life, which can vary from 60 to 1,000 hours; the cost of a replacement bulb; and the cost of maintenance agreements.

Uterine Distention Equipment

There are three commonly used modes of uterine distention: carbon dioxide, LVFs, and Dextran 70 (Hyskon, Medisan Pharmaceuticals, Inc., Parsippany, NY).

Carbon Dioxide

Carbon dioxide is a common distention medium used during office hysteroscopy. It has the advantages of being very safe, providing acceptable clarity (gas does not mix with blood), and of not "gumming up" the valves of the hysteroscope or its lens system. Its major disadvantages are the cost of its delivery system, the occurrence of carbon dioxide bubbles, the flattening out of polyps due to the pressure of the CO_2, and poor visualization in the presence of blood. The physician observes a different image in a CO_2-inflated uterus during diagnostic hysteroscopy than the image observed during operative hysteroscopy performed in a fluid medium. The refractive index of the fluid will magnify the image by about 30%.

Carbon dioxide has several additional disadvantages as a distention medium. First, it can leak through the fallopian tubes into the peritoneal cavity, where it collects under the diaphragm, irritating the phrenic nerve and causing referred pain to the patient's neck and shoulders. Other disadvantages of carbon dioxide insufflation include hypercarbia with resultant acidosis and the rare occurrence of CO_2 emboli. More commonly, carbon dioxide combines with water on the surface of the endometrium to form carbonic acid, a powerful uterotonic agent, which causes the patient to experience very painful labor-like uterine contractions.

Carbon dioxide should be delivered only through specifically designed hysteroscopic insufflators. A laparoscopic insufflator should never be used for hysteroscopy. Hysteroscopic insufflators are low-flow high-pressure machines that typically produce a maximum output of 100 mL/min and are capable of pressures up to 150 mm Hg. A typical "low-flow" laparoscopic insufflator can produce 1,000–10,000 mL/min at 20–30 mm Hg. Under no circumstances should CO_2 be delivered without an approved hysteroscopic metering system. Deaths have resulted when CO_2 was delivered directly from the tank.

When carbon dioxide is used for insufflation, this simple checklist should be followed before each hysteroscopy:

1. Check that adequate carbon dioxide is available for the examination. Most machines have an indicator that tells you how much gas is in the storage tank.
2. Assemble the tubing and the hysteroscope.
3. Turn the inflow valve of the hysteroscope to the full "on" position. The flow should be in excess of 80 mL/min and the pressure should be below 20 mm Hg.
4. Now, with everything assembled, the inflow valve is turned to the full "off" position with CO_2 being pumped out of the insufflator. The pressure should rise above 150 mm Hg and the flow should be 0. This indicates that all the tubing is intact.
5. Finally, if everything is assembled and operating properly, the hysteroscope and diagnostic sheath can be introduced with the carbon dioxide "running."

Low Viscosity Fluids (saline, glycine, sorbitol, lactated Ringer)

Several companies manufacture continuous flow sheaths with diameters of 5.0–6.5 mm. This type of insufflation medium offers numerous advantages. LVFs do not clog valves and can be delivered by a simple gravity-fed system, obviating the need for expensive and complicated hysteroscopic insufflators. By performing both diagnostic and operative hysteroscopy with LVFs, the physician can expect that the images obtained in the office will match those seen in the operating room.

Sound strange? Consider this.

During an office-based diagnostic hysteroscopy performed with a carbon dioxide insufflation system, the physician notes the existence of a submucous, sessile, posterior wall myoma located well within the uterine cavity. The distention pressure of 100 mm Hg allows the physician to see clearly around the fibroid and note that the lateral and anterior walls are free of involvement. The same patient is taken to the operating room 1 month later for removal of this "simple submucous myoma." Using a gravity-fed LVF system (mannitol 5%, sorbitol 3%, or glycine 1.5%), the uterus is not as fully distended as it was with CO_2 insufflation; therefore, all four uterine walls remain in contact with the myoma. Additionally, the myoma now appears 30% larger due to the increased refractive index of the liquid distention medium. The physician, once confident in his or her ability to remove the myoma, is now faced with a sudden unexpected dilemma.

Consider another example of how one can be "surprised" in the operating room. A physician plans to perform an endometrial ablation on a patient with abnormal menstrual bleeding. A previous diagnostic hysteroscopy (in the office), using a carbon dioxide distention system, revealed an anatomically normal uterus. Much to the physician's surprise, a large, flat, sessile polyp arising from the posterior wall is revealed during operative hysteroscopy. The polyp was present during the diagnostic examination but was camouflaged against the posterior uterine wall by the increased intrauterine pressure provided by CO_2. In the LVF environment, it begins to float, revealing the real cause of the patient's menstrual disorder. In the interest of reliable hysteroscopic diagnosis and optimal surgical results, the office diagnostic system should simulate the conditions present during an operative treatment. The use of LVFs to provide uterine distention for both diagnostic and operative hysteroscopy would effectively solve this problem.

Another advantage of LVFs is that they simply "wash" away blood during an acute bleeding episode, often revealing the source. Carbon dioxide distention works poorly under similar conditions. LVFs produce much less intraoperative and postoperative pain, requiring less patient sedation and improved patient participation.

There are also disadvantages to the use of LVFs for uterine distention. Although no expensive insufflation equipment is required, the cost of the individual fluid packs and tubing (approximately $25) discarded at the end of each case must be considered. Distention provided by gravity-fed systems frequently proves inadequate for a large uterus or an obese patient. Attention must be given to the collection of turbid fluid returning from the uterus. A collection system must be used that will safely collect, measure, and contain this fluid for appropriate disposal.

Finally, one must remember that LVF systems do not perfectly simulate what gynecologists may expect at the time of operative hysteroscopy. Most resectoscopes (25 or 26F) provide a flow of 800–1,000 mL/min. Diagnostic systems, by contrast, produce 80–200 mL/min through a 5.0- to 6.5-mm diameter sheath. This results in a relatively turbid view of the endometrial cavity if significant bleeding is present. The larger resectoscope and its concomitant flow generally overcome these minor annoyances.

High Molecular Weight Dextran 70 (Hyskon)

Hyskon is a colorless solution containing 32% Dextran with a molecular weight of 70,000 in a 10% dextrose solution. It is electrolyte free, making it suitable for unipolar electrosurgery (i.e., roller-ball resectoscope). The major advantage of Hyskon is that it is immiscible with blood. It has good optical properties, and a special delivery system is optional. If a Hyskon pump is not purchased, a staff person will have to manually pump Hyskon, because this viscous fluid cannot be gravity fed. The major disadvantages of this method for obtaining uterine distention include Hyskon's notorious ability to obstruct the valves of the hysteroscope and sheath. Lens systems are rendered unusable by "caked-on" Hyskon. It is the most problematic method of uterine distention primarily due to the risk it poses to expensive telescopes and sheaths. Furthermore, there have been rare reports of even small quantities (less than 50 mL) of Hyskon causing severe anaphylactic reactions with vascular collapse. Another rare hazard of Hyskon lies in its ability to cause fluid overload in the office patient. Hyskon exerts considerable osmotic activity. One hundred milliliters left in the abdominal cavity can draw 350 mL of fluid into the peritoneal space. No more than 100 mL of Hyskon should be used during a diagnostic examination.

Pulse Oximetry

A pulse oximeter, suitable for office hysteroscopy, records the patient's oxygen saturation, pulse rate, and will sound an alarm whenever the patient's oxygen saturation drops below 88–90%. All patients receiving midazolam (Versed, Roche Pharmaceuticals, Manati, PR), with or without a narcotic, should be monitored for any signs of early respiratory depression. Pulse oximeters are available today at prices ranging from $500 to $2,000.

Emergency Equipment

Respiratory arrest is the major risk associated with hysteroscopy performed on a patient receiving intravenous sedation. Respiratory arrest occurs when there is enough intravenous sedation to depress the patient's respiration to a life-threatening level and the physician fails to adequately monitor the patient's respiratory function. Astute and vigilant patient observation by a well-trained nurse or medical assistant is the most important factor in avoiding a true emergency. Thankfully, although respiratory arrest is a major risk, it is a very uncommon occurrence. I have sedated over 11,000 patients with midazolam during a variety of office procedures and have not witnessed a single respiratory arrest. Some patients do suffer respiratory depression, which is usually short lived (15–20 minutes) and responds well to gentle stimulation. This is in marked contrast to intravenous narcotics, which can cause profound respiratory depression that may last for 1–2 hours, often requiring intravenous narcotic antagonists and vigorous stimulation.

An emergency kit or cart (Fig. 6.10) should be readily available in the procedure

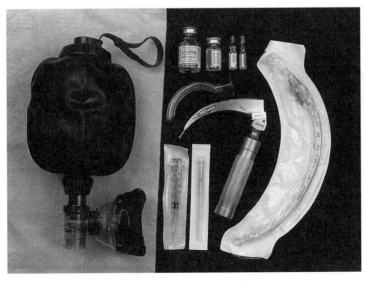

Figure 6.10. Emergency kit.

room. It should have its contents listed on an attached placard, thus providing a dependable method for inventory. The kit must contain an Ambu bag and mask (Ambu, Inc., Hanover, MD); oxygen tank, tubing, and regulator valve; laryngoscope handle and blade; batteries; endotracheal tubes, oral airways, or laryngeal mask airways; intravenous catheters, tubing, and fluids; and syringes and heparin locks and such medications as flumazenil 0.5 mg/mL (Romazicon, Hoffman-La Roche, Inc., Nutley, NJ), naloxone hydrochloride 0.4 mg/mL (Narcan, DuPont Pharmaceuticals, Manati, PR), atropine 0.4 mg/mL, and epinephrine 1:1,000, 1 mg/mL.

Video Documentation

Hysteroscopic documentation may be accomplished in several ways. Intraoperative findings may be recorded with a 35-mm camera or multiple video prints. The entire procedure may be videotaped with or without narration. This method of documentation is especially useful for the patient who prefers sedation and will allow the physician to record "mental notes" regarding patient management issues. Video documentation provides information for patient education, physician communication, physician training, physician comfort, and medicolegal considerations.

Patient Education

A picture is worth a thousand words, and a video image is very helpful in explaining to a patient what a myoma is or why it may explain her symptoms. A patient who has an opportunity to view her diagnostic hysteroscopy has more realistic expectations and will have the information she needs to decide what, if any, surgery she should have. Postoperatively, the video will be a powerful tool for helping the patient understand the findings in her particular case.

Physician Communication

A video tape of a diagnostic procedure provides an excellent method for sharing findings with another physician. The tape, which should always be made available to the patient, provides an avenue for seeking a second opinion, without having to repeat costly procedures. It may also prove to be a superior method of conveying information back to a referring physician. It is the ultimate operative note.

Physician Training

The most important reason for incorporating video documentation into a diagnostic examination is that it forces the physician to develop the eye–hand coordination essential for operative hysteroscopy. Additionally, the novice hysteroscopist will be able to review videotaped diagnostic examinations with a more experienced preceptor. This is a crucial step in developing patient management strategies.

Physician Comfort

The use of a video system will allow the hysteroscopist to get off his or her knees. Examining the acutely anteverted uterus is simplified by the use of an endoscopic video camera.

Medicolegal Considerations

Video prints or other photo documentation should be a permanent part of the patient record. They reflect an honest effort on the part of the physician to convey accurate information to the patient, medical colleagues, preceptors, and referring physicians. In no way can such open and honest behavior compromise the physician in the event of injury. Lawyers will be denied the opportunity to say "Well doctor, if you observed this condition, why didn't you take a picture of it for your records? All we have is your word for it, don't we?"

Staff

A well-trained staff is the "sine qua non" of successful office-based hysteroscopy. Education of physicians and patient care staff in office hysteroscopy should include didactic training, observation of hysteroscopic procedures, and the supervised practice of procedural techniques. Learn it, watch it, do it.

Didactic training courses, offered by several organizations specializing in endoscopy, often provide physicians with an opportunity for hands-on experience and may also supply instruction for patient care staff at reduced rates. After this formal training, the physician and staff trainees should visit an office where hysteroscopy is being performed and observe a team in action. Much can be learned from the exchange of information during the visit, including insights pertaining to equipment purchases and care, office protocols, consent forms, and teaching aids. Finally, when the novice hysteroscopist is ready to begin performing this procedure, he or she should invite a physician-preceptor to supervise the first several cases. This will ensure the completion of a proper diagnostic examination under conditions that optimize patient safety. The preceptor's guidance will be invaluable in shortening the novice's "learning curve" and in assisting in the resolution of problems that may be encountered.

Once diagnostic hysteroscopy is undertaken in an office practice, the untrained staff members must be included in the learning process. The more they know about hysteroscopy, the better is their ability to arrange appropriate scheduling and respond accurately to patient inquiries.

Protocols

Staff members must fully understand the part they play in making the hysteroscopic procedure convenient and informative for the physician and the patient. The receptionist, receiving the initial telephone contact, will arrange for all pertinent records to be sent to the office for review. She will then allow sufficient time for history taking and an initial examination. A receptionist may provide special consideration for patients who travel 1–2 hours to be seen. Some offices schedule a 90-minute appointment to accommodate the needs of the geographically challenged. This allows an initial history and physical, diagnostic ultrasound, and possible hysteroscopy to be performed at a single office visit.

Nurses and medical assistants who assist during the procedure also follow strict protocols before hysteroscopic examination. All equipment and supplies needed for the procedure must be assembled. A checklist is completed for all hysteroscopy equipment to ensure its proper functioning. The nurse will meet with the patient to review her current problem, past medical history, drug allergies, and current medications. Initial vital signs are taken and recorded along with the results of a urine pregnancy test and hematocrit.

Written protocols for each member of the hysteroscopic team should be carefully formulated. Each staff member should take part in perfecting these written protocols. Once protocols are developed, a complete procedural handbook is supplied to each member of the team.

Environment

The patient should experience the sense that all office personnel, including the receptionist, nurse, and medical assistants, are working in concert to make her examination safe, comfortable, and informative. Staff members should speak in "solo voce" about the availability of analgesics, sedation, and all other aspects of the procedure. For example, it is very disruptive and confusing to the patient who asks the receptionist "Will it hurt?" to get the answer "You can handle it, dear," only to hear "You better take the pain medication!" when posing the same question to the medical assistant.

Every attempt should be made to reduce the highly technical atmosphere of the procedure room. The staff must keep the equipment out of the patient's view until the physician is ready to use it. The sight of multiple syringes, tenacula, and scissors only intensifies the patient's anxiety. Music is a helpful addition but not as important as the sound of a reassuring voice explaining what is about to happen.

PATIENT PREPARATION

Successful office hysteroscopy depends on more than the simple coordination of equipment and staff with a carefully developed office protocol. The whole patient must be evaluated, given a thorough history and physical examination, educated about the evaluation process and the procedure, and informed about treatment choices.

Patient Evaluation: Initial History and Physical

The patient may present with any of a variety of problems, including abnormal menstrual bleeding, recurrent pregnancy loss, or infertility. It must be remembered that gynecologists should not promote a particular form of therapy or technology. The emphasis should be on the most beneficial, efficient, and complete care of the patient. This can only be accomplished with a clear understanding of the patient's current medical problems, past medical history, and family medical history. Equally important is an understanding of who the woman is—her personal and social history. She may be experiencing anxiety because she has just started a new job and will have difficulty taking time off from work for medical office visits. She may fear any surgical intervention because of childhood experiences or information about her family members. For example, the patient's mother may have shared her experience of no longer feeling sexually desirable after a hysterectomy. Each woman comes with her own "information packet" that the physician must explore and understand before he or she may offer advice. Completion of the patient history and physical examination, including pelvic sonography, equips the physician to determine which diagnostic examinations will elicit the most information while controlling cost, risk, and patient discomfort.

Laboratory Evaluation

The extent of laboratory evaluation for a particular woman who presents with abnormal uterine bleeding is a lengthy subject that cannot be covered in this text. The laboratory

CHAPTER 6 / DIAGNOSTIC AND OPERATIVE HYSTEROSCOPY

Table 6.1
Postoperative Instructions

1. Get as much rest as you need. Generally, you will feel very sleepy for several hours after receiving intravenous medications. You may experience some nausea *(this should not last long)*.
2. You may eat whenever you feel comfortable doing so.
3. Vaginal bleeding is normal and may last several days after the procedure or taper off to a brownish vaginal discharge. Lack of bleeding should not concern you, especially if you have not had an endometrial biopsy.
4. You may shower or take tub baths whenever you wish.
5. You may resume sexual relations whenever you wish to.
6. You may use either pads or tampons.
7. Under no circumstances are you to drive or operate dangerous machinery for the 12 hours following your procedure if you received intravenous drugs.
8. Please call the office to schedule a follow-up appointments in 1–2 weeks.
9. Report any temperature over 100 degrees Fahrenheit.
10. Call the office if you feel worse tomorrow than you did today.

evaluation for any woman in her reproductive years should always include a hematocrit and a urine pregnancy test. Patients who have clinical stigmata of hypo- or hyperthyroidism should undergo appropriate laboratory screening, including for thyrotropin and thyroxine (free or total). Women with acyclic bleeding or bleeding secondary to a suspected luteal phase defect should undergo a properly timed measurement of serum progesterone. Those patients suspected of an androgen excess disorder, von Willebrands disease, or other bleeding diathesis should be referred for evaluation by a hematologist.

Patient Education

Teaching aids that can supply important information about hysteroscopy should be made available in written and video formats to the patient, her partner, and other concerned family members. A 25- to 30-minute video tape explaining preoperative preparation (laboratory work and meals before the procedure), anesthesia and analgesia, patient participation, requirement for a support person, availability of video prints, postoperative instructions, and a complete review of operative risks, consequences and alternatives should be supplied for home viewing before the patient signs the consent form. A patient who truly understands the procedure and is given an opportunity to ask questions for clarification will become a more knowledgeable participant in the informed consent process as well as the procedure. Additional patient information will be provided in the form of written postoperative instructions when the procedure has been completed (Table 6.1).

Informed Consent

Honest and thorough informed consent is not just a medicolegal requirement but an ethical requirement as outlined by the American College of Obstetrics and Gynecology (Table 6.2). The basis of informed consent lies in the patient's understanding of what procedure is being performed, why it is being performed (i.e., what does she have to gain by it), the reasonable alternatives to the procedure, and an understanding of its risks. Obtaining thorough informed consent is a time-consuming job. It is a rare physician who is fortunate enough to have a staff member to whom this task may be safely and confidently entrusted. Delegation of such responsibility must be carefully made.

Table 6.2
Operative Consent Form for Diagnostic Hysteroscopy

I, _____, do hereby grant permission to Dr. Morris Wortman to perform a procedure known as a diagnostic hysteroscopy. It has been explained to me that Dr. Wortman has suggested this procedure to gain diagnostic information regarding my _____.
I understand that there are other alternatives to diagnostic hysteroscopy which include _____.

It has further been explained to me that it may be necessary for Dr. Wortman to use either local anesthetic agents or intravenous sedation.

There are risks to performing hysteroscopy and to administering intravenous sedatives and anesthetic agents. The risks of hysteroscopy include perforation of the uterus and infection. Also, I understand that the procedure may not yield all the intended information because of poor visualization of the uterine cavity. The risks of sedation include respiratory depression and respiratory arrest. The latter can be life threatening.

In addition, Dr. Wortman will be removing some uterine lining tissue (endometrium) to have it analyzed by a pathologist. I give Dr. Wortman permission to have this tissue removed and analyzed.

I understand the reasons for undergoing this surgical procedure. I also understand the risks and consequences of this procedure. My questions have been answered by Dr. Wortman prior to my signing this consent form. Additionally, I have reviewed the patient teaching videotape entitled: *Hysteroscopy— A Patient's Perspective.*

_____   _____
Signature of patient   Date

_____   _____
Signature of witness   Date

HOW TO PERFORM A DIAGNOSTIC HYSTEROSCOPY

Hysteroscopic examinations should be organized so that they yield the maximum amount of information in the most time-efficient and safe manner. Such procedures produce patient satisfaction and at the same time build the physician's confidence and skills. Furthermore, physicians who contemplate engaging in operative hysteroscopy must first possess a solid experiential foundation in diagnostic hysteroscopy. Successful use of the hysteroscope in diagnosis leads to successful use of the hysteroscope in surgery. Before pilots fly they must first attend ground school.

Procedure

This section reviews my practice of office-based diagnostic hysteroscopy. It is an approach that has been used to successfully diagnose and treat patients in an office setting for more than 10 years and has resulted in a high degree of patient satisfaction and diagnostic accuracy.

Patient Preparation

On the day of the procedure, the patient is required to bring a responsible adult who will drive her home afterward. Although she may drink clear liquids such as apple juice and tea, the patient is directed not to eat 4 hours before the procedure. Before the procedure, the patient's vital signs, urine human chorionic gonadotropin (hCG), and hematocrit are recorded. After disrobing from the waist down, the patient may elect to be sedated. Sedation is never administered until all equipment has been checked and found to be ready for use.

Adequate Analgesia

Paracervical Block Anesthesia

Paracervical block anesthesia provides a moderate amount of anesthesia for the dilation portion of the procedure. Patients and physicians should understand that it provides little, if any, pain control during uterine distention. An injection of Xylocaine 1% is administered with a 25-gauge × 5/8-inch needle mounted on a 2- or 3-inch needle extender. One milliliter is administered on the anterior cervical lip at the tenaculum site. After the cervix is grasped and stabilized, the remainder of the solution is injected at the posterior cervical lip, in the midline, just beneath the mucosa. No more than 10 mL of Xylocaine 1% (100 mg) is administered. When using a small diameter flexible hysteroscope, it may not be necessary to anesthetize the posterior cervical lip.

Intravenous Sedation

Although not required for most hysteroscopic examinations, intravenous sedation is an important option to offer patients. The availability of diazepam and midazolam, "just in case," will help reduce patient anxiety. As one's operative and interpersonal skills improve, fewer patients will request this option. The sedative amnesiac effect of midazolam will allow the physician and office staff an opportunity to adapt to the new technology and routines. A well-sedated patient may allow the physician the additional few minutes needed to obtain a perfect intrauterine view.

Midazolam (Versed), given in a 5.0-mg slow intravenous push, will provide safe and effective sedation for healthy women under the age of 50. Women over the age of 50 should have a heparin lock in place and receive an initial dose of 2.0 mg of midazolam, followed by 1.0 mg every 2–3 minutes until sufficient sedation occurs. Physicians often ask about the proper dose of Versed to produce amnesia. Amnesia correlates very well with two findings: slurring of speech and the perception that room lights are "moving."

Many physicians are reticent to use intravenous midazolam for fear of acute respiratory arrest. Remember, it takes two things to have a respiratory arrest. First, you must have respiratory depression. Second, you must ignore it.

The combined use of midazolam and a narcotic analgesic should be avoided except in the most anxious and uncooperative patients because the combination will work synergistically to increase the risk of profound respiratory depression. On occasion it may be necessary to administer a nonsteroidal anti-inflammatory drug orally, intramuscularly, or intravenously. Ibuprofen or ketorolac may be given 10–60 minutes before the procedure.

If sedative hypnotics or narcotics are used in an office setting, it is vital that a strict office protocol be instituted to address each of the following areas of concern:

- Patient health conditions, which preclude conscious sedation in an office setting (examples are severe cardiac disease, liver or renal disease, massive obesity);
- Training for personnel, which includes cardiopulmonary resuscitation, recognition of respiratory depression, and its management;

- Pulse oximetry;
- Use of intravenous drugs, heparin locks, and so on;
- Use of sedative hypnotic agents and their antagonists;
- Use of narcotic analgesics and their antagonists;
- Patient transportation to and from the office;
- Presence of a support person;
- Maintaining accurate inventory, control, and log sheets of all controlled substances.

Room Preparation for Diagnostic Hysteroscopy

In the operating room, assemble the following equipment for all hysteroscopic procedures. Please note the slight differences in the setup for carbon dioxide hysteroscopy (Fig. 6.11) compared with LVF hysteroscopy (Fig. 6.12).

The following list is a checklist for those responsible for the procedure room setup: single-toothed tenaculum, 30° (or 12°) 4.0 mm diagnostic hysteroscope, open-sided speculum, 10 mL Xylocaine 1% on a 2-inch needle extender, 25 gauge × 5/8-inch needle, Novak curette, and formalin for specimen.

Based on the type of insufflation system, assemble the following: for carbon dioxide, dilators through 24F, Gimpelson tenaculum, and 5 mm diagnostic sheath, and for LVFs, dilators through 26F 5.5 or 6.5 continuous flow sheaths, 500 mL bag of saline, urologic tubing, and collection container.

Check the hysteroflator (CO_2) to see that hoses are intact, that adequate carbon dioxide is in the tank, and that the controls are appropriately zeroed.

Regarding the light source and cables (CO_2 and LVFs), ensure the photo lamp is turned on and warmed up and that cables are attached.

The monitor, camera, and video cassette recorder (CO_2 and LVFs) should all be attached and checked to see that they are in working order. Make sure the video tape is loaded into the machine and check that the video printer is turned on and that sufficient paper is loaded. Also check that the 35-mm camera is loaded with film.

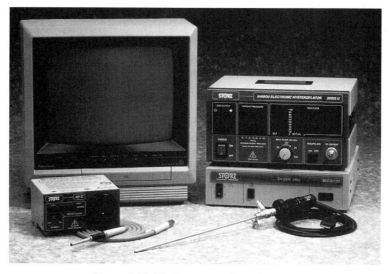

Figure 6.11. CO_2 hysteroscopic equipment.

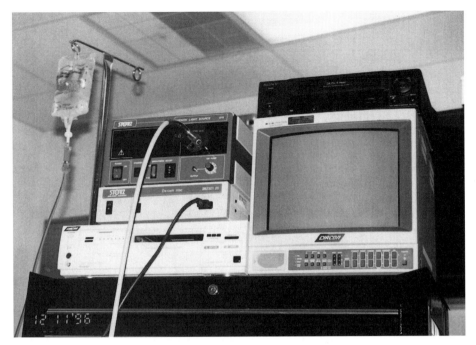

Figure 6.12. LVFs hysteroscopic equipment.

Preoperative Checklist for CO_2

Before beginning the procedure, the camera, hysteroscope, diagnostic sheath, light cord, and gas cord are assembled. The camera is white balanced. At this point, the gas flow is placed in the full maximum flow position. The stopcock to the diagnostic sheath is turned full "off." In this position the pressure should be between 150 and 200 mm Hg and the flow should be zero. This indicates that no leaks are in the system and that there is adequate carbon dioxide to start the case.

The second preoperative check occurs when the valve to the diagnostic sheath is turned "on." The pressure rapidly falls to 10–20 mm Hg and the flow should exceed 80–90 mL/min.

Preoperative Checklist for LVFs

The preoperative checklist for using LVFs for uterine distention consists simply of turning the inflow port to the "on" position and checking that the flow is of good quality (unobstructed) and egresses through the inner sheath. If all preoperative checks are met, then and only then does the procedure begin.

The patient is premedicated with intravenous midazolam, if she so elects. She should place her legs comfortably in the stirrups and lay flat. It is important, especially if CO_2 is used, that the patient not be placed in the Trendelenburg position. Positioning the patient in this manner has been associated with CO_2 emboli and even death. After adequate sedation has been established, a warmed prelubricated speculum is inserted into the vagina. Ten milliliters of Xylocaine 1% are used to complete the paracervical block. At

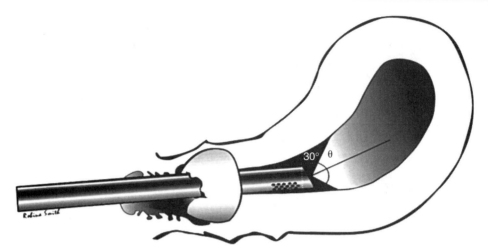

Figure 6.13. Examination of the anteverted uterus. Note that the hysteroscope and sheath are pointed in a 30° "upward" position.

least 5 minutes is allowed to pass before resuming the procedure. The cervix is grasped with a single-toothed tenaculum. After this, the cervix is dilated to a 22 Hank dilator and the assembled hysteroscope (lens, diagnostic sheath, gas tubing, light cord, and video camera) is guided, under direct vision, through the endocervical canal, slowly approaching the fundus. The camera is always held in its "12 o'clock position." For an anteverted uterus, the hysteroscope and sheath are held in a 30° upward position (Fig. 6.13). In the case of a retroverted uterus, the position of the hysteroscope and lens is reversed. With either gas or LVFs, the distention medium should be "running" as the instrument is inserted, allowing the cervix to dilate under the gentle pressure supplied by the medium. Using this approach one can usually anticipate easy access to the endometrial cavity.

If easy access into the canal is not gained, then the diagnostic scope is held in the

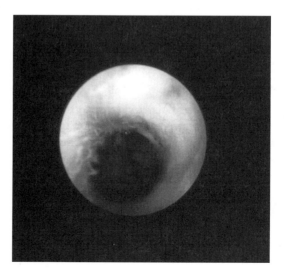

Figure 6.14. Black spot.

cervical canal and one looks for the black spot (Fig. 6.14), which is the view of the fundus through the cervix. If the lens is 30° "up," then you will gain access into the cavity by aiming 30° up and past the black spot. If this concept is difficult to understand, hold a hysteroscope in this position and stare at a wall clock. Center the wall clock in your field. Now stand back and look at where the scope is actually aimed (Fig. 6.15).

If you still have not gained access to the endometrial cavity, consider the following:

1. Overdilating the cervix
   - 24F with a 5.0-mm o.d. hysteroscopic sheath (carbon dioxide)
   - 26F with a 6.5-mm o.d. hysteroscopic sheath (LVFs)
2. Correcting any acute anteversion or retroversion of the uterus
   - If the uterus is acutely anteflexed, push it down with an "abdominal hand"
   - If the uterus is acutely retroverted, use a rectal finger to push it up.

Examine the uterus systematically. Start at the patient's left uterine cornua, then her right cornua, anterior wall, lateral walls, and posterior wall. Finally, examine the cervix.

Always hold the video camera (if you are right handed) in the left hand in the 12 o'clock position. The right hand is firmly attached to the light cord. The cord can be

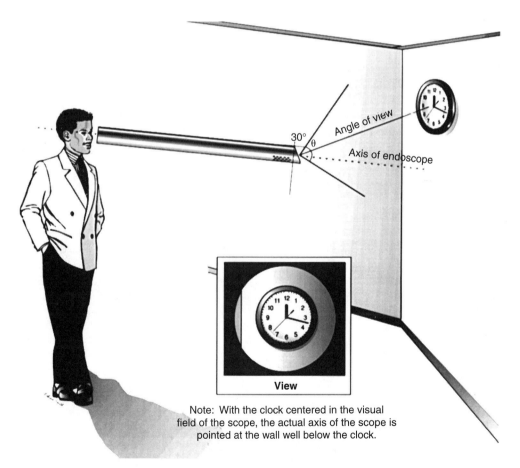

Note: With the clock centered in the visual field of the scope, the actual axis of the scope is pointed at the wall well below the clock.

Figure 6.15. Illustration of the concept of aiming the diagnostic scope.

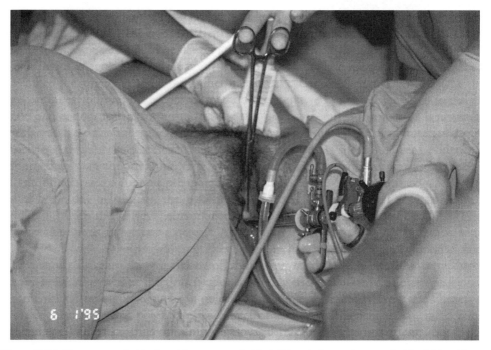

Figure 6.16. The surgeon holds the video camera in his left hand, the endoscope in his right, while an assistant controls the cervical tenaculum.

swiveled back and forth independently of the camera so that orientation is always maintained. Have an assistant (your two hands are already tied up) hold the tenaculum for you. This is exactly the same technique that will be used later on when describing operative hysteroscopy (Fig. 6.16).

If you wish to use a LVF, remember to switch to a continuous flow sheath. Urologic tubing is attached to a 250- or 500-mL bag of an LVF. The other end of the urologic tubing is connected to the inflow port. Allow 20–30 mL of fluid to pass through the system to be certain that your connections are secure and correct. Attach a 10-mL syringe to the "outflow port." Fluid is released as the hysteroscope is passed into an already dilated cervix (6–7 mm as appropriate). When the scope enters the cavity, the syringe is used to create suction at the outflow port. Once the system has been primed, continuous flow should occur readily. The effluent can be collected in a large plastic bucket.

Troubleshooting Problems for CO_2 Hysteroscopy

Lack of pressure—check for the following:

- Gas control is turned off
- Gas tank or cartridge is empty;
- Leak at the gas cord attachment site;
- Leak at the hysteroscope attachment site;
- Crack in the tube;
- Diagnostic sheath is not tightened around scope;
- Cervix is leaking.

Lack of flow—check for the following:

- Lack of gas pressure;
- Plastic gas tubing is kinked;
- Hysteroscope valve turned off or misaligned;
- Internal channel to hysteroscope is blocked (flush out with sterile saline).

"Red out"—check the following:

- Correct any problem leading to low pressure and low flow (see above);
- Rub lens up along the uterus;
- Wash off lens with running sterile water;
- Move the scope to the fundus until you get a "white out" (i.e., you are up against the fundus), then slowly withdraw the hysteroscope, manipulating it as little as possible to prevent bubbles from forming.

Failure to enter the uterine cavity:

- Start with small dilators;
- Overdilate the cervix;
- Consider acute anteversion— abdominal hand;
- Consider acute retroversion—rectal hand;
- Consider anatomic obstruction (septae, fibroids, synechiae).

Troubleshooting Problems for LVF Hysteroscopy

The problem that is unique to LVF hysteroscopy lies in the possible inability to establish a continuous flow of fluid. This results in a very turbid picture. In the event that a continuous flow is not established, the following should be immediately checked:

- Check that the entire system of LVFs is open and that all lines are unkinked;
- Be certain that the tubing is attached properly to the intake and outflow ports;
- Verify that fluid is streaming from the inflow channel of the continuous flow sheath;
- Be certain that the outflow ports or suction of the external sheath are free of blood and debris;
- Check to see that fluid is egressing from the outflow port into the collection container.

If fluid is not egressing from the outflow port consider the following:

- Uterine perforation;
- Hysteroscope has not passed the cervix;
- Hysteroscope is in a functionally small uterus (fibroid, septum, or multiple polyps).

Contraindications to Hysteroscopy

Contraindications to hysteroscopy are few and far between. Known pelvic infections should be treated before hysteroscopy. Heavy uterine bleeding is a relative contraindication. One often has no choice but to hysteroscope some patients in the face of heavy uterine bleeding. The uterus can be "washed out" with a continuous flow of LVF. A recent uterine perforation is a relative contraindication. Hysteroscopic ablations have been done after a known uterine perforation. This kind of procedure should only be performed by someone who knows how to manage this complication and is prepared for laparoscopic guidance. Invasive carcinoma of the cervix would qualify as an absolute contraindication unless microcolpohysteroscopy was being performed for a staging procedure.

Office Hysteroscopy: Complications and Management

Complications of office hysteroscopy are fortunately uncommon. If the use of Hyskon for uterine distention is avoided, severe life-threatening complications are exceptionally rare.

Complications Secondary to Inadequate Sedation or Analgesia

Many patients tolerate office hysteroscopy well without the use of sedative hypnotics or narcotic analgesics. The patient who experiences significant pain will demand "that you get that thing out of me"; move around in an uncontrollable fashion, launching herself off the examination table onto a hard surface; break loose of the straps binding her knees to the stirrups, endangering the integrity of the gynecologist's cervical spine; frighten any remaining patients in your waiting room; and never refer another patient to your office. The frightened and uncomfortable patient will force you to hasten your examination, resulting in an inadequate image of the uterine cavity and an incomplete examination. You might even seriously reconsider why you ever undertook this expensive venture into office surgery. The solution to these problems is to allow the patient, at any time before, during, and after the initiation of the procedure, to choose to be sedated.

Further Complications Secondary to Inadequate Sedation or Analgesia

It is important for the physician to recognize the signs of a severe vasovagal reaction, a rare occurrence among well-sedated patients. They include bradycardia, loss of consciousness, nausea and vomiting, and diaphoresis. The patient experiencing a vasovagal reaction first presents with diaphoresis and nausea. This should alert the physician to check for bradycardia. A persistent heart rate below 60 beats/min calls for the administration of atropine, 0.2–0.4 mg, intravenously. The patient should lie flat, either on her back or her side. Fortunately, most vasovagal reactions are short lived and respond well to conservative management such as the application of cool towels, loosening of clothing, and positioning the patient's body in the manner described above.

Uterine Perforation

Uterine perforation occurs in approximately 1% of all diagnostic examinations. Signs of uterine perforation include inability to distend the uterus; the appearance of a persistent "red-out," if carbon dioxide is used; actual visualization of the perforation, if an LVF system is used; and lack of uterine distention, coupled with the loss of egress of fluid from the outflow portion of the scope. Most perforations are made with cervical dilators and usually occur at the fundus and in the midline. Uterine perforations may be minimized by avoiding the use of dilators unless absolutely necessary and by using short dilators, such as Hegars.

After recognition of a uterine perforation, the patient should be observed for at least 1–2 hours in an office setting. The baseline hematocrit included in the preoperative laboratory work should be repeated at specified intervals based on the patients clinical condition. Transfer to a hospital is indicated if the patient experiences worsening abdominal pain, postural hypotension, or other signs of hypovolemia and hemoperitoneum.

Uterine perforations can generally be managed without laparoscopy. Sequential ultrasound examinations are invaluable in alerting the physician to active intrapelvic bleeding.

Respiratory Depression and Respiratory Arrest

The avoidance of respiratory depression and subsequent arrest is discussed above. Respiratory depression, secondary to the use of midazolam, should be treated only if oxygen saturation drops below 90%. The initial treatment consists of gentle verbal stimulation. Many patients will start to breathe if they are simply asked to. Oxygen should be administered either by nasal prongs or by mask. Further stimulation, if necessary, involves rubbing or gently slapping the palms of the patient's hands or feet. Under no circumstances should a patient be stimulated by pinching or slapping any other region of the body. If the patient does not respond to these maneuvers, 0.2 mg flumazenil should be given by intravenous bolus every 30 seconds until adequate respiration ensues. Do not exceed a total dose of 1.0 mg. The patient should be carefully monitored because flumazenil has a short half-life and more than a single administration may be required.

If narcotic analgesics are used in combination with midazolam, they should be "reversed" before the administration of flumazenil. Naloxone hydrochloride (Narcan), 40 μg, is administered, incrementally, to achieve the desired effect on respiration. Up to 400 μg may be given. This too requires careful monitoring because of its short half-life. Respiratory depression may be minimized by avoiding the combination of a potent sedative hypnotic with a narcotic analgesic (see above). Respiratory arrest should never occur if proper patient monitoring is carried out, using pulse oximetry. In the event of this emergency, naloxone hydrochloride, 0.4 mg (400 μg) is given by slow intravenous push.

Carbon Dioxide Emboli

The occurrence of CO_2 emboli can be catastrophic in an office setting. This emergency manifests itself by the sudden onset of hypoxia and vascular collapse. Prompt recognition and treatment are essential to patient survival. Treatment generally calls for needle aspiration of carbon dioxide and room air bubbles lodged in the right heart. Carbon dioxide emboli occur when examinations are performed, with carbon dioxide insufflation, on a patient who has been placed in a deep Trendelenburg position. This allows the heart to fall below the level of the uterus. Gas becomes entrapped in the uterus as a result of the diagnostic examination. The sudden change from Trendelenburg to a flat or seated position creates a strong pressure gradient, allowing the gas to enter the uterine vasculature. Bubbles of carbon dioxide admixed with air become trapped in the heart, leading to cardiac and vascular collapse if left untreated.

This complication can be avoided if one follows these simple rules. Never perform any diagnostic or operative hysteroscopic procedure with the patient in Trendelenburg. Second, if at all possible, use a continuous flow system that incorporates LVFs. Remember to purge the system of air before entering the uterine cavity.

HYSTEROSCOPIC SURGERY

Abnormal Menstrual Bleeding

Gynecologists have long recognized that many women develop abnormal menstrual patterns at some time in their lives. Young women, having difficulty "getting started," suffer heavy irregular menses. A variety of menstrual abnormalities may affect mature women as they approach the "other end" of the reproductive cycle.

Derangements of menstruation may present with an alteration in cycle length, duration, and intensity of flow. Women may experience a shortening or lengthening of their cycle length, metrorrhagia (intermenstrual bleeding and spotting), or menorrhagia (menses that suddenly become much heavier than previously encountered). The onset of postmenopausal bleeding may signal the presence of endometrial hyperplasia, a polyp, or adenocarcinoma. In all instances, abnormal bleeding is uncomfortable and disruptive both physically and emotionally. Unpredictable or heavy bleeding can create stress and uncertainty in the work place and during social engagements. Severe bleeding can lead to anemia, fatigue, and hemodynamic changes. Even a constant prolonged period of light spotting and bleeding may produce fatigue and restlessness disproportionate to actual blood loss.

Before 1987, women whose bleeding was uncontrolled by medical therapy chose between "living with it" and hysterectomy. Since the FDA approvals of the Nd:YAG laser (1987) for endometrial ablation and the continuous flow gynecologic resectoscope (1989) for electrosurgical ablation and resection, gynecologists have been able to give their patients the option of minimally invasive management of abnormal uterine bleeding.

Most women who undergo evaluation of abnormal uterine bleeding have an anatomically normal uterus or one containing minimal pathology such as benign endometrial polyps. Submucous myomata are present in approximately 20% of the patients referred to me for evaluation of menorrhagia and may also be responsible for recurrent pregnancy wastage and infertility. Most patients with acyclic bleeding (>90%) have no observable anatomic abnormality. This is also the case with most women experiencing postmenopausal bleeding. Although many patients will be satisfied with the results of medical treatment, our quest has been to find an effective minimally invasive surgical technique to manage those patients who do not respond adequately to traditional pharmacologic treatment.

A Quest for Treatment

The search for a minimally invasive treatment for abnormal uterine bleeding has led to two schools of thought. Gynecologists of the "ablation school" sought methods that caused thermal necrosis of the endometrium either by freezing or heating the tissue. The members of the "resection school" preferred to surgically excise the endometrium down to its underlying myometrium. Both schools hoped to produce predictable and lasting amenorrhea or oligomenorrhea accompanied by a minimal complication rate.

Endometrial Ablation

The ablationists trace their origins to Droegmueller's (13) blind technique that used liquid nitrogen to cryocoagulate the uterine lining. Goldrath et al. (8), working with the Nd:YAG laser, sought to coagulate endometrial tissue by heating it beyond the boiling point of water. The laser, approved by the FDA in 1987, gained little popularity because of its expense, awkwardness, and limited effectiveness. The FDA approval of the first continuous flow resectoscope in 1989 provided gynecologists with a unique and inexpensive tool that was adaptable to energy sources already available in most operating suites—the electrosurgical unit (ESU). The 100,000 dollar Nd:YAG laser was eliminated by the

$2,000–6,000 ESU found in virtually all operating rooms. The visual clarity provided by the continuous flow resectoscope far surpassed anything achieved by the simple hysteroscope used with the Nd:YAG laser.

Several studies have reported that endometrial ablation, whether by cryosurgery (14), laser surgery (8), or electrosurgery (10, 15), produced unpredictable results. In vitro studies by Onbargi et al. (16) showed that neither power density nor wave form (coagulation versus cutting current) can be a predictor of the depth of tissue destruction. In the years that followed, Nd:YAG laser treatment was shown to produce an amenorrhea rate of only 25% at 1 year. Electrosurgical ablation with the continuous flow resectoscope and ball-end electrode produced better results, 1 year amenorrhea rates of 40–55%. Endometrial ablation, by any means, fails to produce reliable outcomes. Finally, no tissue sample of endometrium or myometrium is recovered during ablation, detracting from the understanding of underlying clinical problems.

Endometrial Resection

Endometrial removal was first described by DeCherney and Polan (9) using a urologic resectoscope fitted with a wire loop electrode to remove endometrium. Just how much endometrium they removed is not well documented. This work was later taken up by Magos et al. (17), who removed endometrium along with some underlying myometrium, using a technique they called transcervical resection of the endometrium. Tissue was obtained for histologic analysis. The surgical outcomes were poor, as measured by an amenorrhea rate of only 26% at 12 months.

To remedy the shortcomings of the techniques described above, I set out to develop a sound geometric approach to endometrial resection, taking into consideration the unique anatomy of the uterus. It was reasoned that a uniform and substantial depth of myometrium should be excised to prevent endometrial regrowth—an apparent problem already described in previous techniques. EMR is the uniform removal of endometrial and myometrial tissue to a predictable depth. With a 1-year amenorrhea rate of 87%, it has the most predictable outcome yet reported. EMR is defined as the systematic and geometric excision of at least 3 mm of uterine endomyometrium (atrophic) throughout the cavity, except at the tubal ostia, where 2 mm is removed. EMR produces a excellent tissue specimen for histologic analysis that may reveal heretofore undiagnosed adenomyosis and endometrial hyperplasia.

Hysteroscopic Myomectomy

Surgical procedures for myomectomy have evolved on a path parallel to endometrial resection techniques. Various techniques have been described for both the removal or destruction of fibroids. In 1983, Neuwirth (18) reported using a urologic resectoscope for the first excision of symptomatic fibroids. Others (19–23) reported the successful treatment of intractable bleeding by the resection of one or more submucous fibroids using the myoma shaving technique, a laborious and time-consuming task appropriate for only small submucous fibroids.

Thermal destructive methods have included myolysis with the Nd:YAG laser and the VaporTrode (Circon, ACMI, Stamford, CT). The former causes coagulation necrosis of the fibroid, whereas the latter actually vaporizes the tissue with very high current density at the tip of this unipolar electrode. Neither of these techniques produces a tissue specimen. I have reported a series of 75 myomectomies in which three cases of uncertain malignant potential were found. In all three cases, consulting oncologists recommended a total hysterectomy and node dissection. In view of these findings, and similar findings by Corson and Brooks (24) and Goldrath (25), a very good argument can be made for a resection specimen that can be analyzed.

I have reported several new myomectomy techniques that facilitate the more efficient removal of fibroids. These procedures shorten operative time and result in the retrieval of larger fibroids. The first, myoma coring, allows for the removal of cavity filling myomata that would prevent placement of the resectoscope between the uterine wall and the fibroid, making the shaving technique impossible. The second, myoma resection, accomplishes the removal of tissue in large strips rather than in small chips or "shavings," thus reducing surgical time and the danger of fluid intravasation. Incorporation of real-time ultrasound guidance makes it possible to perform the resection of fibroids that have a large intramural component without concern for uterine perforation. Ultrasonography has eliminated the need for laparoscopic "control," an invasive technique for which a role in accident prevention has not been established.

In the remainder of this chapter, the techniques of EMR and myomectomy are explored in great detail. It is my hope that gynecologists will be stimulated to acquire and perfect these techniques and offer minimally invasive alternatives to their patients.

ESSENTIALS OF ENDOMYOMETRIAL RESECTION

Patient Selection

Proper patient selection is the most important step whenever offering any therapy to a patient. The physician who offers minimally invasive surgery to a patient who may well respond to hormonal therapy is doing her the same disservice as the gynecologist performing a hysterectomy where a simple myomectomy would suffice.

Patient selection begins with the careful documentation of medical history. This should include information about cycle length and duration of menses, frequency of pad changes, sleep disturbance, and accompanying pelvic pain and cramps. Any irregular or intermenstrual bleeding should be noted. The interview may also provide an opportunity for the physician to put into perspective some of the patient's concerns about cancer, hysterectomy, and menopause, none of which need be associated with their particular problem.

A careful history should be followed by a directed laboratory evaluation. At minimum, a hematocrit and urine hCG is obtained. When clinically appropriate, thyroid function, coagulation studies, and bleeding time are also evaluated. For patients with acyclic bleeding, a serum progesterone (appropriately timed) and gonadotropin assays are drawn. An initial physical examination and transvaginal pelvic ultrasound are performed. A normal sonogram is followed by an endometrial sampling, whereas the more ambiguous scans will require clarification with sonohysterography and office hysteroscopy. Diagnostic hysteroscopy performed with a continuous flow hysteroscope and LVFs is well tolerated by patients and provides the most useful information for the physician and patient. Patients must have a recent endometrial biopsy and Pap smear. Approximately 70% of my patients have been shown to have an anatomically and histologically normal uterus, as determined by physical examination, ultrasound, diagnostic hysteroscopy, and endometrial biopsy.

The remainder have shown some combination of fibromyomas, endometrial polyps, endometritis, or endometrial hyperplasia.

Patients who complete this initial evaluation are sent home with a booklet and a 35-minute videotape detailing the medical and surgical approaches to the management of intractable uterine bleeding. Experience indicates that patients spend a great deal of time reviewing this information and return for their next appointment knowledgeable about their alternatives.

"Ideal" patients can be characterized as well informed; having cyclical heavy bleeding that may involve clotting, frequent pad changes, and sleep disturbances (nocturhagia), presenting with dysmenorrhea appropriate to menstrual blood loss; having completed childbearing; previously failing on medical therapy; willing to accept some cyclic bleeding as a final surgical result; having no evidence of chronic pelvic pain or pain not explained by the volume of menstrual blood loss; possessing a uterus equal to or less than 12 cm in length as determined by ultrasound examination; and showing no evidence of acute or chronic endometritis, adenomatous hyperplasia, or cancer.

Although I initially avoided pharmacologic preparatory agents, a review of the first 100 outcomes showed no difference in amenorrhea rates at 6 and 12 months between patients treated with a gonadotropin-releasing hormone (GnRH) agonist and ones that were not medically or surgically prepped. However, the use of leuprolide depot was associated with 20% decrease in operative time compared with patients who did not receive any form of medical preparation. Certainly, for the newcomer to hysteroscopic EMR, the use of preoperative leuprolide acetate is strongly recommended.

The Right Equipment

Fluid Infusion System

LVF (mannitol 5%, sorbitol 3%, or glycine 1.5%) is warmed to approximately 39°C by a Level I fluid warmer (Level I Technologies, Marshfield, MA), reducing postoperative hypothermia, and fed from 3-L bags through standard urologic tubing to the resectoscope. The spout of the 3-L bags is held approximately 4 feet above the patient and is adjusted to the minimum height that will allow good distention of the uterine cavity and an intrauterine pressure sufficient to overcome venous and arterial bleeding. Because of the importance of careful tabulation of fluid input and output, it may be necessary to weigh the bags of fluid because they are frequently overfilled by as much as 10%. Although devices are available that measure fluid infusion and output, they are not yet adaptable to a fluid warming system.

Fluid Collection System

Because much of the fluid retrieved during EMR passes though the exocervix, it becomes imperative that a double collection system be used: one for egress of fluid from the cervix and the second for the fluid that passes through the outflow ports of the continuous flow resectoscope. A Urocatcher drape (MDT Castle No. S4004FTB, MDT Corp., Rochester, NY) and supporting hoop (AMATECH accessory S/N 18006, Amatech Corp., Acton, MA) is used to collect all fluid not recovered through the resectoscope and trap the surgical specimen. Fluid passing through the Urocatcher drape and fluid returning from the resectoscope travels through standard urologic tubing to a collection containment system where it is measured and then disposed of.

Video System

Gynecologists wrongly assume that what works well for the laparoscopist will also work for the hysteroscopist. Video cameras that function very well with the larger 10-mm laparoscopes may prove inadequate for the 4-mm hysteroscope. Microdigital cameras are extremely light sensitive and allow the operator superb panoramic viewing with the hysteroscope lens placed at the internal cervical os. Many video cameras have push-button features mounted on the camera head for manual gain control and operation of the videotape recorder. All cases should be video recorded from start to finish, without editing.

Illumination System

Most endoscopists realize the importance of high output light source, preferably xenon arc, and a transmission cord as described in the diagnostic section of the chapter.

Electrosurgical Generators

A standard operating room ESU, such as the Force II (Valleylab, Boulder, CO), should be available to provide 100–200 W of unmodulated (cutting) current and accept a return electrode monitoring pad.

Resectoscope (Lens, Element, and Sheaths)

Selecting a particular resectoscope requires attention to its ergonomic appeal (how it handles, articulates, and disarticulates), its optical characteristics, its durability, and its flow rate. The flow rate will demonstrate not only the effectiveness of the resectoscope in distending the uterus but its ability to clear away debris, bubbles, and blood that collect throughout an operative procedure. A simple test, when selecting or comparing instruments, is to measure its no-load flow rate, a measurement not available from the manufacturer. This number should approximate 1 L/min. The no-load flow rate can be measured by raising the spout of a 3-L bag of LVF 36 inches above the level of the resectoscope inflow port. The inflow port is opened, releasing an LVF into a container or sink under no load. I have tested five different commercially available resectoscopes in the laboratory under a no-load situation. The difference in flow varied from 320 to 960 mL/min, a 300% difference from the worst to the best! The resectoscopes varied from 25F to 30F, and, surprisingly, the larger diameter scopes did not perform best.

The Right Team

Hysteroscopic surgery requires a minimum of four individuals who have established a close working relationship: the surgeon, the anesthesiologist, the scrub nurse, and circulating nurse.

Surgeon

Hysteroscopic EMR is an advanced hysteroscopic procedure. Because there are no clear credentialing guidelines for this procedure, one should consider the surgeon's background, which should, at least, fulfill the AAGL and the ACOG requirements for credentialing in hysteroscopic surgery. This includes a complete didactic and laboratory course in operative hysteroscopy and electrosurgery. Before attempting hysteroscopic EMR, one should have performed at least 50 operative procedures that include endometrial ablation, myomectomies, and polypectomies. A specific understanding of the use of adjuvant agents such as vasopressin and GnRH agonists are imperative. If ultrasound is to be incorporated into hysteroscopic EMR, credentialing of the entire team is essential. Specific training in hysteroscopic EMR should also be considered and should include didactic lectures and a laboratory experience specific for this surgical modality. Proper supervision by an experienced surgeon is imperative. All cases should be reviewed by the supervising physician well in advance of surgery. Finally, the patient should be aware of the training exercise.

In addition to proper training, it is the surgeon's responsibility to clearly understand and define the roles of operating room staff and to be knowledgeable of the intricacies of all operative equipment. After all, the surgeon is not just a "player" but also the "manager" of the team. Additionally, he or she needs to understand the principles of establishing a maximum allowable fluid absorption limit ($MAFA_{limit}$) (see below) and the management of complications related to fluid overload and electrolyte imbalance.

Anesthesiologist or Nurse Anesthetist

The anesthesiologist, in addition to being familiar with the risks and consequences of hysteroscopic surgery, has a variety of other responsibilities in avoiding the complications of hyponatremia, fluid overload, and fatal air emboli:

- Keep fluid administration to a minimum;
- Use normal saline unless some clear contraindication exists;
- Calculate $MAFA_{limit}$ and be aware of fluid absorption throughout the procedure;
- Remain alert to subtle ST-T abnormalities that may develop on electrocardiogram;
- Have a protocol available for treating moderate ($[Na^+]$ 120–130 mmol/L) and severe ($[Na^+]<120$ mmol/L) hyponatremia;
- Avoid placing the patient in Trendelenburg position.

Circulating Nurse

The circulating nurse ascertains the function of all major operative equipment systems. This is done through the use of a master checklist, which is completed for each case. Additionally, he or she carefully maintains I and O (fluid input and output) records, fluid absorption figures, and alerts the operative team to any change in net fluid absorption. Often, the role of the circulating nurse is so demanding that some operating room managers assign two nurses to fulfill the responsibilities of the circulating nurse.

Scrub Nurse

In addition to the usual role of preparing the operative field, the scrub nurse vigilantly observes the operative site, ensuring that all fluid is collected and measured. Frequently, the scrub nurse must alter the use of operative drapes and collection bags so that all effluent can be collected and measured.

The Procedure

Prophylactic Antibiotic

Cefonicid 1 g intravenous Solu-Set (IVSS) intraoperatively will provide adequate antibiotic prophylaxis. Patients who are penicillin allergic should receive doxycycline 100 mg IVSS or gentamicin 80 mg IVSS. Patients with a history of rheumatic heart disease, mitral valve prolapse, artificial heart valves, or septal defects should receive standard rheumatic heart disease prophylaxis.

Establishing the MAFA$_{limit}$

Before beginning any hysteroscopic surgical procedure, the surgical team establishes a MAFA$_{limit}$. This figure is based on the regression analysis of a large number of data points comparing fluid absorption and body mass to serum sodium changes (ΔNa^+). The MAFA$_{limit}$ suggests that a healthy female, without cardiac, liver, or renal disease, may absorb a volume of glycine 1.5% equal to 17.60 mL/kg without experiencing a fall in [Na^+] greater than 10 mmol/L. For instance, a healthy 37-year-old woman weighing 67.3 kg may absorb up to 1,184 mL of glycine 1.5% without concern for symptomatic hyponatremia. Although MAFA has not been analyzed for sorbitol or mannitol, it is still calculated in the same manner.

Once the MAFA$_{limit}$ is established, it is not "renegotiated." In addition, fluid absorption is calculated every 5–10 minutes throughout the procedure. If the MAFA$_{limit}$ is reached before completion of the case, surgery is halted. Because dilutional hyponatremia is a very real risk with the use of nonconductive fluids (glycine 1.5%, sorbitol 3%, and mannitol 5%), a serum sodium is drawn at the start and finish of each case. In the event that net fluid absorption cannot be accurately calculated (e.g., such as when a large amount of liquid is lost in the drapes or on the floor), the procedure should be halted pending the results of a stat serum sodium.

Dilatation

Dilatation can be accomplished by various methods. Townsend (26) recommended the preoperative use of laminaria japonica, a procedure that some older patients find uncomfortable. Adequate dilatation can usually be achieved using standard Hegar dilators. I prefer Hegars because their short dilating surface decreases the risk of a uterine perforation, compared with the longer Pratt dilators. The judicious use of 2- and 3-mm laminaria the day before surgery allows a shorter and less cumbersome operative procedure. One is cautioned, however, that laminaria may not prevent subsequent intraoperative cervical stenosis. Additionally, laminaria occasionally become entrapped, requiring additional manipulation and procedures.

Vasopressin

Vasopressin is routinely injected intracervically before resection. The solution is prepared by diluting 5 units of vasopressin in 40 mL of normal saline. Twenty milliliters of solution is injected at 3 and 9 o'clock, and using a 21-gauge × 1.5-inch needle appears to offer several advantages that are worth considering. First, it causes intense spasm of the myometrial arterioles, allowing one to develop a clinically useful intrauterine pressure without fear of rapid fluid absorption through the myometrial vasculature. Second, this vasospasm decreases intraoperative bleeding and allows excellent visual clarity throughout the procedure. Third, vasopressin appears to diminish operative time and net fluid absorption when compared with control subjects. A study by Phillips et al. (27) even suggests that vasopressin may "soften" the uterine cervix, allowing less forceful dilatation.

Introducing the Resectoscope

It is preferable to avoid the use of obturators in favor of guiding the scope into the uterine cavity under direct vision. An anteflexed uterus requires that the 30° lens be pointed toward the ceiling (light cord "down" on ACMI, Storz, and Olympus models), whereas a retroflexed uterus requires opposite orientation. There are several difficulties that may be encountered at this point in the procedure. The inability to establish a continuous flow may occur in an anatomically normal uterine cavity if the outflow ports become clogged with endometrium, blood, or cervical mucus. There are four other situations that are associated with poor continuous flow: the deeply septated uterus, the small uterine cavity undergoing retreatment, the cavity that contains a large endometrial polyp, and the

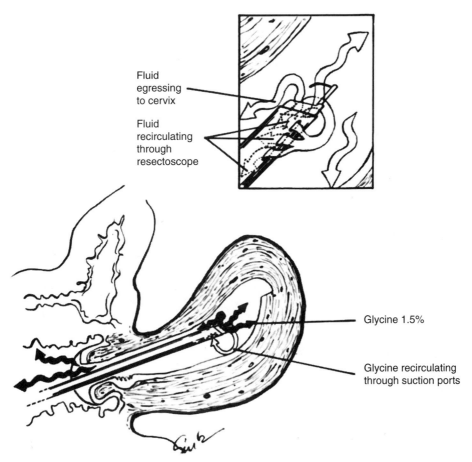

Figure 6.17. Resection of the entire anterior cardinal strip and the endocervical canal. *Dotted line* represents fluid within the resectoscope.

cavity filled with large myomata. In all four of these scenarios, the outflow ports of the resectoscope are likely to become mechanically blocked. This problem is best solved by resecting the anterior or posterior endocervical canal from the internal os to the exocervix, allowing egress to occur from the cervix. In cases demanding a more aggressive approach, the entire anterior cardinal strip (Fig. 6.17) may be resected.

Relative cervical stenosis refers to stenosis that either prevents the introduction of the resectoscope or retards its easy and fluid movement throughout the procedure. Almost all cervical stenosis can be managed in the following manner. If the loop electrode fits into the endocervical canal, it is used to resect the posterior or anterior endocervix just beyond the internal os. This may require a series of two or three sequential (Fig. 6.18) resections, each one resulting in steady progress toward the internal os. In cases of severe cervical stenosis, the loop must be reconfigured before it will slip into the endocervical canal. This is done by bending the entire loop so that it extends obliquely outward (usually 155°) and narrowing the diameter from 8 to 6 mm. In all cases of resection, 100–150 W of pure cutting current is used. In more than 50 endocervical resections, rarely has it been necessary to remove more than the anterior wall. In the limited cases where this has been necessary, the posterior wall has been excised in a similar fashion.

Diagnostic Hysteroscopy

Repeating the diagnostic hysteroscopy is extremely important, especially if the original hysteroscopy was performed with carbon dioxide insufflation. Any "new information" obtained allows one to map out a more appropriate strategy for an individual patient.

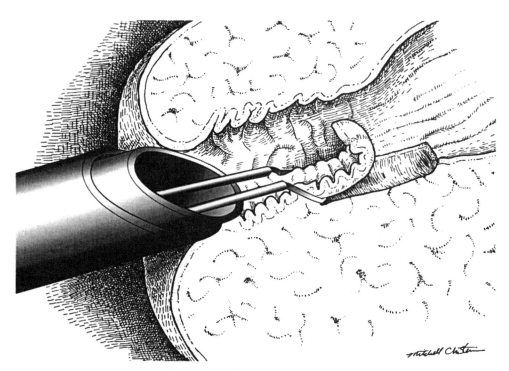

Figure 6.18. Endocervical resection.

CHAPTER 6 / DIAGNOSTIC AND OPERATIVE HYSTEROSCOPY

The Technique of EMR—A Geometrically Sensible Approach

Most cases are performed in power settings that vary from 100 to 150 W of pure cutting current. Blended currents should be avoided because they produce greater tissue "drag." At the power settings noted, the loop electrode easily cuts through the endomyometrium and slides almost effortlessly 5 mm beneath the surface.

EMR begins by extending an 8-mm loop electrode 7–8 mm, as measured by the excursion of the Iglasias working element. The resectoscope is kept in this configuration throughout the entire procedure. Beginning on the anterior uterine wall, using the cervix as a fulcrum, the loop electrode is buried into the endomyometrium to its full 5-mm depth. The entire assembly is moved in unison from the uterine fundus through the endocervical canal. If the cervix needs to be "loosened" or will not allow continuous flow, by egress through it, a 5-mm channel is cut through the endocervical canal. If the cervix is already patulous, the cut can be tapered by slowly bringing the Iglasias working element to its rest position once the internal os has been passed. Next, the posterior wall (Fig. 6.19) is treated in a similar fashion. After completion of these first two steps, the anterior and posterior strips should be separated by a 1-cm thickness of endometrium at the

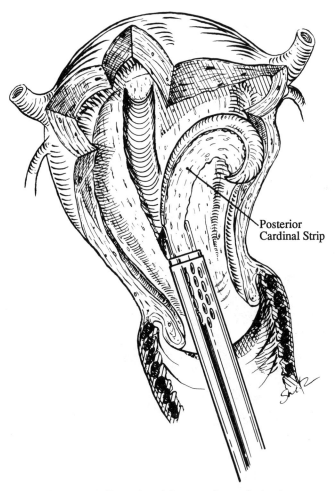

Figure 6.19. Resection of the posterior cardinal strip.

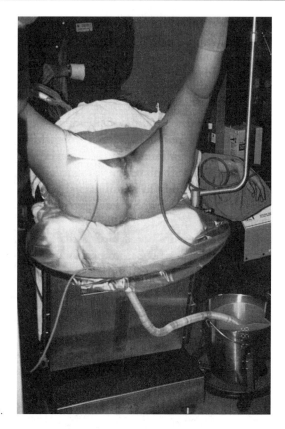

Figure 6.20. Urocatcher drape.

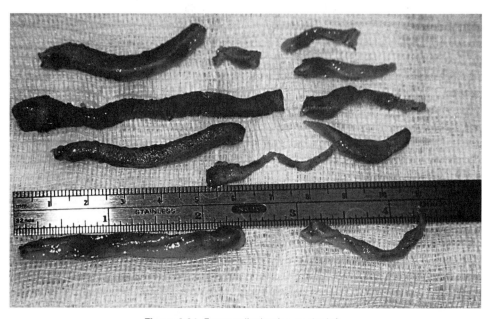

Figure 6.21. Four cardinal strips on the left.

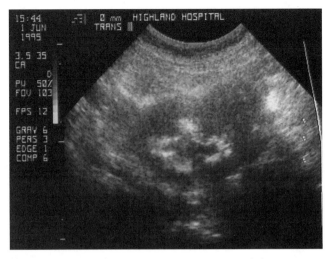

Figure 6.22. Four-leaf clover appearance on panoramic hysteroscopy.

fundus. After removal of the anterior strip, the suction valve is shut, allowing continuous flow to occur by egress from the cervix. All fluid passes through a Urocatcher drape (Fig. 6.20). The lateral walls are dissected starting 5 mm proximal to each tubal ostium. The removal of these four strips of tissue, referred to as the cardinal strips (Fig. 6.21), results in a "four-leaf clover" appearance on panoramic hysteroscopy (Figs. 6.22 and 6.23). The cardinal strips should be 8 mm wide $\times$ 5 mm deep, corresponding to the dimension of the loop electrode, and 6–12 cm in length. The strips are removed by individually trapping them between the resectoscope and the loop electrode. The surgeon is now left with four triangular-shaped pieces of tissue: the anterolateral triangles and posterolateral triangles

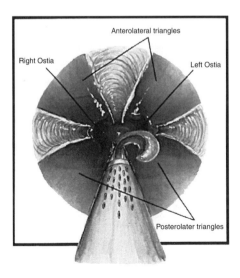

Figure 6.23. Four-leaf clover on ultrasonography.

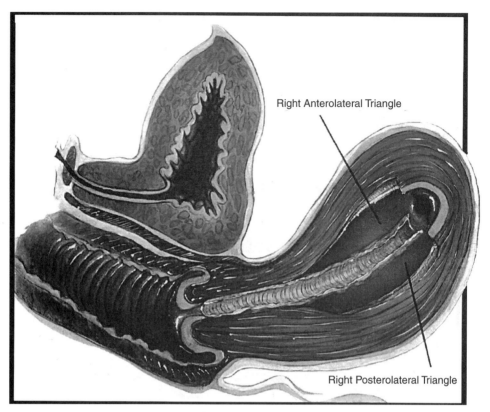

Figure 6.24. Anterolateral and posterolateral triangles.

(Fig. 6.24). These two anterolateral triangles are formed between the anterior cardinal strip and the lateral cardinal strips. Their geometry is the result of ever-shrinking diameters found in transverse sections of the uterus as one progresses from the fundus to the cervix. The posterolateral triangles are formed between the posterior cardinal strip and the two lateral cardinal strips. Each triangle is removed in one to four strips, the number varying with operator experience and the specific geometry of the uterus. Every attempt must be made to avoid successive resections of the same area of the uterus so that only 5 mm is removed throughout the uterus.

After excision of the anterolateral and posterolateral triangles, the uterus will contain endometrium at the top of the fundus and around each tubal ostia. Additionally, there should be a significant amount of "ridge tissue," as demonstrated in Figure 6.25. This tissue must be carefully excised and sculpted to conform to a uniform depth of excision throughout the remainder of the uterine cavity. Only after the ridge tissue is resected should one proceed to the uterine fundus.

The fundus and tubal ostia are excised using a reconfigured loop. A standard 8 × 5 mm electrode is narrowed to 3–4 mm (o.d) and extended so that it forms an oblique angle of 135–160° (Fig. 6.26). This oblique extension of the wire loop electrode allows excision of the tubal ostium to a depth of 2 mm. A novice is well advised to perform this

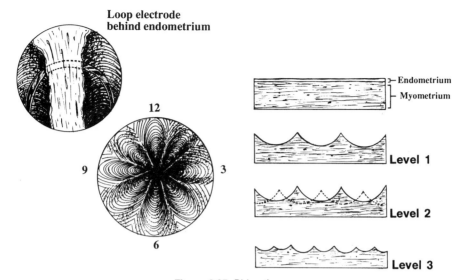

Figure 6.25. Ridge tissue.

excision in stages of 1-mm tissue strips. The loop is then used to sweep transversely across the fundus to remove any remaining endomyometrium to a depth of 3–5 mm.

Once the uterus has been completely denuded of all endomyometrium to a depth of 3–5 mm and at least 2 mm at the uterine cornua, the procedure is complete. The uterine cavity is carefully inspected for any missed strips of endometrium and ridge tissue. Active bleeding may be controlled using the same loop for electrosurgical fulguration. This is accomplished at 100–120 W of coagulation current using a noncontact technique. The tissue specimens are collected (Fig. 6.27), weighed, and sent for histologic analysis.

Postoperative Care

Before the patient is awakened, a serum sodium is drawn. Total I and Os, net fluid absorption, surgical time, power settings, and any intraoperative difficulties are noted. These data are recorded in the nursing notes, the I and O sheets, and in the dictated

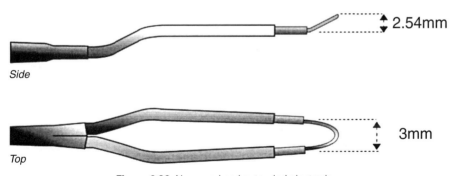

Figure 6.26. Narrowed and extended electrode.

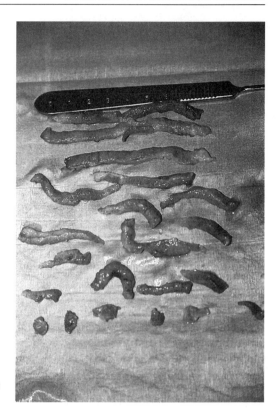

Figure 6.27. The specimen collected for histologic analysis.

operative report. All videotapes are labeled and stored. Patients are given a set of routine postoperative instructions and an appointment for a 2-week office visit.

Other Applications for Endomyometrial Resection

EMR provides at least two other theoretical uses. First, the gynecologist has a method to preoperatively determine the possibility of adenomyosis. This may be accomplished by removing a 5-mm depth of the anterior or posterior cardinal strip. Second, physicians have a technique for accurately sampling the endocervical canal in cases of suspected cervical intraepithelial neoplasm that extends well beyond what can be generally reached with the loop electrosurgical excision procedure (LEEP) technique.

Management and Avoidance of Hysteroscopic Complications

A complete discussion of hysteroscopic surgery must address the complications that can occur and how best to treat and prevent them.

Fluid Overload, Hypoosmolarity, and Hyponatremia

Inattention to net fluid absorption may lead to the most severe complications of hysteroscopic surgery, a cascade of fluid and electrolyte imbalances resulting in hypoosmolarity, hyponatremia, generalized edema, encephalopathy, pontine herniation, and death. Glycine 1.5% (178 mOsm/L) and sorbitol 3% (165 mOsm/L) are both anionic and hypoosmolar compared with human serum (280 mOsmol/L). Excess fluid absorption of these LVFs may be cause dilutional hyponatremia, encephalopathy, fluid overload, and cardiac failure. Additionally, their hypoosmolarity may cause the life-threatening problem of massive generalized tissue edema, pontine herniation, and respiratory center death. Mannitol 5% (280 mOsm/L) is isoosmolar with serum. Although it is anionic and capable of causing significant hyponatremia and generalized edema, its isoosmolarity with human serum make it a more "forgiving" distention medium. Additionally, the diuretic properties of mannitol are an additional benefit to the fluid-overloaded patient. For these reasons, its use has been advocated by several authors, including Dr. Paul Indman.

Avoiding the complication of excess fluid absorption requires a disciplined approach by the entire operating room staff. Strict attention to net fluid absorption must be maintained at all times. I and O measurements should be performed at 5-minute intervals. As the $MAFA_{limit}$ is approached, I and Os should be calculated with the infusion of each liter of fluid. Strict adherence to these rules should virtually eliminate significant hyponatremia or fluid overload. A serum sodium should be drawn after each case. Should the drapes become fluid soaked or large quantities of distention medium suddenly appear on the operating room floor, absorption data should be considered unreliable. The procedure should be immediately halted pending the outcome of serum electrolytes.

Severe hyponatremia (<110 mmol/L) is uncommon and would most likely occur with an inexperienced operating room team, poor attention to I and O records, and long cases requiring large volumes of distention fluid. Arieff and Ayus (28) contend that although men and women are equally prone to develop hyponatremia and resultant encephalopathy, menstruant women are 25 times more likely to die of encephalopathy than men or postmenopausal women who experienced similar serum sodium changes. Importantly, Arieff (29) did report one death after an endometrial ablation that lasted nearly 3 hours and resulted in a serum sodium of 121 mmol/L several hours postoperatively.

With this in mind, one might consider the following policy. With patients of normal renal function whose postoperative serum sodium is 130–140 mmol/L, no treatment is necessary. Restoration of normal serum sodium should occur within 12–24 hours. With patients whose postoperative serum sodium concentration falls between 130 and 120 mmol/L and in whom there is no evidence of encephalopathy, fluid restrictions and furosemide (10–20 mg intravenously) constitute the mainstay of management. Careful I and O records should be kept, and serum sodium should be checked every 4 hours until a level greater than 130 mmol/L is attained. Patients whose serum sodium concentration falls below 120 mmol/L should be treated with hypertonic saline unless there is a clear reason not to do so.

Patients who show clear evidence of encephalopathy (Table 6.3), regardless of their serum sodium concentration, should be treated with hypertonic saline. Before adminis-

Table 6.3
Signs and Symptoms of Hyponatremic Encephalopathy

- Tremulousness
- Dilated pupils
- Decreased oxygen saturation
- Hypothermia
- Grand-mal seizures
- Lethargy
- Clonus

tration of hypertonic saline, furosemide should be administered to prevent circulatory overload. If serum sodium is corrected by 1–2 mmol/L/hr, the risk of central pontine myelinolysis is minimal. The goal should be to correct serum sodium to approximately 130–135 mmol/L but to not exceed 25 mmol/L/24 hr.

The following case study illustrates a problem and resolution. A 42-year-old woman undergoes a hysteroscopic EMR. Her postoperative serum sodium is 112 mmol/L. The patient weighs 100 kg. How should her serum sodium concentration be corrected using a 3% solution of sodium chloride? A 5% solution of sodium chloride?

First, you will need to calculate total body water. Total body water, in most women between 30 and 50 years of age, is approximately 45%. Markedly obese women may have a total body water of 50%. Use the following formula: 100 kg × % body water (0.45) = 45 L total body water.

Second, you will need to determine how many mmol of sodium should be administered per hour. To correct serum sodium from 112 to 130 mmol/L, a total of 1–2 mmol/L/hr or 45 L × 1–2 mmol may be given. If we choose 1.5 mmol/hr, this calculates to 67.5 mmol/hr.

Hypertonic saline is available in 3% (513 mmol/L) and 5% (856 mmol/L). A 3% saline solution would contain 513 mmol/L. A 5% saline solution would contain 856 mmol/L. To infuse 67.5 mmol/hour using a 3% solution, we may calculate the rate of flow set at the infusion pump: desired infusion of sodium in mmol/hr × mL/mmol (desired solution) = desired flow rate of the infusion pump 67.5 mmol/hr × 1,000 mL of 3% sodium solution/513 mmol = 132 mL/hr of 3% sodium solution. To infuse 67.5 mmol using a 5% solution, the infusion pump would need to be determined as follows: 67.5 mmol/hr × 1,000 mL 5% sodium solution/856 mmol = 78.9 mL/hr of 5% saline solution.

Perforation of the Uterus

Perforation can occur with an electrosurgically inactive (or "cold") implement or an active ("hot") electrode. Perforation injuries occur in less than 1% of all hysteroscopic procedures.

An injury with a "cold" or electrosurgically inactive implement may occur during dilatation of the cervix, introduction of the hysteroscope, or during any surgical maneuver that places excessive force against the uterine wall. Such injuries rarely result in a significant secondary injury to the patient. Management involves observation for any signs or symptoms of hemoperitoneum in its early stages. Laparoscopy is rarely indicated in the management of simple traumatic uterine perforation and may expose the patient to the additional risks of a second operation. Most injuries may be prevented by avoiding the use of the longer Pratt or Hank dilators and substituting the shorter Hegar dilator. Additionally, the use of hysteroscopic obturators should be replaced by simple insertion of the resectoscope into the uterine cavity by direct vision. The use of laminaria japonica to accomplish cervical dilation may prevent many injuries that occur as a result of difficult and traumatic cervical dilatation.

Injuries with a "hot" or electrosurgically active electrode present greater concern for life-threatening vascular and visceral injuries to the patient resulting in hemorrhage, sepsis, and death. Fortunately, such injuries are rare and are more likely to occur in the hands of inexperienced surgeons or during the resection of large and complex myomata. Whenever an active electrode perforation is suspected, surgery must be halted immediately.

Management of active electrode perforations is a subject of some debate. Soderstrom (30) stated that immediate laparoscopy or laparotomy should be performed to accomplish meticulous inspection of the bowel and other pelvic contents. Any blanching of tissue should be taken as a sign of thermal injury and should be followed by appropriate resection and repair. The drawback to immediate laparoscopy or laparotomy in a hemodynamically stable patient is that it exposes the patient to the risks of a major operation and may not identify a thermal injury to bowel or bladder in its early stages. Few laparoscopists possess the skill to completely inspect the bowel and identify an area of subtle blanching through the endoscope. A negative laparoscopy immediately after a perforation injury must still be accompanied by clinical vigilance. The patient must be alerted to the signs and symptoms of a bowel perforation that may not develop for a full 2 weeks after surgery. Clinicians are cautioned not to be lulled into a false sense of security in the face of a negative laparoscopy.

Our approach is to observe the patient for any signs of hemodynamic instability. An ultrasound examination should be obtained on the operating room table as a means of following the development of a possible hematoma or hemoperitoneum. In the absence of compelling evidence of hemodynamic instability, the patient should be awakened and allowed to recover in a carefully monitored setting for a period of at least 48 hours. The integrity of the ureters and bladder may be confirmed either by cystoscopy or intravenous pyelography. A Foley catheter is inserted and the patient is followed for the development of fever, hematuria, leukocytosis, abdominal distention, or increasing abdominal pain. Only when the patient has remained quiescent for a period of 48 hours should she be discharged. After hospital discharge, she must be followed carefully for at least 2 full weeks for signs and symptoms of a perforated bowel.

Uterine Rupture

I have observed two cases of uterine rupture with EMR. Uterine rupture occurs with aggressive resection of the myometrium, resulting in an intrauterine hydrostatic pressure that is great enough to overcome the tensile strength of the remaining thin myometrial layer. A rupture may be differentiated from a perforation by the sudden loss of distention pressure that occurs from a defect in the wall of the uterus at some site other than the current operative site. Ruptures are generally small (<1 cm) and may be treated as "cold" perforations as long as the patient is hemodynamically stable. In the two cases, the diagnosis of uterine rupture was made by replaying the surgical videotape and noting that the loss of pressure within the uterine cavity resulted from a defect that occurred at a site remote from the immediate operative site.

Infection

Myometritis is an uncommon complication of hysteroscopic surgery with a variable set of presenting symptoms. At one extreme, patients may present with the rapid onset of fever, chills, and abdominal pain, suggestive of a beta-hemolytic strep. At the other extreme, myometritis may present with subtly increasing bleeding and cramping several weeks postoperatively, accompanied by a low grade fever, leukocytosis, an elevated erythrocyte sedimentation rate, and uterine tenderness. Such patients respond well to antibiotic therapy and may or may not require hospitalization.

Although the benefit of prophylactic antibiotics is unproven in hysteroscopic surgery, common sense would lead one to err on the side of caution on this issue. Some data suggest that vasopressin may also play a role in reducing postoperative infectious morbidity.

Hemorrhage

Intraoperative bleeding during hysteroscopic surgery must be managed by the careful use of vasopressin, coagulation of specific blood vessels, and the judicious management of intrauterine pressure. Rarely, bleeding occurs with such magnitude that tamponade is necessary. In such cases, a Foley catheter is placed into the uterine cavity and filled with 15–30 mL of liquid. After 2 hours, the catheter is removed. The patient may be discharged after an additional hour of observation, providing that bleeding is minimal. Hemorrhage that occurs 1–3 weeks postoperatively could be the presenting sign of an underlying myometritis.

Pregnancy

The pregnancy rate associated with EMR is less than 1%. It is important to explain to all women who have not been sterilized that EMR is not intended as a form of sterilization and that a simultaneous sterilization can be performed at their request.

Hematometra

Hematometra is uncommon in the immediate postoperative phase (first 6 weeks). We have experienced a single case, however, in a woman with preexisting cervical stenosis. The patient presented with increasing abdominal pain and labor-like contractions 2 weeks postoperatively. She had not bled since her second postoperative day. Transvaginal ultrasound examination revealed a large collection within the uterine cavity that was easily evacuated with dilatation and drainage. A large Jackson-Pratt drain was inserted into the uterine cavity, sutured to the cervix, and left in place for 8 weeks. The drain was easily removed by simply cutting the suture. We are currently investigating whether or not routine placement of such drains may have a role in preventing the late development of intrauterine fluid collections.

Results

At the time of this writing, I have performed 255 hysteroscopic EMRs on anatomically normal uteruses, that is, uteruses that contain no fibroids or polyps. The average age of subjects in this series is 39.9 years. Their length of follow up varied from 6 to 66 months. Surgical time averaged 25.5 ± 11.9 minutes and produced a specimen weighing 11.9 ± 5.5 g. Of the women studied, 169 were medically prepared with leuprolide acetate given 1 month before surgery.

One hundred ninety-seven patients were successfully contacted by phone and interviewed by a registered nurse. Of these, 174 (88.4%) reported complete amenorrhea and 16 (8.1%) reported hypomenorrhea, as previously defined by the author. Only six (3.0%) women experienced moderate improvement and one (0.5%) patient experienced no improvement. Ten patients (0.5%) went on to have a second EMR, whereas 5 (2.5%) underwent subsequent hysterectomy.

There have been nine (3.5%) immediate complications in this series outlined in Table 6.4. One patient experienced significant intraoperative bleeding that required uterine

Table 6.4
Immediate Complications of Endomyometrial Resection (n = 255)

	No. of Cases
Uterine rupture	4
Uterine perforation	1
Hyperabsorption	2
Hemorrhage requiring uterine tamponade	1
Inability to complete procedure	1

tamponade with a Foley catheter. She was not transfused but was admitted for overnight observation and did well subsequent to her discharge the following day. There were four uterine ruptures and one uterine perforation. None of these five patients suffered sequelae requiring additional surgery. One patients who suffered a uterine rupture was admitted for observation and discharged the following day. Two additional patients absorbed well beyond their $MAFA_{limit}$. One patient absorbed 1,700 mL in the first 7 minutes of surgery. A laparoscopy failed to reveal a uterine perforation. She was discharged later the same day. A second patient became hyponatremic to 117 mEq/L. She responded well to furosemide, fluid restriction, and observation. She was discharged 8 hours postoperatively with a serum sodium of 134 mEq/L. Finally, one patient with severe cervical stenosis and severe uterine retroversion underwent sonographically guided endocervical resection and EMR. The technical difficulties encountered were so great that her procedure was stopped before it could be completed. She did well postoperatively and reported significant improvement in her menstrual flow.

There were six (2.4%) delayed postoperative complications. One woman presented with a tuboovarian abscess during her seventh postoperative week. She underwent a unilateral salpingoophorectomy and did well. This patient had the only severe complication in this group of patients. There were two cases of confirmed postoperative myometritis and two unproven cases that were treated with antibiotics. Of the two confirmed cases, one presented 2 weeks postoperatively and required hospitalization and intravenous antibiotics. The second case presented on the third postoperative day and involved a woman who had experienced vaginal intercourse after anal intercourse only 24 hours prior. She responded rapidly to oral antibiotics. Finally, one patient in this series developed a pseudomembranous colitis (*Clostridium difficile*) thought to be the result of her prophylactic antibiotics.

ESSENTIALS OF HYSTEROSCOPIC MYOMECTOMY

Patient Presentation

Patients with uterine myomata present to our practice in one of three ways. The first group is comprised of patients with heretofore undiagnosed abnormal uterine bleeding. Some of these patients have a history of severe and acute bleeding that required hospitalization and transfusion. The gynecologist must consider the presence of myomata in the differential diagnosis of near catastrophic (intractable) uterine bleeding. The second group is composed of women who have suffered recurrent pregnancy loss. Finally, the third group constitutes patients with a known "fibroid uterus" and have had hysterectomy offered to them. They present as women seeking a second opinion.

Evaluation of the Patient With Intractable Uterine Bleeding

In a study of 450 patients evaluated for abnormal uterine bleeding, I found that the incidence of submucous fibroids was approximately 20%. Many of these patients had intractable bleeding as well and presented with heavy bleeding that lasted longer than 7 days, required pad changes in the middle of the night (nocturhagia), and led to iron-deficiency anemia that was unresponsive to iron replacement therapy or required hospitalization and blood transfusions. These patients often reported the passage of large clots and moderate to severe dysmenorrhea, although this was an inconsistent finding.

Protocol for Evaluation of Patients With Intractable Uterine Bleeding

The evaluation of patients with intractable uterine bleeding has already been reviewed. Transvaginal ultrasound, sonohysterography, and hysteroscopy will confirm the presence of uterine myomata and clearly differentiate subserous, intramural, and submucous myomata.

Role of Transvaginal Sonography (TVS)

Transvaginal ultrasound should always accompany the physical examination of the patient with abnormal uterine bleeding. Sonography is an inexpensive and noninvasive diagnostic tool that may obviate the need for further testing. For example, the patient with an entirely negative TVS need not undergo sonohysterography or diagnostic hysteroscopy. On the other hand, a patient with a 3-cm calcified fundal myoma, which is clearly intramural and unrelated to the endometrial cavity, needs no further evaluation except for an endometrial sampling. Often, ultrasound will reveal a uterus of such proportion and complexity that serious consideration for minimally invasive surgery cannot be entertained. Conversely, sonography may provide an ambiguous or equivocal clinical picture that requires further clarification. For example, a sonographic image of a centrally located 4-cm uterine fibroid could represent a pedunculated submucous fibroid attached to the fundus by a 1-cm stalk or a submucous fibroid with a large sessile attachment to the fundus, lateral and anterior uterine walls, or a transmural myoma. Further investigation will be necessary to determine the relationship of the fibroid to the endometrial cavity, as well as the extent and location of its attachment.

Role of Sonohysterography

Sonohysterography, or saline infusion sonography (SIS), is especially important in describing a submucous fibroid in terms of the percentage that lies within the endometrial cavity and the location and the size of its attachment point. This procedure, described by Goldstein (31), involves the introduction of a thin, flexible, plastic catheter beyond the internal cervical os. Saline is instilled into the uterine cavity, causing it to distend. The intensely echolucent saline outlines (Fig. 6.28) intrauterine structures such as polyps and fibroids. Additionally, it provides unmatched information regarding the location and extent of the attachment site.

Role of Hysteroscopy

Considering the amount of information available from transvaginal ultrasound and sonohysterography, one may ask, "Why perform hysteroscopy at all?" This question is the

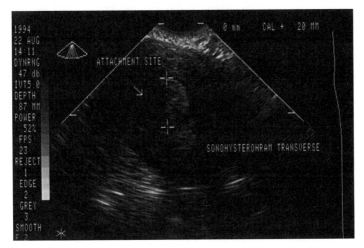

Figure 6.28. Sonohysterogram depicting the fundal attachment site of a small submucous myoma.

subject of active debate. Some would argue that the physician will find no better way of preparing for hysteroscopic myomectomy than by actually visualizing the fibroid to be removed. The supporters of this argument would insist that diagnostic hysteroscopy should be performed to prepare the surgeon by simulating, to the degree possible, the conditions that will exist during actual hysteroscopic myomectomy. However, even the best simulation will result in some intraoperative surprises. The actual size of the fibroid may shrink as a result of several months of pretreatment with a GnRH analogue. The potential space between the fibroid and the endometrial surface may change because uterine distention differs from that noted at the time of the diagnostic procedure. This difference reflects the interplay of general anesthesia, GnRH analogues, increased flow of LVFs through the resectoscope, and the egress of fluid from the cervix. Perhaps a more rational approach would be to reserve diagnostic hysteroscopy for specific indications.

First, whenever confronted with a cavity-filling myoma, diagnosed at the time of sonohysterography, a physician must assess his or her technical ability to meet this challenge. Certain questions must be asked. Will I be able to perform coring, if required? Can I assemble a team for sonographically guided surgery? Would I be better advised to perform a hysterectomy instead?

Second, whenever the physician is faced with an equivocal sonohysterogram, a hysteroscopy must be performed. SIS is easiest to interpret in the presence of a single fibroid. The coexistence of other fibroids, polyps, or a septum will confuse the picture and demand further clarification.

Third, hysteroscopy must be performed whenever SIS does not clearly differentiate the various causes of intrauterine filling defects—myomata, polyps, and retained products of conception. Hysteroscopy is indicated, because subsequent therapy will vary significantly.

Fourth, when there is a history of previous surgery to the cervix (cryosurgery, LEEP, laser conization, repair of an obstetric injury), hysteroscopy should be performed in an attempt to evaluate whether or not the cervix will permit the access to and retrieval of the uterine fibroid.

Evaluation of Recurrent Pregnancy Loss

The medical evaluation of recurrent pregnancy loss is beyond the scope of this book. Patients may present with a history of recurrent spontaneous pregnancy losses or with known intrauterine lesions discovered at the time of sonography, hysterosalpingography, or even hysteroscopy. It is important to remember that most recurrent pregnancy losses are not the result of uterine myomata. Careful attention must be paid to other possible causes before hysteroscopic surgery is undertaken. Additionally, when counseling the patient about to undergo hysteroscopic surgery for recurrent pregnancy loss, it is imperative that she understand that the sequelae of such surgery may include infertility, abnormal placentation, and uterine rupture. The latter has been reported after hysteroscopic myomectomy and resulted in fetal and maternal demise.

Patients with Known Fibroids

Patients with known fibroids often present seeking a second opinion. With few exceptions, the first opinion they received suggested hysterectomy as permanent therapy for their problem. Frequently, their first opinion was well thought out. It is wisest to approach such patients as if one were meeting her for the very first time—without the bias of knowing the name of the original physician or his or her opinion. Whenever possible, insist on looking at the medical record after your initial evaluation. Avoid asking the patient what recommendations have been made to her. Explain to her that avoiding such bias is essential in offering her the very best second opinion.

Patient Selection

Perhaps one of the most difficult challenges that faces the hysteroscopic surgeon is knowing which patients may benefit from hysteroscopic surgery and which will not. Hysteroscopic surgery, to be truly minimally invasive, must not only be associated with acceptable risks and consequences but must also have an acceptably low rate of reoperation. One cannot justify hysteroscopic myomectomy on a 41-year-old woman who has completed her childbearing if there is a 50% likelihood that she will develop a recurrence that might require a hysterectomy within the next 5 years. In such cases, hysteroscopic myomectomy would only serve in delaying an inevitable hysterectomy. Proper patient selection, however, can minimize the likelihood of subsequent surgery. Factors to consider when selecting patients include the following.

Degree of Intramural Extension

Wamstecker et al. (23) instituted a classification system to categorize the degree of intramural extension for submucous fibroids. Pedunculated submucous myomas without intramural extension are classified as type 0. When the submucous fibroid is sessile and the intramural part is less than 50%, the fibroid is classified as type I; with an intramural extension of 50% or more, the fibroid is classified as type II. When more than one fibroid exists, patients are classified according to the fibroid with the greatest intramural extension. Wamstecker et al. showed that the degree of intramural extension is related to the likelihood that multiple procedures will be required to achieve complete resection. Interestingly, the fibroid type (0, I, or II) is less predictive in achieving control of uterine bleeding than whether or not complete resection is achieved. The message here is simple. Choose patients in whom the likelihood of complete resection is greatest. It is wisest in inexperienced hands to avoid transcervical resection of submucous myomas with more than 50% intramural extension because complete resection often necessitates repeat procedures.

Classification of Attachment by Anatomic Site

All other factors being equal, I prefer to avoid resection of fibroids that are attached to the lateral uterine walls and cornual regions of the uterus. These represent the regions of the uterus with the most abundant vascular supply.

Myoma Size and Volume

Most simple fibroids are spherical in shape. It is important to recognize that the volume of a sphere is expressed by the formula $V = 4/3\Pi r^3$. Therefore, the change in volume from a myoma with a 3-cm diameter to a 6-cm diameter can be summarized as a ratio of the radius of each myoma to the power of 3: $\Delta \text{Volume} = 3^3/1.5^3 = 27/3.37 = 8.01$-fold increase in volume. Therefore, merely doubling the diameter of the fibroid resulted in an eightfold increase in volume. For this reason, many gynecologists would consider it imprudent to remove any myoma larger diameter than 4–5 cm.

Multiple Myomata

Most hysteroscopists would agree that the requirement for multiple myomectomies correlates poorly with successful hysteroscopic surgery.

Patient Age

All other factors being equal, better outcomes are directly related to the age of the patient. Patients under the age of 35, at the time of their initial myomectomy, are more likely to require subsequent myomectomy or hysterectomy. Patients over the age of 45 tend to have fewer repeat procedures. In general, the older the patient, as long as she is in good health, the more aggressive one can be in offering her hysteroscopic myomectomy as an alternative to hysterectomy.

Desire for Future Childbearing

Again, all other factors being equal, the woman who has not yet completed her family may warrant hysteroscopic myomectomies that would be deemed less appropriate if the same woman were no longer interested in having children. However, it bears reminding that offering someone hysteroscopic surgery that may result in infertility, abnormal placentation, uterine rupture, and even death requires careful consultation with the patient, her husband, and other important family members.

Patient Weight

Because the $\text{MAFA}_{\text{limit}}$ is directly related to body weight, it is reasonable to assume that, all things being equal, the patient who weighs 200 pounds will be able to tolerate a net fluid absorption (17.6 mL/kg) twice that of a patient weighing 100 pounds. The combination of a large grade 1 myoma in a thin 45-kg woman should alert the gynecologist to plan for either a two-stage procedure or a nonhysteroscopic approach to the patient's problem.

Planning the Operation

In planning to perform complex hysteroscopic surgery, a variety of issues needs to be addressed. In all cases, the physician must focus on two questions: What can be done to make surgery technically easier? What can be done to make it safer?

Medical Pretreatment

The use of a GnRH agonist is extremely useful in converting an otherwise difficult procedure to a relatively simple one. I prefer the use of depot-leuprolide acetate 3.75 mg intramuscularly for 3–4 months before surgery for a single myoma greater than 3 cm in diameter. The effect is not limited to reducing the volume of the fibroid but appears to devascularize the myoma itself, resulting in diminished intraoperative bleeding, improved visual clarity throughout the procedure, and diminished operative time.

Laminaria Tents

The removal of larger myomata is associated with multiple insertions and removals of the resectoscope as individual tissue fragments are excised. Additionally, myomectomy often calls for the introduction of a variety of grasping forceps to dislodge and retrieve large tissue fragments. Because many forceps range from 10 to 14 mm in diameter, cervical dilatation is absolutely essential for the removal of larger myomas. I prefer the insertion of a single 2- or 3-mm laminaria tent the afternoon before surgery.

Vasopressin

The role of vasopressin has already been discussed during hysteroscopic EMR where it is administered as an intracervical injection. During hysteroscopic myomectomy, however, vasopressin may be administered directly into the myoma by injection through an operative port on a continuous flow operative hysteroscope (*not* a resectoscope). I prefer the use of a 30-cm injection needle that tapers to a 23-gauge tip (Reznick Instrument Co., Skokie, IL). In preparation for its administration, a solution of vasopressin is prepared by diluting 10 units in 100 mL of saline. Forty milliliters is used as an intracervical injection. The remaining 60 mL is available for injection directly into the myoma. This is especially useful in the resection of fibroids with a very pronounced superficial vasculature.

Sonographic Guidance

Laparoscopy, an invasive diagnostic technique, has been used by various authors as a method of "control" for cases involving aggressive hysteroscopic myomectomy. Laparoscopy has many pitfalls as a means of hysteroscopic control. It is important to recognized that laparoscopy does not prevent uterine perforations, it merely diagnoses them. Laparoscopy cannot distinguish whether or not an electrode is within 5 or 15 mm of the uterine serosal. Additionally, laparoscopy offers little, if any, guidance on the posterior uterine surface where uterine perforation may result in direct rectal injury. Finally, lapa-

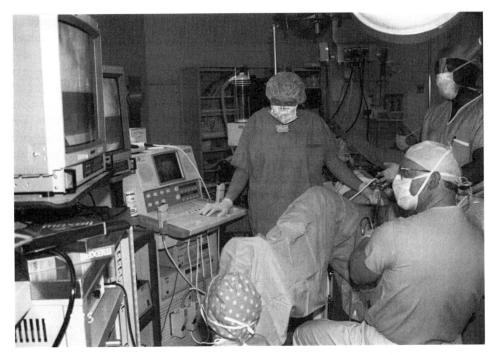

Figure 6.29. Operating room setup for sonographically controlled hysteroscopic myomectomy.

roscopy is an additional operative technique that has the potential to cause injury and also increases the recovery period necessary for hysteroscopic myomectomy. Operative control, using real-time abdominal ultrasound (Fig. 6.29) by an experienced sonographer, will prove invaluable in preventing uterine perforation and aid in such techniques as myoma coring (see below). I insist on sonographic guidance whenever the resection of a type I or a type II fibroid is anticipated.

Two-Stage Procedure

Patients with large or multiple myomata should be cautioned that if the myomectomy cannot be accomplished before the $MAFA_{limit}$ has been reached, it will be halted and completed in a second procedure. The patient will have the option of returning for another procedure at a later date if she is dissatisfied with the outcome of her initial procedure. Planning for a two-stage procedure removes much of the pressure on the gynecologist that can be brought to bear in an operating room environment.

Simultaneous EMR

There is little clinical data available to address the issue of whether women who have completed childbearing and are planning to undergo hysteroscopic myomectomy should be offered simultaneous EMR or some other endometrial ablation technique. In some instances, it would appear neglectful not to offer such a procedure. For instance, consider the healthy 45-year-old mother of five with a large uterine cavity (sounds to 10 cm) containing a pedunculated 2-cm myoma that presents with severe menorrhagia and anemia. One might argue that her menorrhagia may be a function of the large surface area available for endometrial sloughing rather than this small fibroid. It would seem prudent, in this situation, to offer the patient an EMR along with a myomectomy.

By contrast, consider the 40-year-old woman with a history of diabetes, hypertension, ischemic heart disease, and menorrhagia. Her evaluation reveals a solitary 3-cm pedunculated myoma occupying most of her uterine cavity. She would clearly benefit from the safe and quick removal of this fibroid without exposing her to even the slightest additional risk that may occur with simultaneous EMR. Most patients fall somewhere between these extremes. Whether or not to offer a simultaneous endometrial destruction or resection technique will require a thoughtful and honest discussion with your patient as you guide her in assessing the risks and benefits of the contemplated procedure.

Operating Room Setup: Special Considerations for Hysteroscopic Myomectomy

The operating room setup for hysteroscopic myomectomies is identical to that described under EMR (see above). Several important considerations include ultrasound, a continuous flow operative hysteroscope with an injection needle, attention to the greater power settings that may be required for myomectomy, and attention to various hysteroscopic electrodes.

Ultrasound

For cases requiring ultrasound guidance (Fig. 6.29), it is important for the surgeon to have an unobstructed view of the ultrasound screen. Ideally, the sonographer would also have a screen allowing him or her to view the hysteroscopic surgery as well.

After induction of anesthesia, appropriately selected patients undergo a transvaginal examination using a multifrequency vaginal probe (5.5–7.5 MHZ). Fibroids are carefully noted as to their location, size, and relationship to the endometrial cavity. Additionally, measurements are taken of the surrounding myometrium. After this initial examination, a Foley catheter is inserted into the bladder. Sterile saline is infused into the bladder (300–500 mL) so that an anterior acoustic window is clearly evident. Occasionally, when greater clarity of the posterior wall is necessary, a posterior acoustic window may be created by the infusion of 300–500 mL of saline through the cul-de-sac. This may be especially important as the gynecologist and sonographer become accustomed to working together. Although the gynecologist is familiar with the operating room environment, he or she must bear in mind that this is new territory to the sonographer. The creation of acoustic windows often enhances visualization of the uterus and its contents, making the sonographer's vital work somewhat easier. Bear in mind that the sonographer's role is indispensable to the successful outcome of sonographically guided procedures. The sonographer may guide the surgeon away from a possible perforation injury while assisting the surgeon to maintain orientation. Additionally, the sonographer may act as the surgeon's eyes whenever myoma forceps are blindly introduced into the uterine cavity. Real-time ultrasound is an indispensable tool to the hysteroscopist. By developing a close working relationship between the sonographer and the surgeon, a true partnership is formed that benefits the patient by providing a safer and more complete excisional technique.

Operative Hysteroscope

It is helpful, as already noted, to have the ability to introduce vasopressin directly into the fibroid or its stalk. All the major commercial producers of gynecologic resectoscopes also produce continuous flow operative hysteroscopes. These hysteroscopes do not have a "working element" to which a loop electrode is attached. Instead, they have one or more operating channels that allow the introduction of semirigid instruments, laser fibers, catheters for tubal cannulation, or injection needles. I prefer the use of a 30-cm long injection needle (Reznick Instrument Co.). This 23-gauge needle can be introduced directly into the body of the fibroid or its vascular supply.

Electrosurgical Unit

The ESUs found in most operating rooms will produce sufficient power density for the safe resection of a fibroid. Pure cutting current is used, without blending, in settings ranging from 100 to 250 W. Because of the high tissue density of some fibroids, the hysteroscopist may use power settings in excess of 150 W of pure cutting current to effect smooth electrosurgical cutting. The resultant power densities often frighten the novice hysteroscopist and the unfamiliar operating room staff. I have witnessed, operating in many different operating rooms across the northeastern United States, many circulating nurses set an ESU for 200 W of cutting current with the degree of caution familiar only to those who would arm a small nuclear weapon. Most operating room ESUs provide up to 360 W of cutting current, yet most surgeons and operating room personnel have never explored the upper end of the electrosurgical envelope available to them.

For physicians who prefer the use of vaporizing electrodes, settings of 200–250 W of cutting current are not uncommon. Coagulating current is rarely used and is reserved for bleeding that can be controlled with a noncontact fulguration technique. It is important that ESUs are equipped with return electrode monitoring pads. The latter should be applied to clean dry skin.

Specialized Electrodes

A variety of hysteroscopic electrodes must be available to the gynecologists. I prefer standard 8 × 5 mm cutting electrodes with varying angles. Standard cutting electrodes used for the myoma shaving technique vary from 55 to 77°. The myoma resection technique generally uses a 160° electrode, whereas the coring technique is performed with either a 160 or 180° electrode. Other authors prefer the use of vaporizing electrodes. These grooved-barrel electrodes operate under power settings of 200–300 W of cutting current and provide excellent vaporization of tissue. Their disadvantage lies in the fact that no tissue specimen is obtained.

Techniques of Hysteroscopic Myomectomy

Myoma Shaving Technique

The myoma shaving technique (Fig. 6.30) is accomplished when the loop electrode is extended behind a portion of the myoma. Upon initiation of pure cutting current, the loop is drawn toward the operator while the hysteroscope lens remains fixed at some spot proximal to the fibroid. This technique produces small "chips" of tissue that should be individually removed, allowing the surgeon to maintain clear orientation at all times. The technique is very safe and has been performed by numerous authors. Its disadvantage lies in the fact that it is slow and time consuming, making the removal of larger fibroids (>3 cm) a tedious process that may expose the patient to the risk of excessive fluid absorption.

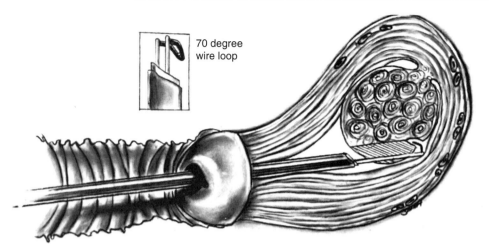

Figure 6.30. Myoma "shaving" technique with 70° wire loop. *Hatch marks*, resected area.

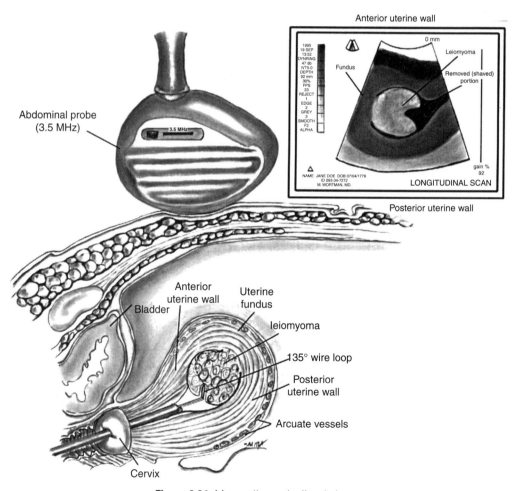

Figure 6.31. Myoma "resection" technique.

CHAPTER 6 / DIAGNOSTIC AND OPERATIVE HYSTEROSCOPY

Remember that in the myoma shaving technique, the endoscope remains fixed while the loop moves from behind the myoma toward the operator.

Myoma Resection Technique

The next technique, in order of complexity, is the myoma resection technique (Fig. 6.31). This technique allows the removal of long strips of myoma and is similar to the technique described for EMR. The electrode used for this technique may vary from 55 to 160°. What distinguishes this technique from the shaving technique is that the electrode is

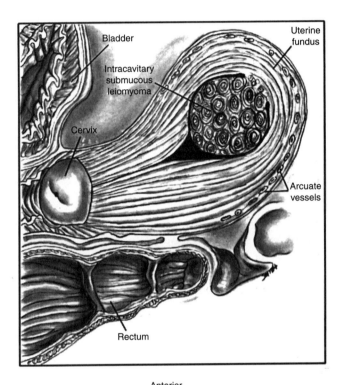

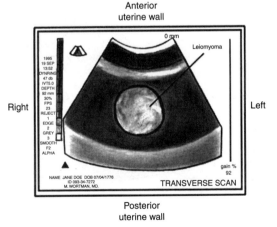

Figure 6.32. Uterus with cavity-filling submucous leiomyoma.

extended to a fixed distance, usually 8–10 mm, while the entire resectoscope assembly moves across the surface of the myoma. This produces long strips of tissue measuring 8 mm wide, 5 mm deep, and 5–6 mm long. This technique allows larger submucous myomata to be removed in long continuous strips, which are removed individually by trapping them between the loop electrode and the distal resectoscope. The major advantages of this technique lies in the efficiency in which larger strips of tissue may be excised.

Myoma Coring Technique

This is used exclusively for cavity-filling myomas (Fig. 6.32) that prohibit the placement of the resectoscope or electrosurgical loop around or behind the fibroid. The myoma surface is infiltrated with dilute vasopressin solution using an operative hysteroscope with a 23-gauge injection needle. A 160–180° loop, guided by ultrasound, is first directed either anteriorly or posteriorly through the myoma surface to a depth of at least 1–2 cm. Next, the loop is swung in the opposite direction using the cervix as a fulcrum (Fig. 6.33). Finally, the loop is withdrawn, producing a loosened core of tissue. Once the core has been excised, a standard resectoscope is used to further excise the myoma core, proceeding from the medial surface of the core to the lateral, anterior, and posterior surfaces of the myoma. After the central core has collapsed, the myoma resection and shaving techniques may be used to remove the remaining fibroid tissue.

ACKNOWLEDGMENTS

I am indebted to many individuals who supplied technical information, patience, encouragement, and wisdom in the preparation of this manuscript. I owe a special thanks to Wayne Kunkel, Margaret Paz-Paltrow, and Eric Paltrow of Karl Storz Endoscopy, USA. They provided much of the technical and historical data that went into the preparation of this manuscript. I thank Robert Quint, Peter Boehlert, and Michael Kesselring

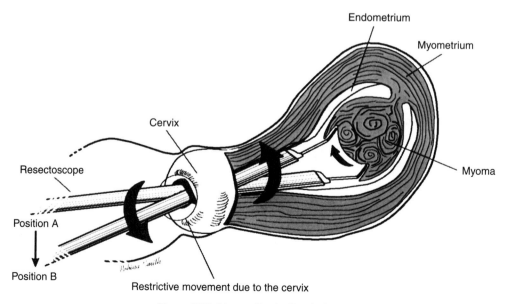

Figure 6.33. Myoma "coring" technique.

from Circon ACMI. Their friendship and guidance have been invaluable. Robina Smith, the medical illustrator who has worked with me for many years, has produced her finest work yet. Amy Daggett-Norton, with whom I have enjoyed 10 wonderful years, has inspired many of the thoughts, techniques, and refinements that are presented in this chapter. Finally, I must thank Deborah McKenzie Bristol. Without her perseverance, gentle smile, and the crack of her whip, this chapter might not ever have been completed.

REFERENCES

1. Fourestier M, Gladu A, Vulimiere J. Perfectionments de l'endoscope medicale. Presse Med 1952; 60:1292.
2. Schroeder C. Uber den Ausbau und die Leistungen der Hysteroskopie. Arch Gynaekol 1934;156:407.
3. Asherman JG. Traumatic intrauterine adhesions. J Obstet Gynaecol Br Emp 1950;57:879.
4. Hepp H, Roll H. Die hysteroskopie gynecologie. 1974;7:166.
5. Hamou J, Taylor PJ. Panoramic, contact and microcolpohysteroscopy in gynecologic practice. J Reprod Med 1983;28:359–388.
6. Inglesias JJ, Sporer A, Gellman AC. New Inglesias resectoscope with continuous irrigation, simultaneous suction and low intra-vesicle pressures. J Urol 1975;114:929.
7. Neuwirth RS, Amin HS. Excision of submucous fibroids with hysteroscopic control. Am J Obstet Gynecol 1976;126:95–99.
8. Goldrath MH, Fuller TA, Segal S. Laser photovaporization of endometrium for the treatment of menorrhagia. Am J Obstet Gynecol 1981;140:14.
9. DeCherney AH, Polan ML. Hysteroscopic management of intrauterine lesions and intractable uterine bleeding. Obstet Gynecol 1983;61:392–397.
10. Lin BL. Transcervical resection (TCR) and endometrial ablation (EA). Jpn J Gynecol Obstet Endosc 1988;4:56–61.
11. Cheslyn-Curtis S, Hopkins HH. The Hopkins rod-lens system. In: Arregui ME, Fitzgibbons RJ, Katkhouda N, McKernan JB, Reich H, eds. Principles of laparoscopic surgery. New York: Springer-Verlag, 1995.
12. Hopkins HH. Optical principles of the endoscope. In: Berci G, ed. Endoscopy. New York: Appleton-Century-Crofts, 1976.
13. Droegmueller W. Cryosurgery in patients with dysfunctional uterine bleeding. Obstet Gynecol 1971:32; 256–258.
14. Zaproprazahn V. Endometrial ablation using a cryosurgical probe. Presented at the 20th Annual Meeting of the American Association of Gynecologic Laparoscopists, 1991.
15. Vancaillie TG. Electrocoagulation of the endometrium with the ball-end resectoscope. Obstet Gynecol 1989;74:425.
16. Onbargi LC, Hayden R, Valle RF, Del Priore G. Effects of power and electrical current density variations in an in vitro endometrial ablation model. Obstet Gynecol 1993;82:912–918.
17. Magos AL, Baumann R, Turnbull AC. Transcervical resection of endometrium in women with menorrhagia. Br Med J 1989;298:1209–1212.
18. Neuwirth RS. Hysteroscopic management of symptomatic uterine fibroids. Obstet Gynecol 1983; 62:509–512.
19. Hallez JP. Single-stage total hysteroscopic myomectomies: indications, techniques and results. Fertil Steril 1995;63:703–708.
20. Goldrath MH. Vaginal removal of the pedunculated submucous myomata. Historical observations and development of a new procedure. J Reprod Med 1990;35:921–924.
21. Wortman M, Daggett A. Hysteroscopic myomectomy. J Am Gynecol Laparosc 1995;3:39–46.
22. Lin BL, Iwata Y, Liu KH. Removing a large submucous fibroid with the two-resectoscope method. J Am Assoc Gynecol Laparosc 1994;1:259–263.
23. Wamstecker K, Emanuel MH, deKruif JH. Transcervical hysteroscopic resection of submucous fibroids for abnormal uterine bleeding: results regarding degree of intramural extension. Obstet Gynecol 1993; 82:736–740.

24. Corson SL, Brooks PG. Resectoscopic myomectomy. Fertil Steril 1991;55:1041–1044.
25. Goldrath MH. Hysteroscopic laser ablation of the endometrium. Obstet Gynecol Forum 1990;4:2–13.
26. Townsend DE. Resectoscope in gynecologic surgery. The Female Patient 1990;15:14–16.
27. Phillips D, Nathanson HG, Meltzer SM, et al. Trancervical electrosurgical resection of submucous leiomyomas for chronic menorrhagia. J Am Assoc Gynecol Laparosc 1995;2:147–153.
28. Arieff AI, Ayus JC. Endometrial ablation complicated by fatal hyponatremic encephalopathy. JAMA 1993;270:1230–1232.
29. Arieff AI. Hyponatremia, convulsions, respiratory arrest, and permanent brain damage after elective surgery in healthy women. N Engl J Med 1986;314:1529.
30. Soderstrom RM. Bowel injury litigation after laparoscopy. J Am Assoc Gynecol Laparosc 1993;1:74.

APPENDIX

Credentialing in Hysteroscopy and Hysteroscopic Surgery: the Center for Menstrual Disorders and Reproductive Choice

Credentialing for any endoscopic procedure that the physician has never performed requires three learning phases.

Phase I: Didactic With or Without Laboratory

The first phase involves an appropriate amount of didactic learning sessions geared to the theory and practical aspects of the technique(s) to be learned. Wherever possible, if appropriate laboratory models do exist, they should be used to facilitate the learning process.

Phase II: Observation

During this phase, the student should observe a qualified surgeon for a minimum of two to three cases. During this period, the student will have an opportunity to ask questions regarding the technical aspects of the surgical technique and those areas that concern patient selection, complication avoidance, and management.

Phase III: Supervised Cases

During the third phase, the student selects at least two cases that have been reviewed by the preceptor. The patient should be informed (in writing) of the student–preceptor relationship. It should be clear that the preceptor assumes medical, ethical, and some legal responsibility for the appropriateness of patient selection, intraoperative management, and management of immediate postoperative complications. The preceptor should also be available for consultation and management of late postoperative complications. During the supervised cases, the student should demonstrate satisfactory knowledge of electrosurgery or laser (as applicable) principles and instrument assembly and disassembly. In addition, the student should have demonstrated satisfactory knowledge of the video system to be used, as well as the use of distention medium and systems. The student should be able to demonstrate knowledge in the area of systems failure and should be able to adequately manage intraoperative and postoperative complications.

Credentialing

The AAGL "Operative Endoscopy Guidelines" represent, at this time, the only statement by a major organized body in gynecologic surgery. These guidelines are rigorous and require a commitment from both the student and the preceptor. They clearly represent what is in the best interest of the profession and what is in the best interest of the patient.

After completing the credentialing process, the student should expect a letter of recommendation from his or her department chairperson attesting to the qualifications of the student to perform hysteroscopic surgery.

As of this writing, the Accreditation Council for Gynecologic Endoscopy (ACGE), an arm of the AAGL, is accepting applications for both hysteroscopic and laparoscopic credentialing. The importance of this council cannot be overstated. It would be prudent for physicians interested in obtaining credentialing through the organization to keep abreast of their latest requirements. Information regarding the AAGL or the ACGE can be obtained directly from The American Association of Gynecologic Laparoscopists,

13021 East Florence Avenue, Santa Fe Springs, CA 90670–4505. Telephone 1–800–554–2245.

American Association of Gynecologic Laparoscopists Operative Endoscopy Guidelines

The AAGL Board of Trustees formally adopted these guidelines at their 20th annual meeting on November 13–17, 1991 at the Sahara Hotel and Casino, Las Vegas, Nevada:

1. Each applicant must be a member in good standing of the Department of Ob/Gyn or Surgery of the institution providing the facilities.
2. Each surgeon must be qualified in diagnostic laparoscopy/hysteroscopy and laparotomy is a prerequisite.
3. Each surgeon must demonstrate evidence of satisfactory training in *each* area of operative endoscopy of which privileges are requested. The hospital may wish to consider the following special techniques: operative laparoscopy (pelviscopy), CO_2 laser, YAG laser, argon/KTP laser, operative hysteroscopy, YAG ablation, electrosurgical ablation, and hysteroscopic resectoscope. Training should include didactic sessions of 10–14 hours that cover the theory and review instruments and safety factors. After didactic training, a "hands-on" laboratory must be incorporated with each participant having at least 2 hours of actual experience. Tissue models should be used.
4. After appropriate training experience, each surgeon should be supervised in the use of these techniques. The supervisor should make recommendations to the department in writing. Between 5 and 10 cases should be documented before competence can be certified for operating alone.
5. Official training during residency with a letter of certification of competence can also act as evidence of training for credentialing.
6. "Grandparenting" in operative endoscopy should be considered if a surgeon is able to document an adequate number of cases in the past year of procedures performed using the appropriate technique (i.e., five cases each of operative hysteroscopy, operative laparoscopy, or of each laser type).
7. If no surgeons on the hospital staff have been credentialed to act as preceptor/supervisors, then two surgeons who have documented adequate hands-on and didactic training must operate together on at least the first 10 cases performed.

Guidelines for Attaining Privileges in Gynecologic Operative Endoscopy (From the Society of Reproductive Surgeons, The American Fertility Society, Birmingham, Alabama)

These guidelines presuppose the following:

1. The applicant is eligible or certified by the American Board of Obstetrics and Gynecology and is a member in good standing in the Department of Obstetrics and Gynecology of the hospital or institution to which the application is being directed.
2. The applicant has been granted privileges or is eligible for privileges to perform diagnostic laparoscopy, laparoscopic tubal sterilization, and/or diagnostic hysteroscopy and has demonstrated competence in these techniques.
3. Privileges will be granted for laparoscopic and hysteroscopic skill levels as outlined above.

The following guidelines are suggested for institutions that grant privileges for gynecologic operative endoscopy.

1. The applicant will request privileges for the use of a specific endoscope (e.g., laparoscope, hysteroscope, or resectoscope), a specific energy source or modality (e.g., electrosurgery, specific wave length laser, or harmonic scalpel), or a designated laparoscopic or hysteroscopic skill level (see above).
2. For each requested privilege, the applicant must submit evidence of the satisfactory completion of the following:
   A. A recognized (Continuing Medical Education accredited) formal didactic course(s) of at least 16 hours duration, which includes a least 4 hours of a supervised laboratory experience. In addition to a pelvic trainer, laparoscopic, or hysteroscopic models, the use of live animal models may be appropriate to gain necessary skills.
   B. Viewing of and/or assistance in several endoscopic operations at the designated clinical skill level.
   C. A preceptorship with a physician who is credentialed to perform the procedures designated at a particular skill level. The preceptor should be recognized in the community-at-large or nationally as someone who possesses the necessary experience and skills to function as a tutor and preceptor. The preceptorship experience should consist of tutoring both as the first assistant and as the principal surgeon. The hospital should provide an appropriate record-keeping system for the credentialing process and the preceptor should verify that the tutorial experience took place. The applicant should provide a case list that should include:
   - Patient's name, medical record number, and date of surgery;
   - Preoperative and postoperative diagnosis;
   - Endoscopic surgical procedure performed;
   - Type of endoscope used;
   - Energy modality used;
   - Outcome and complications of the procedure;
   - The preceptor should provide a letter stating the applicant has performed the requested procedures in a satisfactory and competent fashion.

   It is recommended that at least 5 and preferably 10 procedures be performed satisfactorily under supervision at each skill level before privileges in full are granted.
3. A periodic review of newly granted privileges to individual surgeons should be performed by the parent institution at annual or biannual intervals. Each credentialed physician should provide to the hospital credentialing committee a case list of endoscopic procedures performed and complications encountered during the time interval to be reviewed. Recertification will require demonstration of continuing performance of endoscopic procedures with an acceptable rate of complications.
4. A letter from the director of an approved residency training program can take the place of 2A–C if the required training criteria have been fulfilled during residency.
5. If there are no surgeons on the staff of the parent institution who can act as preceptors, then supervised preceptorships can be arranged by scheduling a number of appropriate cases in conjunction with other interested surgeons and inviting a visiting expert as an appropriate consultant to serve as the preceptor.
6. Any surgeon already performing procedures for which privileges are being requested at the time the credentialing process is initiated will be required to submit a summary of his or her training and practical experience for each endoscopic skill level. In addition, the surgeon will submit to the Chairman of the Credentialing Committee a case list for the past year that contains the same information as in 2C. The committee may grant privileges without completion of all the criteria stated in 2C.
   - Minor adhesiolysis;
   - Partial salpingectomy for ectopic pregnancy;
   - Linear salpingostomy for ectopic pregnancy;
   - Endoscopic surgery for the American Fertility Society (AFS) stage I and II endometriosis.

Procedures requiring additional training (level II):
- Laparoscopic division of uterosacral ligaments;
- Adhesiolysis for moderate and severe adhesion or adhesions involving bowel;
- Laser or diathermy drilling to ovaries for polycystic ovarian syndrome;
- Neosalpingostomy for hydrosalpinx;
- Salpingectomy or salpingo-oophorectomy;
- Endoscopic management of endometrioma and ovarian cystectomy;
- Laparoscopically assisted vaginal hysterectomy;
- Endoscopic surgery for AFS stage III and IV endometriosis;
- Appendectomy.

Procedures requiring significant additional training (level III):
- Pelvic lymphadenectomy;
- Extensive pelvic side wall dissection;
- Presacral neurectomy;
- Dissection of an obliterated pouch of Douglas;
- Bowel surgery;
- Retropubic bladder neck suspension;
- Hernia repair;
- Ureteral dissection.

Stratification of Laparoscopic Procedures

Procedures not requiring additional training (level I):

- Laparoscopic sterilization;
- Needle aspiration of simple cysts;
- Ovarian biopsy.

Stratification of Hysteroscopic Procedures

Procedures not requiring additional training (level I):

- Diagnostic hysteroscopy.

Procedures requiring additional training (level II):

- Endometrial resection or ablation;
- Division or resection of uterine septum;
- Endoscopic surgery for Asherman's syndrome;
- Resection of uterine myomas;
- Fallopian tube cannulation.

From the Society of Reproductive Surgeons. Credentialing in operative endoscopy. Fertil Steril 1994;62.

7. Laparoscopy for Diagnosis or Sterilization

A. JEFFERSON PENFIELD

Laparoscopy for sterilization or diagnosis is the third most frequently performed gynecologic operation in the United States after first trimester abortion and uterine curettage. Current estimates from the Association for Voluntary Surgical Contraception indicate that there are approximately 400,000 laparoscopic sterilizations each year in the United States. The number of diagnostic laparoscopies is unknown, but many hospital operating schedules list more diagnostic than sterilization procedures. An estimated 800,000 to 1 million laparoscopies are being performed each year in American hospitals and surgery centers. When one considers that laparoscopy in America was a rare operation in 1970, its growth in popularity during the past 25 years has been astounding.

Fascination with this elegant procedure has been stimulated by major instrument companies, which continue to offer newer and sometimes better optical systems, operating instruments, and sterilization devices. The American Association of Gynecological Laparoscopists, under the dedicated leadership of Jordan Phillips, MD, developed standards and presented an annual international forum for the sharing of new knowledge.

A major early impetus to outpatient laparoscopy was provided by Frank Loffer and David Pent at the Surgicenter in Phoenix, Arizona. This was shortly followed by the successful teaching program in ambulatory laparoscopic sterilization under local anesthesia at the University Hospital in Chapel Hill, North Carolina, under the leadership of Jaroslav Hulka and John Fishburne. Fishburne is board-certified both in anesthesiology and gynecology, and his publications on techniques and safeguards in the provision of local anesthesia are important resources (1–3).

The development I believe has had the most profound effect on the safety of outpatient laparoscopy under local anesthesia is the introduction of the open technique of abdominal entry by Harrith Hasson at the Grant Hospital in Chicago, Illinois. Hasson designed a cannula and obturator (Eder Instrument Co., Chicago, IL) to be inserted under direct vision for the accommodation of the laparoscope, thus avoiding the blind puncture with needle and trocar (Figs. 7.1 and 7.2). However, this latter technique of closed laparoscopy is still favored by most laparoscopists because of its relative ease and speed of performance. Unfortunately, closed laparoscopy carries with it the risk of major vessel injury. Therefore, access to a vascular surgeon in a hospital operating room within 10 to 15 minutes must be available to manage this serious complication. The only exception to the need to transfer to the hospital in such an event would be if a laparotomy tray is at hand and an anesthesiologist with full-scale anesthesia backup is on site at all times. Then the laparoscopist could perform an immediate laparotomy and tamponade the bleeding vessel while awaiting the arrival of a vascular surgeon to repair the lacerated vessel.

Open laparoscopy, on the other hand, can be safely performed in an outpatient or free-standing surgery without the need for standby general anesthesia or full-scale resuscitation capabilities. Particularly when a single vertical infraumbilical incision is made and

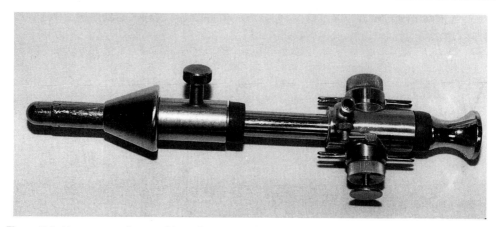

Figure 7.1. Hasson cannula: note blunt obturator, adjustable cone, gas-insufflating stopcock, and suture holders.

an operating laparoscope is used, it is an operation ideally suited to local anesthesia in most instances. This is true for all sterilization and most diagnostic procedures. Prerequisites must include skilled counseling, individualized premedication, and supportive care during surgery.

Gynecologists planning to initiate outpatient laparoscopy services would do well to review guidelines currently being formulated by the American Association of Office En-

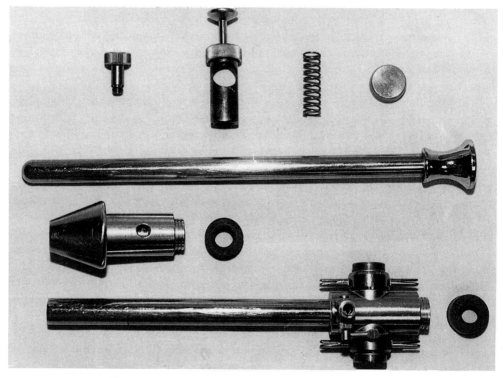

Figure 7.2. Hasson cannula disassembled before sterilization.

Table 7.1
Suggested Instrument List for Open Laparoscopy

6 Hemostats (2 fine-tip)
2 Kelly clamps
2 Allis clamps
2 Baby Kocher clamps
1 Dissecting scissors
1 Hegar needle holder
1 Mousetooth forceps
1 Scalpel with number 15 blade
1 Pair Baby Deaver retractors
1 Pair S-shaped retractors
1 Hasson cannula, 8, 10, or 12 mm
1 Bivalve speculum
1 Single-tooth cervical tenaculum
1 Hulka tenaculum-sound
1 Sargis tenaculum-sound
1 Diagnostic and/or operating laparoscope

Gas or air insufflator with tubing

Light source with fiber optic cable

Grasping forceps

Clips, bands, coagulating equipment, etc.

doscopy, under the leadership of Roosevelt McCorvey, MD, and Beverly Love, MD, of Montgomery, Alabama.

Each practitioner has his or her own preferences, but a set of instruments that has served me during the past 20 years is shown in Table 7.1 and Figure 7.3.

DIAGNOSTIC LAPAROSCOPY UNDER LOCAL ANESTHESIA

When operating under local anesthesia, it is essential to combine skilled use of the laparoscope with gentle manipulation of the uterus by means of such instruments as the Hulka or Sargis tenaculum-sound. In my experience with single-incision laparoscopy, at least two thirds of the ovarian surface may be inspected through the 10-mm operating scope if the adnexa are sprayed with anesthetic solution and the tube, ovary, and utero-ovarian ligament are manipulated with the utmost gentleness. If necessary, of course, one of the lower abdominal quadrants can also be anesthetized and an operating instrument can be inserted through a second incision. This second incision facilitates such procedures as ovarian biopsies, cyst aspirations, and extensive lysis of adhesions, but these operations are usually performed under general anesthesia, because the more extensive manipulations and additional time required would not be tolerated by most patients under local anesthesia. In teaching institutions, where residents are being instructed and more complex procedures are being carried out, most laparoscopies continue to be performed under general anesthesia.

In a general gynecologic practice during the past 22 years, however, I found that almost all laparoscopies, either for sterilization or for the investigation of endometriosis, obscure masses, or pelvic pain, can be performed without difficulty with a 10-mm scope through a single incision under local anesthesia. The hazards, discomforts, and prolonged recovery of general anesthesia are avoided; conversational monitoring of the patient during

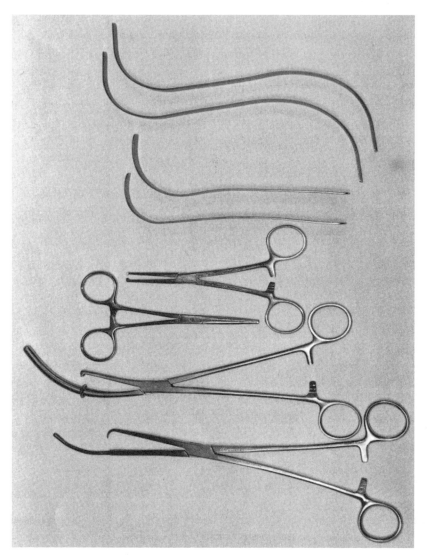

Figure 7.3. Selected instruments for open laparoscopy. Bottom to top, Hulka tenaculum-sound, Sargis tenaculum-sound, Baby Kocher clamps, Baby Deaver retractors, and S-shaped retractors.

surgery reduces her anxiety and provides an earlier warning system for complications that would not be possible if she were asleep; and otherwise obscure sources of chronic pelvic pain may be precisely identified by means of gentle manipulation of specific pelvic structures. These advantages of local anesthesia for the investigation of chronic pelvic pain are illustrated by the following case report.

Patient CM: Chronic Progressive Unilateral Pelvic Pain

CM is a 17-year-old, well-adjusted high school student. Slender and normally developed, she is a competitive member of her school swim team. Menarche occurred at age 11, and since age 12 she has complained of gradually increasing deep right lower quadrant abdominal pain. She has also experienced moderately severe menstrual cramps and, with each period, a moderate increase in the chronic right-sided pelvic discomfort.

From age 13 to 15, repeated examinations by her family physician revealed only right adnexal tenderness. Antiprostaglandins for 3 months, followed by oral contraceptives for 12 months, lessened her menstrual cramps somewhat but failed to relieve her pelvic pain, which began to interfere with her sleep. Her regular swimming workouts did not relieve her discomfort.

I first examined this patient when she was 16 and was immediately impressed by her remarkable maturity and composure. Postmenstrual pelvic examination revealed a normal uterus and a very tender right ovary one and one-half times the diameter of the left ovary, but not cystic. The entire right adnexal area and the right uterosacral ligament on rectovaginal examination were also very tender, but no nodules suggestive of endometriosis were felt. The left ovary, broad ligament, and uterosacral ligament were normal to palpation. A barium enema revealed a normal delicate bowel pattern and normal filling of the appendix. An ultrasound would have been performed, but this case predated its introduction into gynecologic practice.

The above history and findings suggested that differential diagnosis was between unilateral pelvic congestion syndrome and pelvic endometriosis, with no relief from conventional therapy. I therefore recommended laparoscopy. In consideration of the young age of the patient, then 17, I offered to perform laparoscopy in the hospital under general anesthesia. However, the patient and her mother both requested that the operation be done in my office surgery under local anesthesia. This proved to be a fortunate choice because it allowed me to gain far more information than if she had been operated on under general anesthesia.

After initial counseling by one of my nurses, the patient was scheduled for open laparoscopy under local anesthesia in the latter half of her menstrual cycle. On the day of surgery, we gave her 10 mg diazepam (Valium, Roche) by mouth 1 hour preoperatively. On the operating table, an intravenous infusion of 5% dextrose in water was started, and 1 mg butorphanol tartrate (Stadol, Bristol) and 15 mg promethazine hydrochloride (Phenergan, Wyeth) were injected slowly, with an initial test dose, into the tubing.

A pelvic examination was done, a Hulka tenaculum-sound was gently introduced without paracervical block, and the abdominal wall was anesthetized with 8 mL 0.5% lidocaine (Xylocaine, Astra) with 1:200,000 epinephrine. After insufflating about 1 L of nitrous oxide gas, each adnexal area was sprayed with 5 mL additional Xylocaine. The patient remained reasonably alert, comfortable, and communicative throughout the 30-minute procedure. The uterus was normal. The right ovary, although twice the diameter of the left, appeared otherwise perfectly normal without any suggestion of cyst formation. Likewise, the right tube was markedly congested in contrast to the left, the right broad ligament contained large varicosities whereas the left contained none, and the right uterosacral ligament was twice the diameter of the left. Two 1-mm "powder burns" were found in the cul-de-sac, suggesting minimal endometriosis.

A significant additional finding derived from this diagnostic operation was that by gentle manipulation of the right tube, ovary, and uterosacral ligament with the 5-mm grasping forceps, I was able to exactly duplicate the right-sided pelvic pain that was the patient's only complaint. Before surgery I had explained to her that from time to time I would touch or move certain structures in the pelvic cavity. I would not tell her when I was about to do this but would ask her to let me know whenever she felt pain. Accordingly, during the operation and without any signal from me, she notified me of pain each time I manipulated the right adnexal and uterosacral structures but remained silent while I manipulated the left-sided pelvic structures with equal degrees of traction.

Thus, I concluded that this patient had unilateral pelvic congestion syndrome with minimal endometriosis. I placed her on danazol (Danocrine, Winthrop-Breon), 400 mg twice daily, and within 3 months her pain had almost disappeared. The medication was continued for 6 more months, during which time she remained amenorrheic and asymptomatic. Her performance in competitive swimming improved while on the medication, possibly because of pain relief combined with the anabolic effects of danazol. Pelvic examinations after the third month of therapy revealed slight continued tenderness of the right adnexal structures but a marked reduction of the swelling of the right ovary and uterosacral ligament. For the next 18 months, I prescribed oral contraceptives for this patient, and she has continued free of pelvic pain. Pelvic examinations are now completely normal.

The above case report illustrates the fact that it may be possible to arrive at a more precise diagnosis laparoscopically in a case of pelvic pain of obscure origin when one uses local anesthesia in a cooperative patient.

Pain Mapping

The unique advantage of local anesthesia in identifying the source of recurrent or chronic pelvic pain was reported by Martin (4) and by Palter and Olive (5) in patients with normal pelvic examinations. Among these patients are those suspected of having minimal endometriosis but who have not demonstrated any lessening of pain after many months of hormonal therapy. Martin was able to abolish pain from a localized area by injecting a local anesthetic. Studies are underway to determine the efficacy of laser or electrical coagulation of the area in question.

Palter and Olive (5) reported their findings in 11 patients explored with a 1.98-mm fiber optic laparoscope for chronic pelvic pain. These patients had "no clearly identifiable etiology based on clinical examination." There is no mention in the article of transvaginal ultrasound. One would hope this examination was performed before any invasive procedure was contemplated.

Using equipment designed by Imagyn Medical, Inc. (Laguna Niguel, CA), a sheathed Verres needle was introduced and insufflation with carbon dioxide gas was carried out. Most patients complained of crampy dull pain or a sharp burning sensation at the onset of insufflation that the authors claim did not interfere with pain mapping.

In one patient, pain was elicited by probing a "deeply infiltrating sclerotic endometriosis of the rectum at the site of a previous partial resection of the disease. Another had a focus of active endometriosis." A third woman "was sensitive to palpation of an adhesion of small bowel to the anterior abdominal wall that resulted in severe kinking of the bowel lumen." No abnormalities were found in the remaining eight patients. The cost of office laparoscopy under local anesthesia (OLULA) was $1,700 versus $7,500 for operating room laparoscopy.

After reading this article (5), I would like to make some recommendations. First, all patients should have an ultrasound study before an invasive procedure that reveals no lesion in such a high percentage of patients (72% in this small series). Adnexal thickening, hydrosalpinx, or ovarian cysts, for example, are not always palpable but are often diagnosed by transvaginal ultrasound. Second, most patients with symptomatic infiltrating rectal or rectovaginal endometriosis are found to have significant and sometimes exquisite tenderness and thickening upon deep rectovaginal digital examination, particularly premenstrually. Many patients experience dramatic relief from a 6- to 12-month course of intramuscular medroxyprogesterone acetate (Depo-Provera, Upjohn) or danazol (Danocrine, Sanofi Winthrop). If their pain has not begun to lessen by the end of 3 months, then laparoscopy is the logical next step. Third, I recommend either nitrous oxide or room air for insufflation. After carbon dioxide insufflation, the astringent effect of carbonic acid on peritoneal surfaces causes significant discomfort in most awake patients. Therefore, it would seem reasonable to substitute nitrous oxide or room air, which should not cause anything more than mild pressure symptoms. Proponents of carbon dioxide for pneumoperitoneum argue that this gas will not support combustion, whereas nitrous oxide and room air will. However, in practice there have been no reports of problems in cauterizing for hemostasis specifically related to the presence of nitrous oxide or room air.

In summary, I recommend preoperative ultrasound and careful rectovaginal examination before performing microlaparoscopy. I also believe that nitrous oxide or room air is preferred over carbon dioxide.

Feste (6) reported on 36 patients explored with an "optical catheter with an outer diameter of only 1.8 mm (Medical Dynamics, Inc., Englewood, CA)." Most frequent indications for such a procedure are assessment of obscure pelvic pain, evaluation of ectopic pregnancy, and confirmation of endometriosis. In his first 20 cases, performed under general anesthesia, Feste was "encouraged by the nearly 100% correlation between the findings" of the optical catheter with a 10-mm laparoscope. The subsequent 16 patients were operated under local anesthesia.

Microlaparoscopy appears to have a bright future for diagnostic purposes. The disadvantage of somewhat inferior visual resolution is offset by the advantage of a less traumatic abdominal entry and a quicker recovery and healing time.

Increasing experience with microlaparoscopic instruments will undoubtedly result in increasing numbers of OLULA procedures. This may indeed have the paradoxic effect of increasing overall reimbursable costs. It is hoped that overuse of this attractive new technology will not occur.

SINGLE-INCISION OPEN LAPAROSCOPY WITH HULKA CLIP APPLICATION UNDER LOCAL ANESTHESIA

In my own practice, however, most patients who require laparoscopy are those referred for sterilization rather than for diagnosis of obscure pelvic conditions. A detailed description follows of the laparoscopic sterilization method I have come to prefer during the last 17 years, after 6 previous years of coagulation or Yoon band application, which are just as easily performed under local anesthesia (7).

The patient is seen for initial consultation and examination. Existing gynecologic or medical problems are either ruled out or managed appropriately. The nurse-counselor conducts a thorough discussion of the patient's motivation, life, and marital situation, and alternative methods of family planning are discussed. Her partner is welcomed for the discussion if he chooses to be present. Suprapubic minilaparotomy as an alternative sterilization operation may be more appropriate if the patient is reasonably slender with a normal mobile uterus. However, I prefer the laparoscopic approach in the presence of obesity, uterine enlargement, asymmetry, or fixation (see Chapter 8 for further discussion of counseling).

The Hulka clip, designed by Jaroslav Hulka, MD (Chapel Hill, NC) is made of lexan plastic and fitted with a gold-plated stainless steel spring. The patient must be asked specifically if she is allergic to gold, and any history of dermatitis resulting from the wearing of gold jewelry contraindicates the use of the clip. If there is reasonable doubt about allergy to gold, we remove the spring from the clip, bend it open to flatten it, and tape it firmly to the skin of the patient's forearm for 24 hours. If there is no positive skin reaction, we use the clip. Trathen and Stanley (8) reported the occurrence of sterile bilateral adnexal abscesses in one patient a few months after Hulka clip sterilization. She was found postoperatively to be allergic to gold chloride solution in skin testing.

When it is agreed that the patient is a suitable candidate for the Hulka clip, she is scheduled for surgery at any point in her menstrual cycle, care being taken to ensure that she continues with her birth control method preoperatively. There is no need to discontinue oral contraceptives for a month; the risk of postoperative thrombosis is negligible after a relatively nontraumatic procedure. If the patient is wearing an intrauterine device, it may be safely left in place until the day of surgery, unless she has current evidence of endometritis with abnormal bleeding, discharge, or tenderness, in which case the device should be removed to permit preoperative resolution of the endometritis.

On the day of surgery, the patient is instructed to limit herself to a light liquid breakfast. When she arrives she may benefit from an oral tranquilizer such as 5 or 10 mg Valium. She signs an operative permit. An intravenous infusion of 5% dextrose in water is started. Stadol, 1 mg, and 15 mg Phenergan are injected into the intravenous tubing slowly, with a preliminary test dose of about one tenth of the total, to immediately recognize an idiosyncratic reaction. Stadol is a highly effective nonnarcotic analgesic without the risk of respiratory depression unless the dose injected exceeds 4 mg, and Phenergan is an antihistamine that potentiates the effect of analgesics. Phenergan has, in addition, an atropine-like effect, thus preventing vasovagal reactions in most patients. Some surgeons prefer to give an intravenous narcotic such as 50 mg meperidine hydrochloride (Demerol, Winthrop-Breon) or 0.1 mg fentanyl citrate (Sublimaze, Janssen) along with 0.4 mg atropine sulfate. Others add 10 mg Valium or 5 mg Versed, either of which is safe and highly effective if given very slowly. However, profound reactions from intravenous Valium have been known to occur, and our experience has shown that intravenous Valium may reduce inhibitions in certain patients, making them somewhat uncooperative and difficult to manage.

After the medications are injected, I re-examine the patient again to rule out possible pregnancy or pelvic abnormality. A preliminary dilatation and curettage is unnecessary except in certain cases of recent-onset abnormal bleeding.

If the patient has accidentally conceived within the preceding 10 weeks, she may request a presterilization pregnancy termination. With additional appropriate counseling and informed consent, a vacuum and standard curettage procedure is readily carried out under paracervical block immediately before the laparoscopy. Otherwise, paracervical anesthesia is unnecessary before laparoscopy. Although the introduction of the uterine tenaculum-sound may result in mild cramps for about 30 seconds, subsequent gentle manipulation of the uterus causes very little discomfort.

After I introduce and attach the Hulka or Sargis tenaculum-sound, I demonstrate to the patient what she may feel when I move the uterus during the operation to expose the tubes and other structures. It is wise to prepare the patient in this way; she will rapidly lose confidence in her surgeon if he startles her by causing unexpected pain.

The skin of the midabdomen is washed with Betadine (Providone-iodine, Purdue Frederick) soap and solution, a pool of full-strength Betadine solution is left standing in the umbilical fossa for 2 to 5 minutes, and the patient is draped exactly as in the hospital operating room.

With the surgeon fully capped, masked, gowned, and gloved, up to 10 mL of a local anesthetic solution of 0.5% Xylocaine with 1:200,000 epinephrine is injected by increments into the infraumbilical tissues (Fig. 7.4). A 23- or 24-gauge needle is used, and if

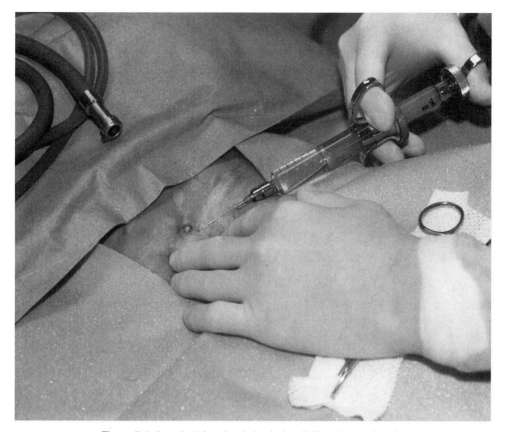

Figure 7.4. Anesthetizing the abdominal wall. Note Luer-Lok syringe.

the injections are given skillfully, the patient will feel no pain beyond the first few "pinches."

Since 1980, Dr. Hasson and I have used a vertical infraumbilical incision in all cases, following the initial informal recommendation of Richard Soderstrom, MD, of Seattle, Washington. This incision permits far better exposure than a transverse incision, an advantage of particular importance in obese women. Each tissue layer is injected with the anesthetic solution, not exceeding a total of about 10 mL (Fig. 7.5). After the skin incision is made, the scalpel is dropped down to the fascia (Fig. 7.6) and the intervening layer of fat is opened by spreading the tips of a Kelly clamp. The fascia, being exposed by the nurse with the aid of Baby Deaver retractors, is anesthetized, grasped, and elevated with small Kocher clamps (Fig. 7.7). Although Hasson incises the fascia transversely, I prefer to continue the incision in a vertical fashion, again for the sake of better exposure (Fig. 7.8). This fascial incision must be made slowly and meticulously, attempting to leave the last few fascial fibers intact. Otherwise, the incision may inadvertently extend through adherent peritoneum into underlying bowel (Fig. 7.9). This accident has been reported to me several times and probably represents the most serious risk of open entry into the abdominal cavity. Bowel laceration should be a rare complication of open laparoscopy. The opening through the fascia may be completed by forcing open the jaws of a curved Kelly clamp. This opening should be just large enough to accommodate the Hasson cannula.

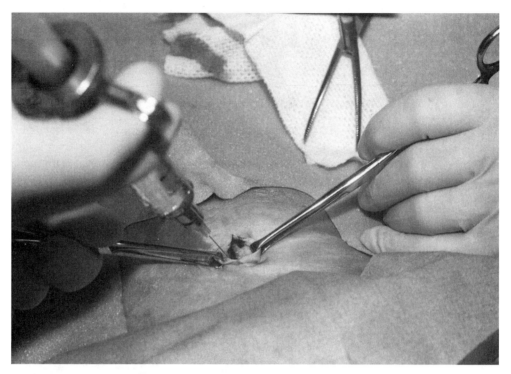

Figure 7.5. Injection of local anesthetic into fascia.

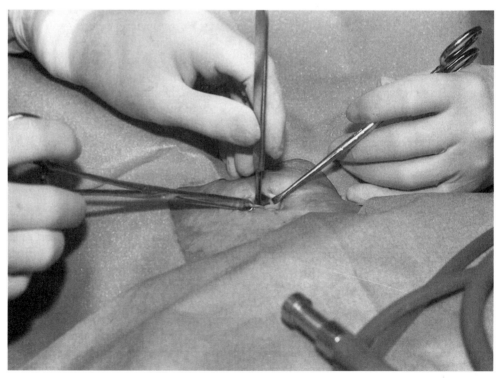

Figure 7.6. Scalpel "dropped" down to fascia.

CHAPTER 7 / LAPAROSCOPY FOR DIAGNOSIS OR STERILIZATION

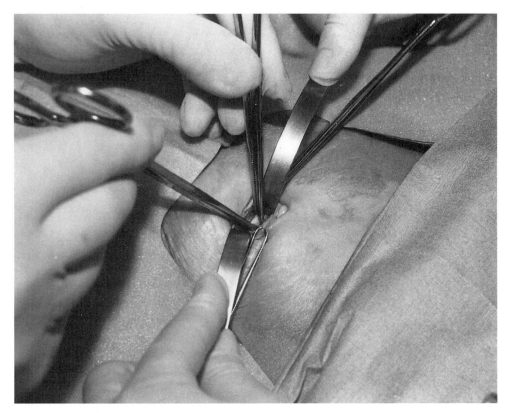

Figure 7.7. Fascia elevated with small Kocher clamps.

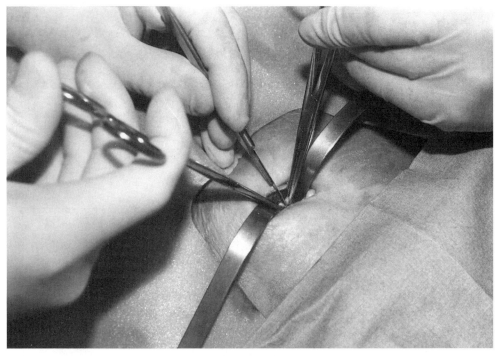

Figure 7.8. Vertical incision through fascia (try to leave deeper fibers intact).

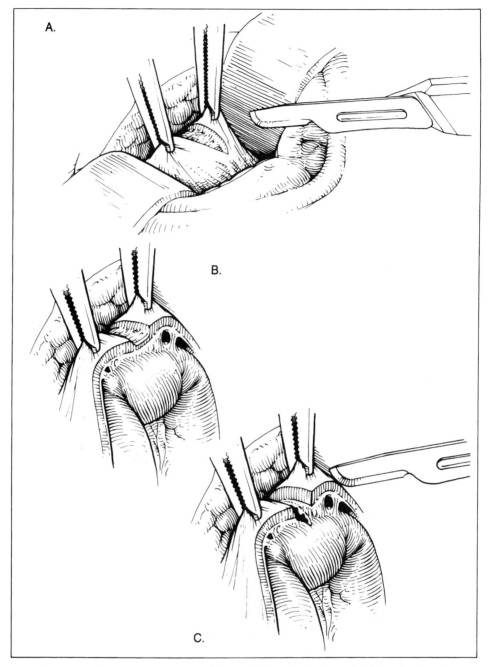

Figure 7.9. A. Vertical incision through fascia. **B.** Bowel adhesions. **C.** Incision into bowel.

At this point, in about 50% of cases, the surgeon discovers that he or she has entered the peritoneal cavity. If not, the fat can be cleared away and a fine hemostat gently dropped through the peritoneum. Only occasionally is it necessary to elevate the peritoneum with clamps and incise between them with a scalpel. Either before or after entry through the peritoneum, a strong polyglycolate suture should be placed in each fascial edge for the purpose of later fixing the cannula in place.

As the assistant exposes abdominal contents by means of the small Deaver or S-shaped retractors, the surgeon inserts the cannula and attaches the fascial sutures firmly to the cannula suture holders (Fig. 7.10). The obturator is removed, and the gas tubing is attached to the cannula stopcock.

Which gas should be selected for insufflation? The practical choices are carbon dioxide, nitrous oxide, or room air. From 1972 to 1974, I used carbon dioxide, but I noted that most patients complained of abdominal discomfort, presumably from the carbonic acid that forms when carbon dioxide strikes peritoneal fluid. For the next 9 years, I used nitrous oxide; this resulted in no peritoneal irritation and was satisfactory in all other respects. Finally, in 1985, after exposed to simpler techniques in Bangladesh, I decided to try room air, which has worked well for many years in the developing world where tanks of any kind of compressed gas are scarce. I chose an electric pump (Hagen Jet Stream, Hagen Corp., Mansfield, MA) designed for aquarium use. With the use of room air for pneumoperitoneum for the next 8 years, we noted no difficulty nor any increase in patient discomfort during surgery or afterward. The pump is equipped with an air filter.

Because the aquarium pump delivers air at a higher rate than the gas insufflator, I squeeze the Hasson cannula trumpet valve partially open when beginning the insufflation and gradually allow it to close for more rapid delivery after the patient has adjusted to the mild initial discomfort. An adequate pneumoperitoneum is produced within 30 seconds. The distal lens of the scope may be cleared with sterile contact lens solution. The laparoscope is introduced promptly (Fig. 7.11). If the lens fogs up, it can be cleared by

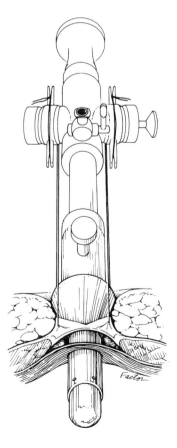

Figure 7.10. Hasson cannula in place.

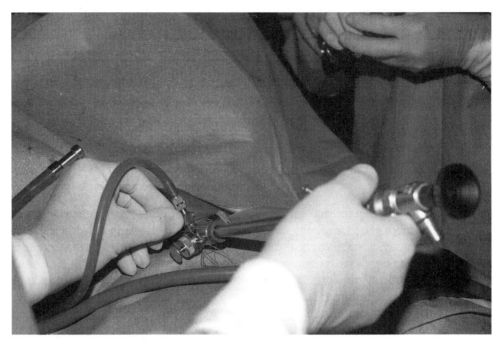

Figure 7.11. Laparoscope introduced through Hasson cannula.

gently stroking the moist bowel serosa. It is unnecessary to monitor the volume of air because only the amount needed to visualize the pelvic organs is insufflated.

After notifying the patient, I slowly tilt the table into a moderate degree of Trendelenburg (head down) position. I ask the patient to breathe in and out to allow the bowel to fall at least partially out of the pelvic cavity. I then manipulate the tenaculum-sound gently through the sterile drape to bring the uterine corpus forward to expose the fallopian tubes. It may be necessary to tilt the corpus to one side or the other and even to twist the uterus slightly to inspect the adnexa. This maneuver is made possible by the firm attachment of the tenaculum-sound to the upper cervix.

Each tube is now sprayed with 5 mL 0.5% Xylocaine with 1:200,000 epinephrine in preparation for the sterilization procedure. After the spring clip (Wolf Co., Rosemont, IL) is loaded into the Hulka clip-applicating scope (Wolf Co.), it is essential before introducing the scope that the surgeon operate the upper ram to test clip function and spring performance.

One clip is applied to the midportion of each tube. In some cases it is advisable to grasp the tube gently with the clip itself and slowly draw it upward in an effort to visualize the fimbria (Fig. 7.12). This step may also assist in bringing the tubal isthmus into a better position for clipping. Whenever possible, the round and utero-ovarian ligaments should be separately identified.

Occasionally, a fold of mesosalpinx will mimic the tube, and one of my colleagues informed me that one of his patients conceived because this fold was mistakenly clipped. Rarely, one tube is congenitally absent.

Frequently, filmy adhesions between bowel or omentum and abdominal wall or pelvic organs hide the tubes. Usually it is possible to maneuver the end of the scope past or through these adhesions. On the other hand, dense thick adhesions may bury the fallopian

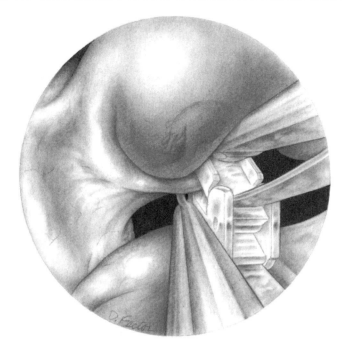

Figure 7.12. Mobilization of tube with clip.

tubes so that no laparoscopic procedure is possible. However, one advantage of the clip is that even a 1-cm length of exposed proximal tube may be sufficient to allow for clipping.

The clip must be applied as nearly as possible at right angles to the fallopian tube. The tube should be teased as far as possible into the crotch (angle) of the open clip, which is closed slowly by means of the upper ram. The lower ram is then advanced to push the spring forward. This maneuver should proceed smoothly and easily until the lips of the spring snap into place. It is most important not to push the spring in too hard with the lower ram because excess pressure may dent the back of the spring, weaken its tension, and distort its position. Subsequently, the clip may become dislodged and slip off the tube.

Occasionally with single-incision laparoscopy, it is difficult to apply the clip at right angles to the tube. If this is the case and the clip after application is seen to be in a markedly diagonal position, then a second clip should be applied at a more favorable angle no more than 0.5 cm from the first (Fig. 7.13). Likewise, if the first clip has not fully encompassed the tube, a second one will provide added assurance. Some laparoscopists, including the late Richard Kleppinger, MD, of Reading, Pennsylvania and Tibor Engel, MD, of Denver, Colorado, routinely apply two clips to each fallopian tube. It remains to be seen if this practice will lower the long-term failure to below the usually reported rate of three to five per thousand patients.

By spraying each tube with anesthetic solution, I found that most patients experience no pain from clip application. Some, however, notice a momentary "pinch," and a few complain of moderate "menstrual cramps" that subside in a few minutes.

It is important not to dislodge the clip as it is released from the applicator. To reduce this possibility, the surgeon should practice the maneuvers of clip application and release on a rubber band or cord before performing his or her first clip application.

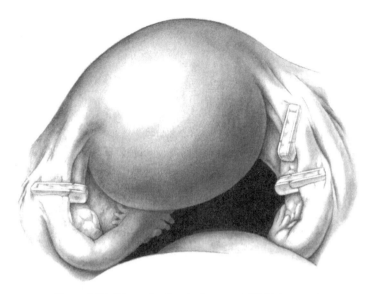

Figure 7.13. Clip application. Left, correct. Right, incorrect.

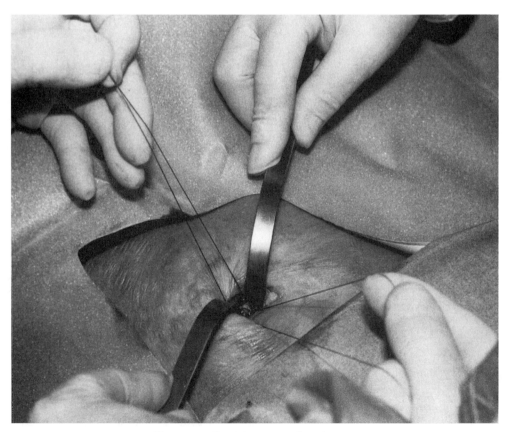

Figure 7.14. Fascial sutures before closure.

One advantage of clip sterilization is that, unlike Falope ring application, it carries no risk of mesosalpingeal bleeding. Therefore, coagulation backup is unnecessary.

Before withdrawing the operating laparoscope, the surgeon should further explore the cul-de-sac, ovaries, and abdominal cavity. The liver edge, gall bladder, and appendix can be inspected.

It is useful to have an operating scope available with a wider angle of vision to better delineate any suspected abnormality. I found in my own practice that the 10-mm Wolf operating laparoscope not only provides a broad field of vision but also, with a grasping forceps in place, is most useful in gently moving a portion of omentum or stripping away filmy adhesions that may be obscuring tubes or ovaries.

After completing the laparoscopy and removing the scope, the patient should remain in the Trendelenburg position with the cannula open to permit escape of as much air (or gas) as possible from the peritoneal cavity (9). This minimizes the volume of subdiaphragmatic air (or gas) that often causes annoying chest and shoulder pains for several days postoperatively.

After removing the cannula, the fascia may be closed by tying together the corresponding ends of each holding suture, drawing up the combined sutures, and tying together the opposite ends (Figs. 7.14 and 7.15). If necessary, additional interrupted sutures may be placed to close off a fascial defect and repair an actual or potential umbilical hernia. Finally, the skin may be closed with two subcuticular polyglycolate sutures, and a small dressing is applied.

After resting for 5 minutes on the operating table, the patient is helped into the sitting position. If she is not dizzy, we walk her to the recovery bed where she rests for at least 1 hour. The nurse monitors her condition at intervals. We give her a sheet of postoperative instructions (Fig. 7.16) and a prescription for oral pain medication such as Tylenol 3

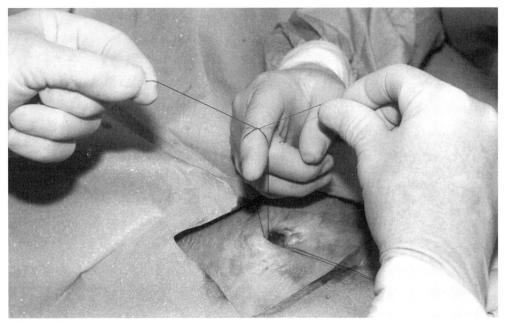

Figure 7.15. Tying fascial suture ends before fascial closure.

A. Pat Doe, M.D., P.C.
1234 Fifth Street
New York, New York 13201
(555) 321-1234

LAPAROSCOPIC STERILIZATION OR MINILAP STERILIZATION

Post-Operative Instructions:

1. Return home with a companion and take it easy today and tomorrow. Eat lightly today. You may shower or bathe the day after surgery. No heavy lifting or strenuous exercise for one week.

2. You may experience "menstrual" cramps, gas pains or shoulder aches for a day or two. Take two pain capsules or aspirins every four hours if needed. You may use an ice pack during the first 12 hours after surgery if necessary.

3. Slight bleeding or drainage may occur from the incision for a day or two. Replace dressing as needed. Usually no dressing is required after 24 hours.

4. It is normal for your abdominal wall to be tender and bruised for a few days.

5. Slight vaginal bleeding may occur for a day or two. (You may use tampax or external pads).

6. You are "safe" immediately, but we suggest you delay intercourse for a few days until your discomfort and bleeding have ended.

7. Your stitches need not be removed. They will dissolve or drop out after a few weeks.

8. This operation will not affect your menstrual cycle nor your hormone levels. Your sex drive will not be decreased.

9. Please call us any time for pain, fever, or if you have any questions.

A. Pat Doe, M.D.

Figure 7.16. Postoperative instructions.

CHAPTER 7 / LAPAROSCOPY FOR DIAGNOSIS OR STERILIZATION

A. Pat Doe, M.D., P.C.
1234 Fifth Street
New York, New York 13201
(555) 321-1234

TO:

DATE:

1. Have you had a normal period since surgery?_____

2. After recovering from surgery, have you had abdominal or pelvic pain?_____

3. Have you had a fever at anytime since surgery?_____

4. Have you needed to visit a doctor because of a post-operative problem?_____

   Please comment_____

   _____

5. Were you pleased with our service?_____

   Comment if you wish:_____

   _____

   _____

   _____

   _____

   _____

   _____

                                                A. Pat Doe, M.D.

Figure 7.17. Follow-up questionnaire.

(McNeil), 2 tablets, with a caution not to exceed two doses a day. Most patients are ready and eager to leave the surgery within 1 hour to rest at home. The nurse then takes the patient either on foot or in a wheelchair out to a waiting car with the patient's companion as driver.

On the day after surgery, we telephone each patient at home to learn of any problems and to review instructions. The patient is asked to make a return follow-up appointment in our office or with her personal physician. Two months after surgery, we send each patient a questionnaire (Fig. 7.17) with a self-addressed stamped envelope for her reply.

In summary, the Hulka clip is an effective device because its application involves no risk of mesosalpingeal bleeding, it obliterates only 5 mm of tubal lumen, and is therefore ideal if the patient is subsequently accepted as a candidate for tubal reconstruction. Finally, its application under local anesthesia causes minimal discomfort.

OTHER LAPAROSCOPIC STERILIZATION TECHNIQUES

Other methods that may be readily performed under local anesthesia include Filshie clip application, silastic band application, and tubal coagulation. Each of these methods, if properly carried out, is equally effective, with a failure rate of 1/1,000 cases each year for 3 to 5 years.

The Yoon silastic band during and after application may cause somewhat more pain because of ischemia of a longer segment of tube. A thick tube may require "milking" before it can be encompassed by the band. Tubal transection is a recognized risk of band application; coagulation backup is a wise precaution with this technique.

Bipolar tubal coagulation continues to be the leading method of laparoscopic sterilization in North America. It is the easiest method to learn, and the risk of burning bowel is minimal if care is taken to avoid bowel contact with the coagulating forceps. A longer segment of tube is destroyed, thus reducing the success rate of tubal reconstruction. If performed under local anesthesia, tubal coagulation will result in only a few seconds of sharp pain. Lingering ischemic pain does not occur because the sensory nerve fibers are destroyed.

COMPLICATIONS OF OPEN LAPAROSCOPY FOR DIAGNOSIS OR STERILIZATION

These complications include perforation of the uterine fundus with the tip of the tenaculum-sound, injury to bowel, postoperative abdominal wall hematoma, and postoperative wound infection.

Perforation of the Uterine Fundus

This possibility is minimized by initial sounding of the cervical canal and uterine cavity to determine their exact relationship and by slow and cautious introduction of the tenaculum-sound in the predetermined direction. If the tip of the sound is seen at laparoscopy to protrude through the fundus, the corpus should be moved with extreme gentleness and the operation completed with dispatch. Bleeding from such a perforation is usually slight and will almost certainly cease after removal of the tenaculum-sound. The sound should be removed under laparoscopic visualization and the site of puncture watched for at least 30 seconds to be sure that active bleeding does not continue. If bleeding does not subside, suturing of the uterine puncture may be required either by laparotomy or laparoscopically through an accessory port.

Bowel Injury

This is most unlikely if all of the above-listed precautions in traversing fascia and peritoneum are observed. One of my early patients had an adherent loop of bowel, and I made a small incision into the intestinal serosa; I found that it was possible, under continued local anesthesia, to enlarge the fascial incision, isolate the loop of bowel, and repair the laceration with a fine polyglycolate suture. Appropriate irrigation and postoperative antibiotic therapy is necessary in such a case. If the laceration extends into the bowel lumen (Fig. 7.9C), management should include repair, irrigations, wound closure, and possible admission to the hospital for overnight observations and intravenous antibiotics.

In September 1984, in an effort to determine the incidence of bowel laceration during open laparoscopy, I gathered information by telephone interview from 18 board-certified gynecologists in the United States, all of whom had abandoned closed laparoscopy in favor of the open-entry technique to avoid needle or trocar injuries to bowel and major vessels (10).

Six bowel lacerations were reported in 10,840 open laparoscopy cases. Four were recognized and repaired immediately, and no patient experienced any postoperative morbidity. Indeed, in one patient who was under general anesthesia, the surgeon elevated the fascia, cut vertically between the clamps through the entire thickness of the fascia, and found himself looking into bowel lumen. He promptly extended the fascial incision inferiorly, isolated the injured loop of intestine, and repaired the laceration. Saline irrigations were carried out, the incision was closed, and the patient received antibiotic prophylaxis to ensure a benign recovery.

In two of six cases, the bowel injury was not recognized at surgery. One patient developed fever and increasing pain on the third postoperative day. Intravenous antibiotics were given, and at laparotomy a scalpel laceration of the ileum was found and repaired. Prompt recovery occurred. The second patient experienced an abrupt onset of abdominal pain on the eleventh postoperative day. At laparotomy, a pin-hole perforation of the ileum was found and oversewn. Recovery was uneventful.

Abdominal Wall Hematoma

This is a rare complication with either open or closed laparoscopy, but I have seen a large paraumbilical hematoma develop after each entry technique. In both cases the estimated volume of the hematoma was over 500 mL, but spontaneous resorption occurred within 2 weeks in each patient. Broad-spectrum antibiotics were given in each case, and early discomfort was easily managed with mild analgesics. One would expect that hidden bleeding would be more likely after the blind introduction of the needle or trocar, but the rarity of this complication is probably due to the absence of large paraumbilical vessels.

The one patient in my practice who developed the hematoma referred to above was an obese woman who had a chronic dry cough from smoking three packs of cigarettes daily. During the open entry technique, an unusual amount of traction was needed to expose the fascia. No fresh bleeding was noted at surgery, and the patient returned home comfortably 1 hour after her operation. However, she was out of bed repeatedly during the next several nights to care for her hyperactive 2.5-year-old child, who enjoyed jumping on her mother's abdomen and traumatizing the fresh incision.

On the ninth postoperative day, she visited the hospital emergency room, where a large abdominal hematoma was diagnosed. Because the hematoma had been present for several days without apparent enlargement or suppuration, I decided to study the natural resolution of her problem. For the next 5 days I examined her daily in the office, taking careful measurements of her hematoma to be certain that further enlargement did not occur. Initial measurements of the lateral limits of the hematoma, in relation to the umbilicus, were two finger-breaths above, three below, and five to the left. Black and blue discoloration extended deep into the left flank.

For 2 days, a small amount of thick fluid blood emerged from her incision, which then promptly sealed over. The hematoma proceeded to shrink noticeably each day until at the end of 2 weeks it virtually disappeared.

At no time did the patient experience fever or sepsis. With constant cajoling, I succeeded in persuading her to cut her cigarette consumption to one pack a day and control her child's desire to jump on her abdomen. It is unlikely that immediate wound exploration and surgical evacuation of the hematoma would have accelerated her recovery. However, under less bizarre circumstances, a fresh hematoma of over 500 mL, diagnosed in the first few days after surgery, should be evacuated and the incision closed with a drain.

Postoperative Infection of the Abdominal Incision

The umbilical fossa is difficult, if not impossible, to sterilize. For this reason the vertical incision described above should in most cases be made through the inferior rim of the umbilicus, thus avoiding the fossa itself. However, in any patient with extreme abdominal obesity, safe entry requires incision directly through the umbilical pit. Whether or not the fossa is incised, careful preoperative cleansing with cotton swabs and Betadine scrub and wash should be carried out. When the patient is on the operating table, Betadine liquid should be poured into and left standing in the umbilical fossa for 4 to 5 minutes while the surgeon is preparing for surgery and draping the patient.

When a patient experiences drainage from an incision between 5 and 15 days postoperatively, the material is usually a small discharging seroma or liquefied fat. In either case, we found on several occasions that the drainage is sterile on culture. This occurs because the umbilical region is poorly vascularized and fluid collections within the incision may not be absorbed into the circulation and therefore eventually drain to the outside. A daily 5-minute hot pack until the drainage subsides is usually adequate for treatment. On the other hand, a classic wound infection with fever, marked tenderness, and purulent drainage is rare. It may require open drainage and debridement. I have only seen one such case in my practice. The patient developed an abdominal wall abscess 1 week postoperatively that required hospitalization, intravenous antibiotics, and full surgical exploration, including inspection of the entire length of small bowel and colon to rule out bowel injury. An incisional drain was left in place for several days. Abscess cultures grew out anaerobic micrococci. In retrospect, we surmise that the infection was precipitated in part by the first-time use of an inadequately sterilized cannula.

CONCLUSION

For patients who can cooperate and relax sufficiently to be examined while awake, laparoscopy may be performed under local anesthesia for sterilization, diagnostic survey, or pain mapping. Particularly in the outpatient setting, I encourage the open entry technique to eliminate the possibility of major vessel injuries from needle and trocar (11). Although some gynecologists also perform double-incision laparoscopy under local anesthesia, the single-incision approach is more easily tolerated and entirely adequate for most of the above procedures.

Success with operative laparoscopy under local anesthesia depends on careful patient counseling, appropriate preoperative medications, continuous supportive communication with the patient during surgery, and gentle precise surgical technique.

REFERENCES

1. Fishburne J. Laparoscopy. Baltimore, MD: Williams & Wilkins, 1977.
2. Fishburne J. Office laparoscopic sterilization with local anesthesia. J Reprod Med 1977;18:233–234.
3. Fishburne J. Anesthesia for outpatient laparoscopy under local anesthesia (OLULA). Presented at the First Master's Course in OLULA, Tuskegee Institute, Tuskegee, AL, May 1996.
4. Martin D. Commentary. Presented at the First Annual Meeting of American Association of Office Endoscopy, Tuskegee, AL, May 1996.
5. Palter S, Olive D. Office micro-laparoscopy under local anesthesia for chronic pelvic pain. J AAGL 1996;3(3):359–364.
6. Feste J. Outpatient diagnostic laparoscopy using the optical catheter. Contributions to Ob/Gyn 1995; 40:54–63.
7. Poindexter AN III, Abdul-Malak M, Fast JE. Laparoscopic tubal sterilization under local anesthesia. Obstet Gynecol 1990;75:5–8.
8. Trathen WT, Stanley RJ. Allergic reaction to Hulka clips. Obstet Gynecol 1985;66:743–744.
9. Hulka JF, ed. Biophysics and physiology. In: Textbook of laparoscopy. New York: Grune and Stratton, 1985.
10. Penfield AJ. How to prevent complications of open laparoscopy. J Reprod Med 1985;30:660–663.
11. Penfield AJ. American Association of Gynecological Laparoscopists Report: prevention and management of laparoscopic complications. Santa Fe Springs, CA: American Association of Gynecological Laparoscopists, 1977.

8. Suprapubic Minilaparotomy

A. JEFFERSON PENFIELD

In this operation, the lower abdominal cavity is entered through a 2- to 4-cm transverse incision located 1 to 3 cm above the pubic hairline. The usual purpose of minilaparotomy is to perform tubal sterilization, but the incision may also permit certain operations for the correction of incidental or unanticipated abnormalities, such as removal of pedunculated myomata, excision of small adnexal tumors, aspiration of ovarian cysts, and salpingotomy or salpingectomy for tubal pregnancy.

Minilaparotomy tubal ligation is the leading method of female sterilization in Japan, Thailand, and other Far Eastern nations and in most developing nations of the world. It is also widely practiced in China, but in that nation of over 1 billion people, the pressure of population growth and a strong national family planning policy are currently promoting the simpler if somewhat less effective method of obliterating the tubal lumen by transcervical injections of phenol mucilage.

"Minilap," as it is familiarly termed, requires only standard surgical instruments and no specialized surgical skills. It is easily and economically adaptable to an outpatient setting (1, 2).

Speidel and McCann (3) presented an analysis of 2,820 cases of minilaparotomy gathered by the International Fertility Research Program from participating centers around the world. Surgical difficulties were reported in only 10% of the procedures and complications in only 1.6%. The most common difficulties reported were bowel-bladder-omentum interference, adhesions and difficulty opening the peritoneum. The most common complications were tubal bleeding, bowel or bladder injury, and uterine perforation. Seventy-five percent of the operations were performed under local anesthesia.

In North America, outpatient suprapubic minilaparotomy for tubal sterilization continues to be "upstaged" by laparoscopy, for at least three reasons:

1. It is contraindicated in any woman with marked lower abdominal obesity.
2. Unlike laparoscopy, it does not permit thorough pelvic and abdominal exploration.
3. It has not achieved the status or sophistication of laparoscopy, which is a fertile field for sponsorship by instrument companies intent on promoting newer and sometimes better instrumentation.

Nonetheless, as an effective, safe, and low-cost operation for nonobese women, suprapubic minilaparotomy for sterilization deserves more recognition than it receives.

MINILAPAROTOMY UNDER LOCAL ANESTHESIA

Many gynecologists resist the idea of entering the abdominal cavity under local anesthesia because they believe that local anesthesia cannot provide sufficient pain relief, the operation will take longer, manipulations will be restricted, and the bowel will get in the way. They claim that their patients would be too frightened by the prospect of being awake for surgery and by the possibility of pain. However, 23 years of experience with this operation in my own practice revealed that these objections, although occasionally expressed, were easily dispelled. I have performed approximately 800 minilaparotomy tubal ligations under local anesthesia in a private office surgery and more than 100 teaching cases by invitation elsewhere in the United States and abroad. We demonstrated that local anesthesia is entirely adequate for most patients, provided there is good counseling and communication and the surgeon is gentle and meticulous in technique.

When I was learning how to perform the operation in 1976, there were a few patients who experienced more pain than I would consider acceptable today. The past 18 years, however, have taught me many things that I would like to share with my readers. I suggest seven prerequisites for consistent success with minilaparotomy tubal ligations under local anesthesia:

1. Skilled preoperative counseling by a nurse or other professional, preferably 2 to 4 weeks before surgery. The counselor should encourage the patient to invite her husband or partner to participate in the discussion;
2. Adequate patient motivation;
3. Preoperative pelvic examination to rule out pelvic abnormalities and to ensure reasonable ability to relax;
4. A restful nonthreatening operating room environment;
5. A warm, relaxed, supportive manner on the part of operating room personnel;
6. Appropriate preoperative oral or intravenous medications selected for analgesic and tranquilizing properties;
7. Gentle handling of instruments and tissues.

Prerequisite 1: Preoperative Counseling

The patient's husband or partner should be invited (with the patient's consent) to participate. If the patient is estranged or contemplating divorce, it may be wise to delay the surgery until she is in a more stable living situation.

Initial counseling is usually best undertaken by the nurse or other professional, preferably the same one who will be present in the operating room. Although additional counseling should be offered by the surgeon after the initial examination of the patient, the nurse can usually empathize better for the preliminary counseling and information session. The counselor must stress that sterilization should not be considered reversible and that it is intended to be a permanent form of contraception. The patient should be informed about vasectomy as an alternative and about all modern reversible contraceptive techniques. It is unwise to assume that the patient already knows about the options open to her. Obviously, such counseling is essential regardless of what form of anesthesia is contemplated, but it is especially important to develop optimum rapport with the patient when one is contemplating local anesthesia for an intraperitoneal procedure. Some patients are frightened or skeptical at the prospect of what they regard as a major abdominal operation under local anesthesia, particularly if it is to take place in an outpatient or freestanding surgical unit. Friends or advisers may have planted the seeds of anxiety in their minds. Whenever appropriate, the counselor should point out that the operation is safe, the discomfort minimal, and the patient will not face the risks and immediate postoperative discomforts of general anesthesia. Otherwise, her postoperative recovery will be the same, regardless of anesthesia.

It is also important for the patient to be informed that rare accidents such as bowel or bladder injury can occur during the operation but that most such injuries can be repaired immediately without additional anesthesia. The consent form used is shown in Figure 8.1.

A. Pat Doe, M.D., P.C.
1234 Fifth Street
New York, New York 13201
(555) 321-1234

Date_____

CONSENT TO TREATMENT

I have been informed by the above named doctor(s) of the risks, possible alternative methods of treatment, and possible consequences involved in the treatment by means of _____

_____

_____

for _____

_____

Understanding this, I hereby authorize the above named doctor(s), or whomever he (they) may designate, to administer such treatment to me (or _____

_____).
     Name of patient, if minor

  I understand that the risk of pregnancy following a sterilization is less than ½ of 1%.

    Signed _____
        Patient or person authorized to consent for patient

Witness _____

Figure 8.1. Consent form.

Prerequisite 2: Adequate Patient Motivation

The decision for permanent sterilization is obviously a major one, heralding a profound change in the patient's self-image. It is important for the counselor to make certain that this is the patient's own decision, that she has not been coerced, and that she has developed an equanimity regarding the permanence of her decision. The counselor should help the patient to resolve her anxieties regardless of the anesthetic technique. If the counselor fails to do so, an operation under local anesthesia can be as stressful as it would have been under general anesthesia. It is also generally true that the higher the patient's level of anxiety, the lower her pain threshold.

Concerning motivation, it is obvious that we must exclude at once some patients who have made a firm and unshakable decision to be put to sleep. If, on the other hand, the patient has an open mind, her candidacy for local anesthesia is often strengthened by positive experiences of her friends and by the support of the gynecologist.

In my opinion, it is both unwise and unfairly confusing to the patient to offer her the choice of anesthesia method. It may suggest to her that her gynecologist is unsure. A reasonable woman will surmise that the surgeon will recommend a method that he or she is comfortable with and believes is most desirable in that patient's particular case.

Prerequisite 3: Preoperative Pelvic Examination

The operation should not be attempted under local anesthesia if the uterus is fixed in retroversion, if it is enlarged or asymmetric with cornual myomata, if there is adnexal fixation or an unexplained mass, or if the corpus cannot be felt through an obese lower abdominal wall after elevating the uterus from below. Even under general anesthesia, these conditions are likely to require that the minilaparotomy incision be extended to a point where the surgeon is performing regular laparotomy.

An equally important finding during the pelvic examination is the patient's ability to relax. Most well-prepared patients, if approached with courtesy and gentleness, relax well for examination. Therefore, there is every reason to expect they will relax equally well during surgery under local anesthesia. On the other hand, an occasional patient will be so tense that she cannot be examined satisfactorily while awake. She will require general anesthesia. So too will the severely retarded patient who cannot lie still or cooperate at all.

Prerequisite 4: A Restful Nonthreatening Operating Room Environment

It is difficult for the patient to be calm and relaxed in a hospital operating room, where she is surrounded by anesthesia machines, resuscitation devices, cardiac monitors, floodlights, and the hustle and bustle normally associated with major surgery. Even the most skilled counselor is unlikely to succeed in allaying anxieties in such an environment. Although minilaparotomy under local anesthesia is an intraperitoneal procedure, it does not require the trappings of major operations. Rather, it calls for a quiet subdued setting, preferably outpatient or free standing, with small focused spotlights instead of glaring overhead lamps. Anesthesia machines, monitors, or superfluous hardware in the outpatient operating room may alarm the patient and are not needed.

Prerequisite 5: Warm, Relaxed, Supportive Personnel

I recall one instance in 1976 while I was learning the procedure and using the main hospital operating room. We prepared the patient for the elaborate machinery she would see but could not protect her from the somewhat sullen and dubious attitude of the anesthesiologist, who was slightly offended that he was not being used to his fullest. Neither could we prevent the operating-room nurse from acting in an overly solicitous manner, hovering over the patient and repeating to her over and over that she really would be alright, that she should not worry, and that she could ask for help (e.g., more anesthesia) any time she needed it. Although the operation was completed without complication, the experience was an unhappy one for all concerned.

Ideally, the nurse-counselor in the outpatient operating room should be the same one who initially interviewed and counseled the patient during her preoperative visit. It is hoped that a warm bond is established that will greatly facilitate surgery. The manner of the counselor should be confident, relaxed, supportive, and not overly solicitous. If the patient does not wish to talk, simply holding her hand may be sufficient.

Local anesthesia for minilaparotomy is generally unpopular in university hospitals, where there is hands-on teaching of residents. In these institutions, small quiet outpatient surgery units should be available, and turnover of nursing personnel should be kept to a minimum.

Prerequisite 6: Appropriate Preoperative Analgesic and Tranquilizing Medications

Once the patient is on the operating table, one of several drug combinations may be injected intravenously. Among effective combinations are meperidine with midazolam, fentanyl with midazolam, and butorphanol with promethazine. My current choice is 1 to 2 mg butorphanol (Stadol, Bristol) with 15 mg promethazine (Phenergan, Wyeth) injected slowly into the intravenous tubing after an initial test dose to rule out hypersensitivity or an idiosyncratic reaction. Stadol is a nonnarcotic analgesic with virtually no depressive effect on respirations even at three times the recommended dose, and Phenergan is a potentiating agent with sedative and anticholinergic properties. Additional medication may be injected during the operation but is seldom necessary.

Prerequisite 7: Gentle Handling of Instruments and Tissues

From the introduction of the speculum and uterine tenaculum-sound or other elevator to the retraction of fascia, peritoneum, and fallopian tubes, the surgeon must exercise utmost gentleness. Ideally, 30 to 60 seconds should elapse between injection of the anesthetic solution and the incision of each tissue layer. Once in the peritoneal cavity, it is obvious that bowel or omentum should be manipulated as little as possible, or preferably not at all.

Although it is not a prerequisite, it is desirable that the short stocky patient with a history of premenstrual abdominal bloating should be scheduled during the first one half of her menstrual cycle. Otherwise, it may be difficult during surgery to manipulate the uterine fundus away from surrounding edematous loops of bowel.

Table 8.1
Suggested Instrument List for Minilaparotomy Tubal Ligation

```
4 Hemostats
6 Kelly clamps
2 Allis clamps
2 Baby Babcock clamps
1 Dissecting scissors
1 Hegar needle holder
1 Mousetooth forceps
1 Metzenbaum scissors
1 Scalpel with number 10 blade
1 Pair Army-Navy retractors
1 Pair Eastman-Richardson retractors
1 Bivalve speculum
1 Single-tooth cervical tenaculum
1 Hulka tenaculum sound
1 Sargis tenaculum sound
```

MINILAPAROTOMY TECHNIQUE

Most instruments used are standard for any laparotomy (Table 8.1 and Figs. 8.2 and 8.3). For the sake of clarity and simplicity, minilaparotomy tubal ligation is presented here step by step.

1. The patient is placed in dorsolithotomy position with her legs comfortably supported in knee-stirrups (Fig. 8.4).
2. A gentle careful pelvic examination is carried out, and the bladder is catheterized if the patient has failed to void preoperatively. Pelvic tumors or inflammation are ruled out. If

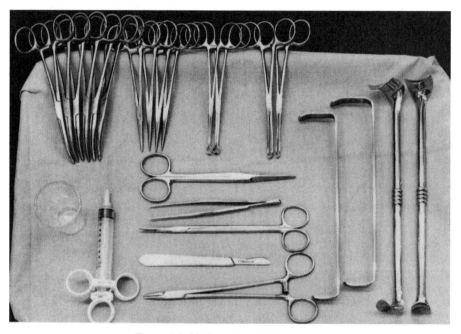

Figure 8.2. Minilaparotomy instruments.

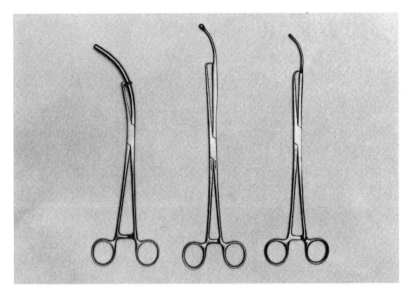

Figure 8.3. Tenaculum-sounds for uterine elevation. Right, two Hulka tenaculum-sounds. Left, Sargis tenaculum-sound for patulous cervix or postabortal uterus.

transient recent dysfunctional-type bleeding has occurred or if there is any suspicion of early intrauterine pregnancy, a preliminary vacuum or standard curettage under paracervical block may be carried out with proper preoperative counseling and consent. A dilatation and curettage should not be routine, however, because such a practice constitutes unnecessary surgery.

3. The cervix is grasped with a single-tooth tenaculum and a uterine elevator is inserted, with preliminary sounding of the internal os if there is the slightest question concerning the cervicouterine axis. Extreme gentleness is mandatory, not only to minimize uterine cramping but also to reduce the chance of fundal perforation. My choice of uterine elevator is the Hulka tenaculum-sound or the wider diameter Sargis tenaculum-sound in the postabortal patient.

   Comment: One gratifying safeguard of minilaparotomy under local anesthesia is that if the patient is going to faint from a drop in blood pressure or experience other features of a severe vasovagal reaction, she will probably have done so by this stage of the procedure. In the absence of severe cardiovascular disease, such a reaction will invariably subside in 2 to 3 minutes and the minilaparotomy itself can be carried out with only a remote chance that a recurrent vasovagal episode will occur, particularly if 0.4 mg atropine sulfate is injected intravenously.

4. The surgeon, standing beside the patient where he or she can speak comfortably with her, should grasp the handle of the tenaculum-sound and gently elevate the fundus of the uterus up against the abdominal wall, while explaining to the patient exactly what he is doing. At the same time, the surgeon should gently palpate the elevated fundus through the abdominal wall with the fingers of the other hand (Fig. 8.5) and tell the patient that this mild discomfort is about all she will feel during the operation, in addition to the initial "pinches" as the local anesthetic is injected.

5. The patient is prepped and draped.

6. With full sterile precautions, local anesthetic solution is injected into the subcutaneous tissues. We use 0.5% lidocaine with 1:200,000 epinephrine injected by means of a Luer-

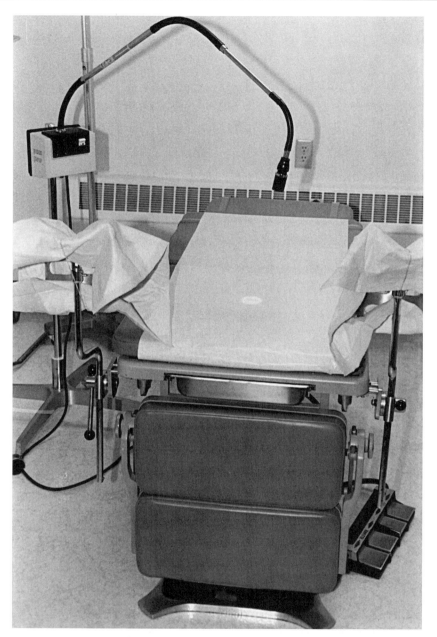

Figure 8.4. Operating table and spotlight.

Lok syringe through a 1.5-inch 25-gauge hypodermic needle (Fig. 8.6). If properly done, the patient will feel no discomfort beyond the first injection, because all subsequent injections are made through previously anesthetized tissues. A volume of 10 mL of solution is adequate for the entire thickness of the abdominal wall. The epinephrine in the solution produces a relatively bloodless surgical field and retards the systemic absorption of the anesthetic agent.

7. A transverse incision is made 1 to 3 cm above the public hairline. The incision is between 2 and 4 cm in length, depending principally on the degree of obesity. Although marked

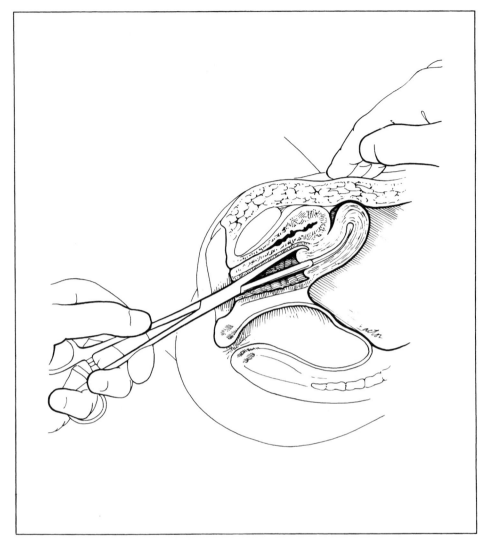

Figure 8.5. Palpation of elevated fundus.

obesity sufficient to render the elevated uterine fundus nonpalpable is a contraindication to minilaparotomy under local anesthesia, some obese patients will have a convenient crease in the lower abdominal wall through which the elevated fundus can be easily palpated. These patients are satisfactory candidates for the operation, but they will require an incision at least 4 cm long.

8. Small Richardson retractors are inserted to separate the subcutaneous fat from the fascial surface.
9. Additional anesthetic solution is injected beneath the fascia (Fig. 8.7).
10. The fascia is opened with a scalpel in a transverse direction, with the length of the incision corresponding approximately to the length of the skin incision.
11. An injection of 2 or 3 mL anesthetic solution is made into the midline between the rectus muscles.
12. With a Kelly clamp, the rectus muscles are separated in the midline, and the Army-Navy retractors are repositioned to separate the muscles.

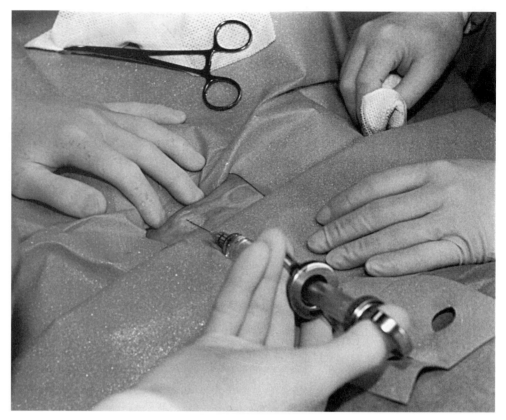

Figure 8.6. Local anesthetic injected radially.

13. A few milliliters of additional anesthetic solution is injected into the posterior rectus sheath, which is cleaned of intervening fat with the aid of the Kelly clamp.
14. The posterior sheath, which is generally loosely fused to the parietal peritoneum, is picked up with two Kelly clamps, superiorly and inferiorly (Fig. 8.8). The clamps are released and reattached once or twice to be certain that no underlying bowel is included in either clamp.
15. The peritoneal cavity is entered in a standard laparotomy manner, "tenting" the tissues in a preliminary step with the handle of the scalpel and then incising with great caution in a transverse direction.
16. With the aid of the two Army-Navy retractors and one or two Richardson retractors, the omentum, bowel, bladder, and uterine fundus can be adequately visualized. I found that self-retaining retractors are not satisfactory because they produce more discomfort and unavoidably cause forceful retraction of tissues in unnecessary directions. Individual retractors, on the other hand, can be maneuvered gently and precisely in the proper direction.
17. After notifying the patient, I lower the head of the table slowly into a moderate Trendelenburg position.
18. The patient is asked to take a deep breath and then breathe out. This action will allow the omentum and bowel to fall out of the pelvic cavity.
19. At this point, the surgeon should grasp the handle of the uterine elevator and gently elevate the fundus.

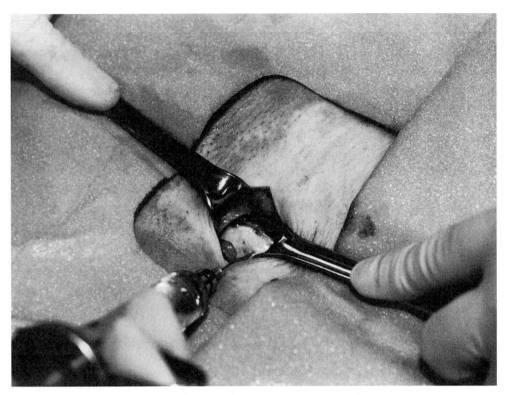

Figure 8.7. Injection of anesthetic beneath fascia.

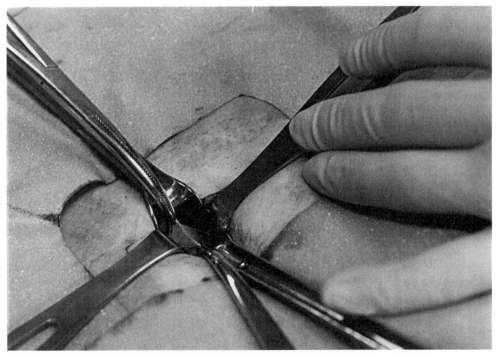

Figure 8.8. Elevation of parietal peritoneum.

20. If the above maneuvers have not resulted in exposing the fundus from beneath bowel and omentum, the surgeon may gently tease away omentum or intestine to expose the fallopian tube at its point of entry into the uterine cornu.
21. As soon as the surgeon catches a glimpse of the proximal tube, he or she should immediately inject 2 mL anesthetic solution into the tube or mesosalpinx. Then, having identified the uterine insertion of the adjacent round ligament, the surgeon can gently grasp the proximal tube with a Baby Babcock clamp and bring it into better view. At this point, the surgeon may release the handle of the uterine elevator and regrasp it only when ready to expose the opposite tube.

    Comment: On rare occasions, with an obese or tense patient, it may be necessary for the surgeon to reach behind the cornu to gently grasp a proximal tube that he or she has been unable to expose. To further facilitate this maneuver, it may be helpful to inject the round ligament with anesthetic solution and elevate it just enough to expose the point of insertion of the tube.
23. With the tube anesthetized and gently elevated in its midportion (isthmus) by means of two Baby Babcock clamps, the sterilization procedure may be carried out. I prefer a modified Pomeroy ligation, using a 1–0 plain catgut suture placed through an avascular portion of the mesosalpinx, tied around one limb of the tube and then around both limbs, followed by a second plain catgut tie and excision of the tubal knuckle (Fig. 8.9).

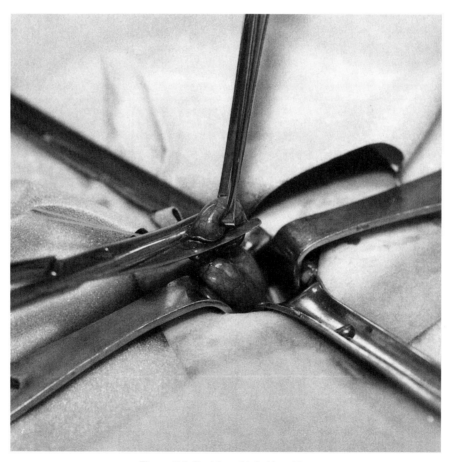

Figure 8.9. Excision of tubal knuckle.

24. When both tubes are ligated and careful inspection of the knuckle stumps reveals no fresh bleeding, an attempt should be made to examine both ovaries if possible. This is relatively easy to accomplish in a slender patient. In my experience I have been able to visualize at least one half of each ovarian surface in about 50% of patients.
25. Before closing the abdomen, excess air should be expressed by gentle pressure through the drapes covering the abdominal wall. The patient should remain in Trendelenburg position until after this maneuver is completed and, indeed, until after the peritoneum is closed, so that air under the diaphragm is more likely to escape from the peritoneal cavity. It is our impression that these measures have resulted in fewer complaints of postoperative chest and shoulder pain.
26. Peritoneum, fascia, and skin are closed in a standard manner. Suture material is optional. My current preference is for 3–0 polyglycollate, because this suture material is hydrolyzed rather than being digested, thus resulting in minimal tissue reaction.
27. A dry dressing is applied, and in 5 minutes most patients are ready to sit up with assistance and walk escorted to the recovery room where they should rest for an hour.

COMPLICATIONS: PREVENTION AND MANAGEMENT

Vasovagal Reaction

Vasovagal reaction refers to a complex of signs and symptoms resulting from a disturbance of the autonomic nervous system. Mild reactions consist of bradycardia and diaphoresis (sweating). Patients with more severe reactions progress to dizziness, hypotension, syncope, and convulsions. Any stressful situation, physical or emotional, may give rise to a vasovagal reaction. Syncope and convulsions may even accompany or follow minor surgical procedures such as intrauterine device (IUD) insertions, particularly in the woman who has been suppressing her anxiety. Fortunately, in a woman with normal cardiovascular function, such a reaction is always self-limited, and spontaneous recovery will occur without special treatment.

In relation to minilaparotomy under local anesthesia, any woman who states that she is especially subject to fainting spells should receive 0.4 mg atropine sulfate, preferably intravenously, immediately before surgery.

Without such a history, either atropine or a mildly anticholinergic drug such as Phenergan should be administered preoperatively, together with an analgesic agent. If a severe reaction occurs and a stable recovery does not follow within 1 to 2 minutes, a supplemental dose of 0.4 mg atropine should be given immediately.

In my practice, a mild vasovagal reaction occurred in about 10% of our minilaparotomy patients. Reactions have progressed to syncope and convulsions in less than 1% of cases. I observed all gradations of vasovagal reactions in a higher percentage (about 15%) of patients undergoing IUD insertions, probably because we normally do not inject a preinsertion anticholinergic agent.

Our minilaparotomy patients who experienced vasovagal reactions have done so during the preliminary maneuvers of uterine sounding and tenaculum-sound attachment. After such a reaction, the threshold for a second reaction is higher unless the patient has a recent history of epileptic seizures. Such a patient should be given 10 mg diazepam intravenously just before surgery. When scheduling an epileptic patient for surgery, it is a good idea to have a preoperative consultation with a neurologist or anesthesiologist who could supervise anticonvulsive therapy.

Uterine Perforation

The possibility of this accident should be far less with minilaparotomy than with dilatation and curettage in a postmenopausal woman with a stenotic internal os and an atrophic uterus. Nonetheless, patients for minilaparotomy may be vulnerable because of acute uterine retroflexion or difficulty in accurate sounding of the internal cervical os.

Most such perforations are preventable by gentle, painstaking, unhurried introduction of a well-lubricated sound through an internal os whose exact location and direction may take a minute or more to discover. Would a paracervical block facilitate this maneuver? Between 1972 and 1976, I routinely administered paracervical block to all patients before minilaparotomy or laparoscopy. No blocks have been administered to these patients since that time because I found that paracervical block not only does little to reduce uterine cramps in these patients, but has no apparent relaxing effect on the internal os, contrary to its strikingly beneficial effects in reducing pain and relaxing the internal os in patients presenting for abortion. Consequently, I abandoned paracervical anesthesia except in those patients who required operative abortion as a preliminary procedure before laparoscopy or minilaparotomy.

Forceful introduction of the sound or the intrauterine manipulator may result in perforation either at the level of the internal os or through the uterine fundal wall. Fortunately, most such perforations are midline, either anterior or posterior, and therefore unlikely to be associated with heavy bleeding. Usually they are not recognized until noted at the time of minilaparotomy or laparoscopy. When the instrument is seen to have perforated the wall of the uterus, the surgery should be completed with gentleness and dispatch, the uterine manipulator withdrawn, and the site of perforation observed for continued bleeding. Normally, suturing the perforation is unnecessary, because bleeding will almost always promptly subside.

Bladder Laceration

This accident is most likely to occur in an obese woman with a distended bladder. Unless the obese patient has a well-defined lower abdominal crease through which the elevated uterine fundus can be easily felt, lower abdominal obesity is a relative contraindication to minilaparotomy. Unless one is certain that the patient has voided immediately before surgery, she should be catheterized.

These two lessons were forcefully brought to my attention on one occasion in 1978. The patient was a stocky moderately obese diabetic woman who claimed to have just emptied her bladder. Unfortunately, some delays were encountered in starting her intravenous infusion and in preliminary maneuvers. I did not suspect the presence of a full bladder during my preoperative pelvic examination. She was prepped and draped, and the suprapubic tissues were injected with 0.5% lidocaine with 1:200,000 epinephrine. After incising transversely through the skin and a 4-cm depth of fat, the anterior rectus fascia was reached and additional anesthetic solution was injected. With the aid of small Richardson retractors, the fascia was exposed and incised transversely. Army-Navy retractors were used to separate the rectus muscles, and the search for the peritoneum began. All tissue layers were obscured by fatty infiltration. I was unable to identify precisely the peritoneal layer, but of equal importance was my failure to recognize that her bladder had become markedly distended. Quite predictably, although I carefully elevated what appeared to be fatty peritoneum, my next transverse incision resulted in a copious outpouring of urine; I had traversed the thinned-out distended bladder wall.

With a little extra retraction and clearing away of the overlying fatty tissues, it was remarkably easy to demonstrate the extent of the laceration and repair it with a single layer of continuous fine catgut suture. The patient appeared to be unaware of any discomfort during the bladder repair. Therefore, no additional local anesthetic was required. A straight catheter was introduced to provide continuous bladder drainage, the peritoneum was located and incised, and a modified Pomeroy tubal ligation was carried out. I closed the abdominal incision without a drain and replaced the straight catheter with an indwelling Foley catheter that was attached to a leg bag for periodic emptying during the first week postoperatively. The patient returned home 1 hour after surgery with a prescription for a urinary antibiotic. A week later she returned and the Foley catheter was removed. Thereafter, she experienced no further difficulty.

Some urologists recommend drainage of the space of Retzius after such an accident. This patient's prompt wound healing and benign postoperative course suggest that such a precaution is unnecessary.

Because of difficulty in exposure and tissue identification, lower abdominal obesity is a relative contraindication for minilaparotomy.

Bowel Laceration

I have never witnessed this accident during minilaparotomy. Its likelihood is minimized by preliminary "tenting" of the peritoneum as described in step 15. Nonetheless, bowel laceration is probably somewhat more likely during minilaparotomy than during a regular laparotomy, simply because of restricted visualization. One would anticipate a greater risk in the presence of dense adhesions of bowel to peritoneum. When the patient's history suggests such adhesions, I usually select open laparoscopy as the preferred approach for sterilization, mostly because additional peritubal adhesions may also be present that would make mobilization of the fallopian tube too painful for minilaparotomy under local anesthesia. It is much easier to avoid, displace, or penetrate adhesions with the aid of the laparoscope.

During minilaparotomy, if the bowel wall is accidentally incised, prompt recognition and repair is highly desirable. Copious irrigations and antibiotics should ensure benign recovery. For a fuller description of bowel injuries, see Chapter 7.

Mesosalpingeal Bleeding

Mesosalpingeal bleeding occurs only if a vessel is lacerated by the hypodermic needle during the injection of anesthetic, excessive traction is placed on the fallopian tube while attempting to mobilize it, or a vessel is punctured by the suture needle during the tubal ligation procedure. With adequate exposure, it is very easy even under local anesthesia to clamp and ligate such a bleeder. However, this remedy is usually unnecessary because a tie around the tubal knuckle almost always stops the bleeding.

Failed Procedure

There were two conditions that prevented me from completing tubal ligation during minilaparotomy: the presence of dense adhesions that restricted mobilization of the tubes and the finding of extreme dextrorotation of the uterine corpus, where the left tube was easily ligated but the right tube was inaccessible. In the first case, after consulting with the patient, I closed the incision and performed an immediate open laparoscopy under local anesthesia. With the laparoscope I was able to circumvent the adhesions and clip the tubes. The second patient also agreed to an immediate laparoscopy under local. With the grasping forceps of the operating scope, I was able to bring out the right tube from behind the uterus. I then replaced the operating scope with a clip-applicating scope and applied a Hulka clip across the proximal right tube near the cornu.

These experiences demonstrate the desirability of having immediate laparoscopic backup when performing minilaparotomy.

Wound Hematoma

The use of an anesthetic solution containing 1:200,000 epinephrine has not in my experience predisposed to postoperative rebound bleeding and hematoma formation. All active arterial bleeders must, of course, be clamped and ligated, but I have encountered such bleeders in less than 10% of cases.

Superficial small hematomas usually drain or resorb spontaneously and should require no treatment other than hot wet packs, applied twice daily. Larger hematomas should be suspected if the patient complains of increasing incisional pain during the first 24 hours after surgery. The volume of trapped blood should be estimated. If it appears to be in the neighborhood of 500 mL or more, then surgical evacuation, suturing of bleeders, and secondary wound closure is carried out.

Wound Infection

This should be a rare complication, becoming evident between 3 and 10 days postoperatively and characterized by pain, tenderness, swelling, and possible fever and discharge. As with open laparoscopy, spontaneous wound drainage usually represents the discharge of a seroma or liquefied fat that is found to be sterile on culture. Although gentle probing and assisted drainage may speed healing on occasion, antibiotics are unnecessary. Diagnosed wound infections, on the other hand, unless undergoing spontaneous resolution, require antibiotics effective against staphylococci, and even debridement, irrigations, and frequent dressing changes during the delayed healing period. I always place my minilaparotomy incision 1 to 3 cm above the pubic hairline to avoid infected hair follicles that might initiate a wound infection. As with any laparotomy, the incidence of wound infections is minimized by skin cleansing and asepsis, sterile technique, gentle handling of tissues, avoidance of unnecessary clamping or coagulation of small bleeders, and the use of polyglycolate sutures for persistent bleeders and for wound closure; this material dissolves rather than being digested and thus causes minimal tissue reaction.

CONCLUSION

Minilaparotomy tubal ligation is admirably suited to an outpatient or free-standing location and can be carried out under local anesthesia in almost all cases. If properly performed, it is probably safer than most first trimester abortions, which carry a greater risk of uterine hemorrhage or perforation. Most patients who have had both procedures tell me that minilaparotomy is also associated with less discomfort and stress than is abortion, although minilaparotomy wound healing causes discomfort during the postoperative period. The operation has been criticized because it does not allow for a panoramic view of the pelvic organs, and it is contraindicated in the patient with lower abdominal obesity. Clearly, in the presence of lower abdominal obesity or obscure pelvic abnormalities, laparoscopy is to be preferred. For the reasonably slender patient with a mobile uterus who requests sterilization, however, I personally prefer the certainty and safety of the direct visual approach of suprapubic minilaparotomy under local anesthesia.

REFERENCES

1. Association for Voluntary Surgical Contraception International. Minilaparotomy under local anesthesia: a curriculum for doctors and nurses. New York: AVSC, 1993.
2. Darney P, Horbach NS, Korn AP. Protocols for office gynecology. Cambridge, MA: Blackwell Science, 1996;5:108–125.
3. Speidel JJ, McCann MF. Minilaparotomy—a fertility control technique of increasing importance. Adv Planned Parenthood 1978;13:42–57.

9. *Outpatient Female Sterilization*

A. JEFFERSON PENFIELD

By the year 1980, almost 100 million men and women worldwide were surgically sterilized, 13 million of them in the United States (1). In 1983, approximately 600,000 tubal sterilizations and 400,000 vasectomies were performed in the United States (2). Since then, accurate figures are not available, but the numbers of these operations performed annually appear to have leveled off.

Suprapubic minilaparotomy tubal ligation was the first outpatient female sterilization operation to be performed on a large scale. It was pioneered 30 years ago in Japan and Thailand and has since become firmly established as a major technique that is easily performed under local anesthesia.

American gynecologists took little initiative in the provision of female sterilization services until the introduction of the laparoscope from Europe in the early 1960s. The emergence of this technology coincided with a rising public demand, and outpatient laparoscopic procedures were then performed by Clifford Wheeless at Johns Hopkins, Frank Loffer and David Pent at the Phoenix Surgicenter, and Jaroslav Hulka at the University of North Carolina at Chapel Hill. Beginning in 1970, these men demonstrated that unipolar laparoscopic tubal coagulation procedures could be carried out in ambulatory surgical units mostly under local anesthesia.

During the past 20 years, in an effort to reduce the risks of burning bowel and other organs, safer methods have been introduced, including bipolar coagulation and the application of bands and clips.

The greatest advance in the safety of laparoscopic sterilization, however, was the adoption of the open entry technique of Harrith Hasson (3), thus eliminating the risk of needle and trocar injuries to bowel and major vessels. Chapters 7 and 8 describe how open laparoscopy and minilaparotomy have been adapted to a private office surgery.

FEMALE STERILIZATION PIONEERS

The concept of surgical sterilization has been in existence for about a century and a half. In 1842, James Blundell at Guy's Hospital in London suggested that "if you intercept the contact between the semen and the rudiments, you insure sterility. . . ." He advised that a portion of each tube be removed either at cesarean section or by interval suprapubic minilaparotomy. There is no record as to whether he actually performed the operation (4).

In 1880, Samuel Smith Lungren in Toledo, Ohio performed the first recorded tubal ligation in America, after a cesarean section. "It was the intention," writes Lungren, "first to remove both ovaries during the operation [an accepted sterilization method of the time] but decided, after mature consideration, that the risk would be lessened and the same result would be accomplished by tying both Fallopian tubes with strong silk ligatures about 1 inch from the uterus" (5). The operation was performed immediately after the patient's second cesarean section, not so much to satisfy the woman's wish of no more children but to protect her from the risk of a possible third cesarean section, which in the 19th century was a dangerous operation with a high incidence of mortality from hemorrhage or sepsis.

In fact, tubal sterilization was seldom countenanced by American obstetricians until the 1950s, when hospital sterilization committees, challenged by family planning advocates such as Guttmacher in Baltimore, Buxton in New Haven, and Barnes in Cleveland, began to accept indications other than grand multiparity or serious medical or psychiatric disorders.

Then, beginning in the early 1960s, came the flood of enthusiasm for both male and female sterilization. The reasons for increasing popularity of tubal ligation, varying in degree around the world, include the following:

1. The acceptance of the principle of small families (e.g., zero to three children);
2. The changing status of women, including a higher rate of employment of women away from home in industrialized societies and the desire of women for education and self-fulfillment;
3. Diminished need in developed nations to rely on children for work on the farm or for economic support of elderly family members;
4. Higher cost of living and higher costs of raising and educating children;
5. Greater requirement for job-related mobility for families in industrialized society;
6. Urban congestion followed by population control imposed externally or from within;
7. Diminishing tolerance for imperfect methods of birth control;
8. Increasing liberal attitudes of both the public and the medical profession, particularly gynecologists;
9. Improved safety, availability, and technology in the field of tubal sterilization.

This chapter deals principally with clarification of the last-listed reasons of safety, availability, and technology.

CURRENT METHODS

I briefly survey current proven techniques (Fig. 9.1), with emphasis on the increasing use of ambulatory facilities.

Laparoscopic Methods

These are most popular in technologically advanced nations. Single-incision techniques are particularly appropriate if laparoscopy is performed under local anesthesia. The open entry technique, developed by Hasson (3), which eliminates needle insufflation and trocar insertion, is a safer operation. In my opinion, it remains the entry method of choice in free-standing units where emergency laparotomy for repair of major vessel injuries may be impossible. In almost all cases, local anesthesia with premedication is entirely adequate for sterilization by open laparoscopy (see Chapter 7).

Unipolar Tubal Coagulation

This operation has been largely replaced by the safer bipolar method. With the unipolar technique, meticulous care is required to avoid bowel burns. In addition, the excessive amount of tubal destruction produced by unipolar coagulation markedly reduces success in later reconstructive efforts. However, the operation is singularly reliable, with a failure

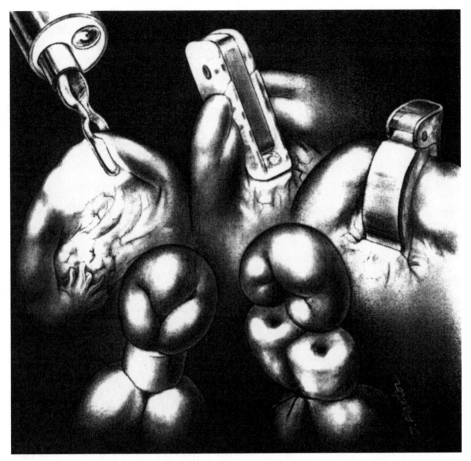

Figure 9.1. The five leading techniques of tubal sterilization. Reading clockwise from top left: Kleppinger bipolar coagulation, Hulka clip application, Filshie clip application, Pomeroy ligation, and Yoon band application.

rate lower than most other methods. Another advantage is that unipolar current is more effective than bipolar in coagulation of retracted bleeding vessels.

Bipolar Tubal Coagulation

A survey of 1,024 members of the American Association of Gynecological Laparoscopists (AAGL) concerning 1982 practice (6) revealed that the bipolar technique was the one most frequently used (64% of cases). This preference for bipolar coagulation has continued to the present time. In 1993, for example, a survey of AAGL membership showed that the incidence of bipolar coagulation had only dropped to 57% (7) (Table 9.1). In bipolar coagulation, an operation pioneered by Kleppinger (8) and Rioux (9), the region of isthmic destruction is largely confined to the tissues between the blades of the coagulating forceps. The electrical current does not depend on dissipation through body tissues to a ground plate. Rather, the current passes directly from one blade through the intervening tissue to the opposite blade and back through the intrinsic grounding of the

Table 9.1
Laparoscopic Sterilization Methods and Complications Requiring Laparotomy: Membership Survey by the American Association of Gynecologic Laparoscopists 1993

Method (%)	Closed or Open (%)	Anesthesia (%)	Complications (n)
Bipolar, 57			
Falope ring, 28	Closed, 92	General, 92	Diagnostic, 5
Hulka clip, 11	Open, 8	Local, 8	Sterilization, 1
Unipolar, 4			

From reference 7.

generator in a continuous circuit. Thus, organs lying close to the fallopian tubes are not threatened. Each tube should be coagulated in two or three adjacent isthmic locations, sparing the proximal 2 cm.

The continuing popularity of bipolar coagulation is due to three principal factors. First, it represents a natural transition from unipolar coagulation. Although the contained circuitry requires that generators be modified or replaced and bipolar instruments purchased, the precautions and techniques are basically unchanged. Second, it is the easiest method of laparoscopic sterilization to perform and to teach. Finally, there is an assumption among many gynecologists that a thorough coagulation of each tube provides a more reliable permanent closure than the application of mechanical rings or clips. However, there is no evidence to support this assumption. The fact that subsequent attempts at surgical reversal are less likely to succeed because a 2- or 3-cm length of each tube has been destroyed may have fostered the false assumption of greater reliability.

It is now well recognized that severing the tube after any form of coagulation, although it may reduce the chance of later recanalization, appears to actually increase the chance of subsequent tubal pregnancy. This is because a proximal tubal fistula is more likely to form, which allows the sperm to pass through into the peritoneal cavity. An ovum may be fertilized subsequently in either the ipsilateral or contralateral distal tubal stump.

The late Dr. Richard Kleppinger, who designed the most widely used bipolar forceps (Richard Wolf Co., Vernon Hills, IL), told me in conversation that he did not ordinarily coagulate the tubes of younger women, where there is a significant potential for later regret, but generally reserved this procedure for women over 30. He preferred the Hulka clip for younger women because this device obliterates a much shorter segment of tube, thus improving the potential for later reconstruction.

Hulka Clip

This carefully engineered device (10) is manufactured by the Richard Wolf Company. It is a lexan plastic clip with teeth on the inner surface of each jaw that fit into recesses in the opposite jaw. The clip is 3 mm in diameter and is held shut by a gold-plated stainless steel spring that is checked on the assembly line for a tension of 90 g. This spring is advanced forward into a locked position after the tube is grasped by the clip. Gradual obliteration of the tubal lumen occurs during the 48 hours after application of the clip. Thus, immediate severance of the tube, which would result in a high failure rate, is avoided. (For further details regarding proper application of the Hulka clip, see Chapter 7.)

Falope Ring

The Falope ring was invented by Im Bae Yoon of Johns Hopkins and is manufactured by KLI (Philadelphia, PA). It is a silastic rubber band that is loaded onto the inside of two cylinders and then fired by the outer cylinder of the applicator onto a knuckle of fallopian tube that has been drawn up into the inner cylinder by a pair of grasping tongs (11). If the band is applied under local anesthesia, such as 1% lidocaine, sprayed or injected, or 5% lidocaine jelly applied to the tubes, then cramps secondary to tubal ischemia are reduced or eliminated.

In contrast to the use of the Hulka clip, the application of the Yoon band or Falope ring destroys a 2- to 3-cm length of the tube. This makes it a less desirable method from the standpoint of possible later tubal reconstruction.

A thickened tube may require "milking" by the tongs before it can be drawn into the inner cylinder of the applicator. The tube may be severed accidentally during attempted application, in which case additional bands can be applied to the severed tubal ends. However, in expert hands, Falope ring application has proven to be as safe and effective as any other method.

The introduction of the Falope ring to practicing gynecologists in 1972 as the first effective mechanical device undoubtedly accounts for its more frequent use relative to the Hulka clip, which appeared on the market some 4 years later.

Filshie Clip

This device, a titanium-silicone-rubber clip which has been used in Britain and Europe for more than 15 years and more recently in Canada, was finally conditionally approved by the U.S. Food and Drug Administration in 1996. Full approval awaits the selection of a U.S. manufacturer. In the meantime, the British manufacturer, Femcare, is making arrangements for imports and distribution in the United States (C. Carrignan, personal communication, 1996). The Filshie clip promises to rival the Hulka clip in effectiveness. Filshie (12) reported on an initial series of 5,700 women sterilized by means of his clip. The first 540 British women were followed from 5 to 17 months. Among these, there was one method failure (an ectopic pregnancy) and two operator failures, resulting in intrauterine pregnancies.

Like the Hulka clip, the diameter of the Filshie clip is only 3 mm. Unlike the Hulka clip, which gradually obliterates the tubal lumen in 48 hours by means of spring tension, the silicone rubber lining the inner surface of each hinged jaw of the Filshie clip swells up within its locked jaws. Thus, the tubal lumen is gradually obliterated by a totally different mechanism. However, neither clip will sever the tube by immediate high compression.

It is claimed by some that the Filshie clip can more reliably encompass a thickened tube as, for example, in a postabortal patient. This supposed advantage over the Hulka clip has not been proven. Indeed, in my own practice, in postabortal cases I never had difficulty in fully grasping the tube with the Hulka clip for adequate closure. Occasionally, to be sure, I applied a second clip on one tube when I realized the first clip had been applied obliquely. If a thickened tube is encountered, I found that it is possible by gentle initial stretching, using the clip itself as a grasping forceps, to narrow its diameter slightly to better encompass the tube within the jaws of the clip.

Mechanical devices for tubal closure, including the clip and the band, are likely to gain in popularity because there is concern about the unnecessarily destructive procedure of tubal coagulation.

Minilaparotomy Tubal Ligation

This operation refers to bilateral tubal sterilization, usually by a Pomeroy-type tubal ligation but sometimes by clip or band application, through a small suprapubic incision. If the operation is done immediately after delivery, the incision should be higher, in the periumbical region. With premedication, the operation can be performed under local anesthesia. It is technically considerably more difficult in patients with lower abdominal obesity or intractable anxiety. Such patients may require general or conduction anesthesia or may be better served by a laparoscopic approach (see Chapter 8 for details regarding counseling and technique).

Minilaparotomy continues to be the leading operation for female sterilization in China because of the slow acquisition and cautious deployment of laparoscopic techniques. Minilaparotomy is almost the exclusive method of female sterilization in Bangladesh, where it is beginning to reduce the rate of population growth because of the successful continuing efforts of the Bangladesh Association for Voluntary Sterilization, funded in large part by the U.S. Agency for International Development (AID).

Minilaparotomy has been adapted to outpatient settings in the United States. Three such programs are illustrative.

Lee and Boyd (13) reported on 208 patients operated on under local anesthesia between 1976 and 1978 at Silas B. Hays Hospital, Fort Ord, California and at the Walter Reed Army Medical Center. Standard operating room equipment was used, and the average operating time was 31.8 minutes. The authors point out that lower abdominal obesity and fixed uterine retroversion are relative contraindications.

In 1978, Planned Parenthood of Baltimore, Maryland under the leadership of Frances Trimble, Medical Director, established a minilaparotomy tubal ligation service modeled after a previously initiated Planned Parenthood program in Nashville, Tennessee. In April 1985, I had the privilege of visiting the center in Baltimore and observing minilaparotomy operations performed by Courtland Robinson and his nursing staff. All patients were scheduled for surgery in the first one half of the menstrual cycle to avoid luteal phase pregnancies and all patients had fasted for the preceding 8 to 12 hours. Atropine, diazepam, and fentanyl were injected intravenously, and 1% Xylocaine without epinephrine was used for local infiltration. It was clear that without a vasoconstrictor, there was a slight delay in controlling bleeding from the incision. This minor inconvenience was counterbalanced by the assurance that no rebound bleeding would occur postoperatively. A modified Pomeroy ligation procedure was carried out, and each patient rested for 1 hour in reclining outdoor-type lounge chairs before going home.

This program was gradually phased out in the early 1980s because of the preference of practicing gynecologists for laparoscopic sterilization. The current Medical Director, Paul Blumenthal, is planning to initiate a Falope ring sterilization service at the Baltimore Planned Parenthood Center within the next year (P. Blumenthal, personal communication, 1996).

In 1979, 1 year after the initiation of the Baltimore service, Planned Parenthood of New York City launched a carefully planned minilaparotomy clinic in the Margaret Sanger Center under the leadership of Enayat Hakim-Elahi, Medical Director, and Al Moran, Executive Director. Over 200 operations were performed. However, the requirement of standby anesthesia and ambulance services presented cost feasibility problems that led to suspension of the clinic.

Although there were positive responses from each community, the experiences of these three innovative programs illustrate some procedural limitations and pitfalls.

OUTPATIENT, FREE-STANDING FEMALE STERILIZATION SERVICES IN THE UNITED STATES

Despite the demonstrated feasibility of the simpler, less costly service of minilaparotomy both in the United States and throughout the world, the more elegant and universally applicable laparoscopic approach is far more popular in most technologically advanced centers worldwide.

The enormous bias in favor of general anesthesia for outpatient as well as inpatient laparoscopic sterilization in the United States can be explained at least in part by the fact that most gynecologists ask their patients which anesthetic they would prefer. When given the choice, anxious patients frequently opt for what they assume to be the more pain-free alternative, without consideration of the greater risk and postoperative discomforts associated with general anesthesia. As discussed more fully in Chapter 1, most gynecologists receive little or no residency training in the use of local anesthesia and therefore are likely to be less enthusiastic about it.

It has been our experience in Syracuse that the substitution of open laparoscopy under local anesthesia without general anesthesia standby is a safe and satisfactory alternative. Open laparoscopy for outpatient sterilization was also favored by Dr. Shaio-Yu Lee in Boston. During the past 20 years at the Brookline Pre-Term Clinic, Dr. Lee used the open entry technique in over 6,000 consecutive cases. Ten patients were scheduled every other Wednesday. In 10 to 15% of these patients, the procedure was performed immediately after first trimester surgical abortion. Preoperative Fentanyl, 0.075 mg, and Valium, 5 mg, was given intravenously, and the abdominal wall was infiltrated with 20 mL of 0.5% Xylocaine. Carbon dioxide was insufflated after insertion of the abdominal cannula, and the tubes were injected with 2% Xylocaine before bipolar coagulation. No serious complications occurred. Currently, all insurance carriers, including Massachusetts Health (which handles Medicaid), are paying the full fee of $1,200 minus a small copayment in some cases (C. Damaro, personal communication, 1996).

Pre-Term in Boston began offering contraceptive services and pregnancy terminations 20 years ago. After the murder of a staff worker by an abortion protestor at the Boston Planned Parenthood in December 1995, the two women's surgical services joined together to form one of the leading programs in North America. Maximum security systems were installed, and an armed guard screens every visitor and patient for proper identification. Patients receive expert counseling. Transvaginal sonography is available to rule out abnormalities in any patient and to guide procedures when indicated. Thirty to 50 early terminations are carried out under local anesthesia 6 days a week. Dr. Mary Briggs is continuing the sterilization service initiated by Dr. Lee. Presently, Dr. Briggs performs open laparoscopy and bipolar tubal coagulation under local anesthesia with video monitoring (A. Osborne, personal interview, 1996).

A fourth clinician who continues to be well pleased with open laparoscopy under local anesthesia in the office setting is Fred Schnepper of Chula Vista, California. He has reported this year on his experience with 813 cases operated between December 1979 and September 1996. In 811, the procedure was successfully completed. There were only two failed laparoscopies, one because of extreme obesity and one because of extensive small bowel adhesions. There were no major complications, and no patients required hospitalization. Equally satisfactory results were obtained with bipolar coagulation, the Hulka Clip, and the silastic band (14).

LESSONS FROM ABROAD: LAPAROSCOPY IN DEVELOPING NATIONS

This section examines four established programs (15). How successful have they been? What lessons may we learn from them?

Dr. Kanti Giri, working out of Kathmandu, Nepal, developed a team of surgeons in the early 1970s who set up rural laparoscopic coagulation camps in Nepal where as many as 92 female sterilizations were performed in 1 day.

In the mid–1970s, Dr. Virgilio Oblepias of Manila organized Tilamsick ("spark" or "spatter") projects in which a team of doctors and nurses loaded their equipment into trucks and traveled to remote villages where one to three surgeons carried out 80 to 100 laparoscopies a day in assembly-line style. Dr. Oblepias found that the laprocator, a low-cost single-incision silastic-band applicator, was a useful instrument. His patients preferred laparoscopy to minilaparotomy because the procedure was faster, the recovery was faster, and the wound was smaller (21). Unfortunately, the Philippine sterilization program was severely curtailed during the administration of Corazon Aquino because of insufficient government funding, but recent reports indicate that it is flourishing once again (C. Carrignan, personal communication, 1996).

Dr. Rohit Bhatt of Baroda, India organized laprocator camps between January and March 1979 in the state of Gujarat. One surgeon, three residents, and one nurse performed 80 to 100 operations a day. A total of 5,287 procedures were performed. Patients were sedated with 100 mg intramuscular oxycodone and 10 mg diazepam. Atropine, 0.6 mg, was also injected preoperatively. Complications included 54 uterine perforations, 15 tubal transections, and 5 mesosalpingeal bleeders. No laparotomies were required; no deaths were recorded (16).

Two principal problems threaten these efforts to provide mass sterilization to the exploding population in India. The first and most ominous problem is the increase in hepatitis and human immunodeficiency virus infections from postsurgical infection and multiple sexual contacts. The second problem is the difficulty in establishing reliable equipment maintenance centers, an effort largely supervised by Johns Hopkins Program for International Education in Gynecology and Obstetrics (JHPIEGO) (C. Carrignan, personal communication, 1996).

Dr. Arunee Fongsri in Chiang Mai, North Thailand during the late 1970s would gather her laparoscopic coagulation equipment together and "set up shop" in a hill-tribe village for 2 or 3 days to perform 20 or 30 sterilization operations under local anesthesia (17).

The success of these four representative programs was due to the enthusiasm, energy, and skills of the surgeons and nurses, as well as to harmonious teamwork with paraprofessionals. The projects would not have been conceived without initiation by the Association for Voluntary Sterilization in New York and the JHPIEGO nor implemented without funding provided by U.S. AID (18).

Efforts such as the above have served as inspirational pilot projects that have generated ongoing local government sponsorship of desperately needed sterilization services. Unfortunately, many such projects are set up for a day or two and then vanish. Facilities are only marginally adequate. Postoperative complications go unrecorded and frequently untreated.

What happens, on the other hand, when physicians from rural areas are trained in laparoscopy and return to their local centers with high technology equipment? The experience in Thailand is of interest.

Dr. Kamheang Chaturachinda of Bangkok analyzed the results of the distribution and use of large numbers of U.S.-funded laparoscopes throughout Thailand; 10,000 cases of laparoscopic sterilization performed between 1974 and 1977 were reviewed. Depending on the skills of individual surgeons, wide variations in the incidence of major complications were noted, from 1 in 3,500 cases in the North to 1 in 100 cases in the Northeast. These complications included bowel burns, bleeding requiring laparotomy, major vessel injuries, and death. Four patients died, two from peritonitis secondary to bowel burns, one from a trocar injury to a major vessel, and one from cardiac arrest after bolus injection of meperidine and diazepam (19).

However, Dr. Chaturachinda's severest criticism of this effort emerged from his discovery that continued use of the laparoscopes was astonishingly low. In a typical rural center, nine procedures would be performed per month. By 1977, 40% of the physicians who had initially trained in a 3-week course at Ramathibodi Hospital had dropped out of the program. The three main reasons cited by Dr. Chaturachinda were that they encountered a life-threatening complication, they were promoted to a higher administrative position, and they experienced malfunction of equipment. The equipment maintenance problem was only partially relieved by establishing a maintenance center in Bangkok. Dr. Chaturachinda concluded that for reasons of safety and cost, minilaparotomy makes far more sense in rural areas of developing countries. He looks forward to the day when Thailand can support its own programs of sterilization. He estimates that the cost of laparoscopy versus minilaparotomy technologies is 18 to 1 (20).

I believe that modern laparoscopic methods may in the future have a continuing impact in rural areas of developing countries only if they are set up in properly equipped hospitals or clinics. Facilities such as these are at present mostly restricted to urban areas. Such services, whether urban or rural, will flourish over the long run only if there is strong leadership with minimal government direction, dedicated surgeons and nursing personnel, and a stable consistent time schedule.

The sterilization center under Dr. Oblepias at the Mary Johnston Hospital in Manila is a good example of a flourishing urban facility. The sterilization unit under Dr. Arunee Fongsri at the Christian Medical Clinic in Chiang Mai, Thailand did provide high quality minilaparotomy and laparoscopy services while it operated. These two units, however, have been unable to adequately serve the far-flung rural areas of their countries. Neither the Philippine nor the Thai governments have provided sufficient transportation to bring large numbers of rural patients into these centers and to return them to their homes. Both Dr. Oblepias and Dr. Fongsri have attempted to meet the rural need by taking their equipment with them and setting up sterilization clinics. These makeshift assembly-line services are gallant attempts to meet the rural need. However, they cannot provide optimum care and emergency backup, and satisfactory postoperative follow-up is impossible. Insofar as laparoscopy is concerned, makeshift sterilization clinics are extremely vulnerable to equipment breakdown. Accidents, delays, and suffering resulting from such deficiencies would most certainly discourage potential patients.

Until developing nations choose to build well-equipped clinics or hospitals in rural areas, sterilization needs are probably better met by minilaparotomy centers such as those established by the Bangladesh Association for Voluntary Sterilization. In the meantime, those women who because of obesity or pelvic pathology are unsuitable candidates for minilaparotomy could be transported to urban laparoscopy centers by bus.

During the years of waiting for adequate rural sterilization services, Depo-Provera (medroxyprogesterone, Upjohn) programs should be further expanded in developing countries. These are highly successful programs in which large groups of fertile women, sometimes whole villages in a day, receive intramuscular injections of Depo-Provera, 150 mg every 3 months, to ensure reliable contraception until sterilization services become available.

OTHER METHODS OF TUBAL STERILIZATION

This review has shown that laparoscopy and minilaparotomy are firmly established as the two major approaches worldwide to female sterilization. Vaginal approaches never gained wide acceptance, although they are practiced in a skillful manner by a number of leaders in the field.

Vaginal Tubal Ligation

Brown and Schanzer (21) in San Antonio, Texas reported on an active ambulatory vaginal tubal ligation program using premedication and local anesthesia. They do not believe that limited visibility, immediate postoperative coital discomfort, and the occasional vaginal vault infection constitute significant drawbacks.

Hartfield (22) in New Zealand reported on 485 patients sterilized under local anesthesia by the vaginal route. With the flat retractor placed along the posterior vaginal wall into the pouch of Douglas, each tube was grasped with long artery forceps and 2 mL 0.5% bupivacaine was injected into the tubal wall and mesosalpinx. Each of the four leading mechanical methods of tubal sterilization were used with essentially equal success. These methods were the Pomeroy in 173, the Falope ring in 135, the Hulka clip in 91, and the Filshie clip in 86. Routine prophylactic antibiotics were not given. Postoperative mild pelvic infection occurred most frequently in the Pomeroy cases (2.8%), probably because of greater manipulation, but also in 1.4% of the Falope ring cases. No postoperative infection occurred in the Hulka or Filshie clip patients.

The vaginal route may be the one of choice in the obese patient. The major contraindications are the presence of dense pelvic adhesions or significant uterine enlargement.

Culdoscopic Tubal Ligation

Wynter (23) reported on 1,138 cases of culdoscopic tubal ligations under local anesthesia in Kingston, Jamaica. Some authorities were concerned with adnexal adhesions or postoperative vault infection in some patients (24). Nonetheless, Wynter has performed an invaluable service for the women of the West Indies.

Interest in culdoscopy, however, has rapidly waned worldwide because of the advent of laparoscopy and its ability to provide a far better panoramic view of both pelvic and abdominal contents (see Chapter 10).

Laparoscopic Tubal Thermocautery

Valle and Battifora (25) and Valle (26) reported on their laparoscopic technique of "shielded thermocautery." In this operation, thermal coagulation of the fallopian tube is accomplished by means of a thermocautery hook that retracts the tube into a Teflon cannula. Great safety is claimed because of the absence of electrical current. Although 570 patients have been reported, with 100 followed for more than 3 years without a pregnancy, the technique is not widely accepted. One drawback is the large secondary incision required to introduce the Teflon cannula.

Transcervical Methods

Transcervical methods of female sterilization are theoretically attractive because they avoid abdominal incisions. They are all presently experimental in nature, however, and none have achieved the uniformly high success rate of laparoscopic and minilaparotomy methods. Nonetheless, these transcervical methods may be refined in the future for possible use by paraprofessionals in countries with serious problems of overpopulation. Among the methods of transcervical sterilization are the following:

1. "Blind" injection of phenol mucilage into the tubes. Chinese physicians claim a 99% rate of bilateral occlusion after 3 months. This is the highest reported success rate of any of the transcervical methods.
2. Hysteroscopically directed injection of catalyzed liquid silicone into the fallopian tubes (27). This method requires great technical skill and is inappropriate in 15 to 20% of women. Reversibility has not been demonstrated.
3. Introduction of a tissue adhesive, methylcyanoacrylate, through a specially designed device to occlude the tubes (28). Clinical experience has been insufficient to determine success rate.
4. Introduction transcervically of quinacrine pellets or quinacrine-tipped intrauterine devices to expose the tubal lumina to this cytotoxic agent, which causes focal epithelial necrosis (29).

What is the current status of these methods? Liquid silicone and methylcyanoacrylate have been abandoned because of technical problems and high failure rates. Quinacrine as a chemical tubal cauterant is no longer used because of reports of carcinogenicity in animals, and there have been no further reports from China on the effectiveness of intrauterine phenolmucilage (C. Carrignan, personal communication, 1996).

SPECIAL CONSIDERATIONS

Community need must be carefully assessed and local health department regulations must be reviewed. The gynecologist must objectively evaluate his or her own skills and enthusiasm for outpatient surgery. The desirability of peer review and certification must be analyzed, particularly in relation to reimbursement of facility costs by insurance carriers. Details of informed consent are of the utmost importance (30). Sound judgment should be exercised in the exploration of risks with the patient in a nonthreatening manner.

The outpatient facility must have laparotomy capabilities if closed laparoscopy is to be performed. Disaster preparedness and periodic recertification of the gynecologist and his or her nursing staff in cardiopulmonary resuscitation are essential precautions.

An up-to-date detailed discussion of certification and reimbursement is found in Chapter 13 by Dr. Paul Allen.

LEGAL STATUS OF FEMALE STERILIZATION

In the United States, voluntary sterilization is legal in all 50 states, even though fewer than a dozen have specific statutes dealing with sterilization. The legality of voluntary sterilization has been confirmed during the 1970s by court decision, by opinions of State Attorneys-General, by the inclusion of sterilization services in state-funded health care services and by the existence of numerous statutory regulations of the operation, all of which presupposes its legality. (7)

However, when federal funds are used to pay for sterilization, prohibitions exist for minor and mentally incompetent patients. Sterilization regulations enacted by the U.S. Department of Health, Education, and Welfare in 1979 include the following requirements when federal funds are used. These requirements remain unchanged to the present day:

1. Approved consent form detailing alternatives;
2. A 30-day wait between consent and sterilization;
3. Consent not acceptable if patient is seeking abortion;
4. Patient must not be under 21, mentally incompetent, or in a correctional institution;
5. Hysterectomy may not be selected as the method of sterilization if that is the principal reason for its performance.

Even when federal funds are not involved, many hospitals enforce similar regulations that practically prohibit the availability of sterilization to mentally incompetent individuals. Protracted court requirements, court orders, and 30-day waiting periods required to contest such court orders represent obstacles and delaying tactics on the part of some hospital administrators to rid themselves of this problem and its possible legal consequences. When mentally incompetent patients can cooperate for examination, however, sterilization procedures may be safely and conveniently performed under local anesthesia in private outpatient surgical units. My own practice is to insist that our patients have at least a partial understanding of the procedure. We require that an informed consent document be signed by the patient as well as by a parent or guardian of the patient.

By protecting a mentally incompetent woman from pregnancy by sterilization reduces the anxiety by her parents that she will be taken advantage of and produce a child that she cannot take care of.

PREGNANCY RATES AFTER STERILIZATION

Peterson et al. (31) reported on the risk of pregnancy after tubal sterilization. They presented a multicenter U.S. study of 10,685 women followed for 8 to 14 years after surgery. Methods used, in descending order of frequency, were the Falope ring (3,329), bipolar coagulation (2,267), postpartum partial salpingectomy (1,637), the spring clip (1,595), unipolar coagulation (1,432), and interval partial salpingectomy (425).

The overall pregnancy rate 10 years after sterilization was 1.8%. The highest incidence of failure occurred after spring clip and bipolar cases, probably largely on the basis of faulty technique or inadequate coagulation. In the case of the clip, the tube must be stretched out before application and the device must fully encompass the tube at right angles.

PREDICTIONS FOR THE FUTURE

In general, screening of candidates for sterilization will improve. Increasing knowledge of factors that predispose to patient regret will diminish abuse of this most valuable technique of fertility control. The shift toward mechanical methods of tubal closure will continue; use of the Hulka and Filshie clip will increase to equal or surpass use of the Falope ring.

The number of free-standing and office surgery settings for performing female sterilization as an outpatient procedure will slowly but steadily increase. Because of lower cost and reduced requirements for specialized surgical skills, some of these services will concentrate on suprapubic minilaparotomy, but laparoscopy will continue to be overwhelmingly favored where the technology and skills are available. There may be a gradual shift toward open rather than closed laparoscopy as the preferred technique of entry in outpatient surgeries.

Innovations in female sterilization are reaching a plateau. Vaginal tubal ligation methods will continue to have a small number of proponents. Hysteroscopic introduction of silicone tubal implants and transcervical injection of methylcyanoacrylate, quinacrine, and phenol mucilage are experimental methods that will continue to reflect an ongoing if thus far unsuccessful effort to improve effectiveness and simplicity.

CONCLUSION

Elective female sterilization in the United States has become the most popular method of birth control after the woman reaches the age of 35 or after her family is complete. Since 1970, American women in increasing numbers have had their fallopian tubes coagulated, banded, clipped, or ligated. In the foreseeable future, there will be a marked decline in the introduction of new techniques. However, there will be a better understanding of current practices, with increasing use of mechanical methods, open laparoscopy, local anesthesia, and outpatient surgical settings.

REFERENCES

1. Peterson HB, Lubell I. Sterilization: a worldwide epidemiologic view. In: vanLith DAF, Keith LG, vanHall EV, eds. New trends in female sterilization. Chicago, IL: Year Book Medical Publishers, Inc., 1983.
2. Penfield AJ. 1 and 2: Trends in sterilization: the American experience. In: vanLith DAF, Keith LG, vanHall EV, eds. New trends in female sterilization. Chicago, IL: Year Book Medical Publishers, Inc., 1983.
3. Hasson HM. Open laparoscopy vs. closed laparoscopy: a comparison of complication rates. Adv. Planned Parenthood 1978;13:41.
4. Siegler A, Grunebaum A. Endoscopic female sterilization. Santa Fe Springs, CA: The American Association of Gynecologic Laparoscopists, 1983.
5. Lungren SS. A case of caesarian section twice successfully performed on the same patient. Am J Obstet 1881;14:78.
6. Phillips JM, Hulka JF, Hulka B, Cates D, Keith L. American Association of Gynecologic Laparoscopists, 1976 Membership Survey. J Reprod Med 1978;21:3–6.
7. Hulka JF, Phillips JM, Peterson HB, et al. Laparoscopic sterilization: American Association of Gynecologic Laparoscopists 1993 membership survey. J Am Assoc Gynecol Laparosc 1995;2:137–138.
8. Kleppinger RK. Female outpatient sterilization using bipolar coagulation. University of Sydney: Bulletin of the Post-Graduate Committee in Medicine, 1977:144–154.
9. Rioux JE. Sterilization of women: benefits vs. risks. Int Gynecol Obstet 1979;16:488.
10. Hulka JF. Spring clip sterilization. In: Textbook of laparoscopy. New York: Grune and Stratton, 1985.
11. Yoon IB, Poliakoff SR. Laparoscopic tubal ligation: a follow-up report on the Yoon ring methodology. J Reprod Med 1979;23:76.
12. Filshie GM. The titanium/silicone rubber clip for female sterilization. Br J Obstet Gynaecol 1981; 88:655–662.
13. Lee RB, Boyd JAK. Minilaparotomy under local anesthesia for outpatient sterilization: a preliminary report. Fertil Steril 1980;33:129–134.
14. Schnepper F. Sterilization by open laparoscopy in a private office. J Am Assoc Gynecol Laparosc (in press).

15. Penfield AJ. Laparoscopy in rural areas of developing countries. Presented to the Science Committee, Association for Voluntary Association, New York, January 1983.
16. Oblepias V, Bhatt R. Country reports. In: Burkman RT, Magarich RH, Waife RS, eds. Surgical equipment and training in reproductive health. Baltimore, MD: Johns Hopkins Program for International Education in Gynecology and Obstetrics, 1980.
17. Fongsri A. Viewpoints of physicians from around the world. In: Penfield AJ, ed. Female sterilization by minilaparotomy or open laparoscopy. Baltimore, MD: Urban & Schwarzenberg, 1980.
18. Ravenholt RT, Wiley AT, Glenn DN, Speidel JJ. The use of surgical laparoscopy for fertility management overseas. In: Phillips JM, ed. Endoscopy in gynecology. Downey, CA: American Association of Gynecologic Laparoscopists, 1978.
19. Chaturachinda K. The use of the laparoscope in rural Thailand. J Gynaecol Obstet 1980;18:414–419.
20. Chaturachinda, K. Viewpoints of physicians from around the world. In Penfield, A. J (ed) Female Sterilization by Minilaparotomy or Open Laparoscopy, Urban & Schwarzenberg, Baltimore, MD, 1980.
21. Brown HP, Schanzer SN. Female sterilization: an overview with emphasis on the vaginal route and the organization of a sterilization program. Littleton, MA: John Wright, PSG Inc., 1980.
22. Hartfield VJ. Female sterilization by the vaginal route: a positive reassessment and comparison of four tubal occlusion methods. Aust N Z J Obstet Gynaecol 1993;33:408–412.
23. Wynter H. The development of outpatient culdoscopic sterilization in Jamaica. Kingston, Jamaica: University of the West Indies, 1977.
24. Koetsawang S, Bhiraleus P, Rachawat D, Kiriwat O. Comparison of culdoscopic and laparoscopic tubal sterilization. Am J Obstet Gynecol 1976;124:601.
25. Valle RF, Battifora HA. A new approach to tubal sterilization by laparoscopy. Fertil Steril 1978;30:415–422.
26. Valle RF. Laparoscopic tubal sterilization by shielded thermocautery 1980. Read before the American Association of Gynecological Laparoscopists (AAGL) International Congress on Female Endoscopic Sterilization, Williamsburg, Virginia, July 21, 1980.
27. Reed TP, Erb RA, deMaeyer J. Tubal occlusion with silicone rubber: update 1980. J Reprod Med 1981;26:534–537.
28. Neuwirth RS, Richart RM, Stevenson T, et al. An outpatient approach to female sterilization with methylcyanoacrylate. Am J Obstet Gynecol 1980;136:951–953.
29. Goldsmith A, Laufe LE, King TM. Discussion: Research and clinical experience with quinacrine. In: Zatuchni GI, Sheton JD, Goldsmith A, Sciarra JJ, eds. Female transcervical sterilization (PARFR series on fertility regulation). Philadelphia, PA: Harper and Row, 1983.
30. Gonzales BL. Counseling for sterilization. J Reprod Med 1981;26:538–540.
31. Peterson HB, Xia Z, Hughes J, et al. The risk of pregnancy after tubal sterilization: findings from the U.S. Collaborative Review of sterilization. Am J Obstet Gynecol 1996;174:1161–1170.

10. *Additional Gynecologic Operations Under Local Anesthesia*

A. JEFFERSON PENFIELD

In addition to uterine curettage, operative abortion, hysteroscopic procedures, laparoscopy for sterilization or diagnosis, and minilaparotomy tubal ligation, a large number of gynecologic procedures can be readily performed under local anesthesia. For the gynecologist with the necessary skills, equipment, and support staff, these operations are adaptable to the office surgery with safety, convenience, and economy. Indeed, the feature of increased safety of local versus general anesthesia should be emphasized to each patient, and the more rapid and comfortable recovery after the use of local anesthesia should be stressed. Only in exceptional situations should general anesthesia be necessary. These situations include unmanageable apprehension or severe mental retardation in a hyperactive or uncooperative patient.

In the outpatient operating room, standing floor or wall-mounted spotlights are preferred over large glaring ceiling lights. Some gynecologists prefer headlights, but everyone else is in the dark each time the surgeon looks away, thus diminishing their usefulness. A portable battery-powered flashlight must always be ready, and one of the staff should be assigned to check its proper functioning at least once each month. It is useful to have an adjustable operating table equipped with adjustable padded knee stirrups to allow the patient to relax completely during the procedure. The dimensions of the operating room should be a minimum of 10 by 15 feet, about one and a half times the size of an average examining room. If the room is too small, support personnel are crowded, the patient may feel claustrophobic, and surgical contamination is more likely.

Small-caliber hypodermic needles should be used for injection of local anesthetic solutions. I found 24- or 25-gauge needles satisfactory for infiltration, but 30-gauge needles are better for certain procedures, such as anesthetizing the hymen or the dome of an exquisitely sensitive Bartholin duct abscess. For most operations, the patient should feel only one or two injections because it should be possible to administer all additional anesthetic through previously anesthetized regions.

Although chloroprocaine or mepivacaine are favored by some gynecologists for their prolonged duration of action, I continue to prefer 0.5% lidocaine with 1:200,000 epinephrine because of its unmatched safety record and superior spreading characteristics. The epinephrine produces a relatively bloodless operating field and retards systemic absorption of the anesthetic agent. Lidocaine without epinephrine should be substituted if the patient is hypertensive.

Knowledgeable assistants should be skilled in providing gentle traction to maximize exposure. Meticulous hemostasis is of particular importance because excessive sponging and searching for retracted vessels are poorly tolerated by the awake patient.

An unusually apprehensive patient will benefit from diazepam or midazolam, 5 to 10 mg given intravenously preoperatively, preceded by an initial test dose of 1 mg. An analgesic anticholinergic combination such as 1 mg butorphanol and 15 mg promethazine may then be given from a second syringe. These medications are particularly effective before the incision, drainage, and packing of abscesses that may be extremely tender. In general, however, preoperative medications are unnecessary for any other operation described in this chapter.

VULVAR AND VAGINAL BIOPSIES

Single or multiple excisional biopsies of condylomata, polyps, nevi, or small cysts of the vulva or vagina are easily accomplished under local anesthesia. For each lesion, the patient should feel no more than one or two needle pricks. Within 1 minute of the injection of the anesthetic, the tumor may be elevated by an Allis clamp or thumb forceps and excised with a wide margin of surrounding skin or mucosa by means of a scalpel or curved Metzenbaum-type scissors. Fine polyglycolate sutures are recommended for skin or mucosal closure because they are gradually hydrolyzed, cause virtually no tissue reaction, and do not require removal.

INCISION AND DRAINAGE OF VULVAR OR SMALL VAGINAL ABSCESSES

Because anesthetizing the dome of an abscess further increases existing tissue fluid tension and causes a sharp momentary increase in the already existing pain, the patient may benefit from a preoperative intravenous analgesic such as butorphanol or meperidine.

After a gentle wash with povidone-iodine solution, a small amount of anesthetic solution is injected through a 30-gauge hypodermic needle into the thin layer of skin or mucous membrane covering an abscess that has previously failed to drain despite repeated hot soaks.

The tissues surrounding the abscess should also be anesthetized, with great care being taken to avoid entering the abscess cavity. Antibiotics are unnecessary in these cases because the infection is already well localized. After waiting 1 to 2 minutes, the abscess is lanced with a pointed scalpel blade, and the incision in the dome is enlarged as appropriate. If the patient has had several recent abscesses in the same location, a complete blood count and a 2-hour postprandial blood sugar level should be obtained to rule out anemia, inappropriate white cell responses, and diabetes mellitus. The pus from a recurring abscess should be sent immediately to the laboratory for culture and antibiotic sensitivities.

Deep abscess cavities may require packing with iodoform gauze to prevent roofing over and recurrent suppuration. The pack should be removed in 3 to 5 days if it has not already dropped out during the course of postoperative sitz baths.

Suburethral abscesses must be approached with great caution because they may indeed be infected urethral diverticulae. Preoperative urethroscopy may be indicated in such cases.

INCISION AND DRAINAGE OF BARTHOLIN DUCT CYST OR ABSCESS FOLLOWED BY MARSUPIALIZATION OR INSERTION OF A WORD CATHETER

A recurrent or enlarging Bartholin duct cyst, whether infected or not, may require incision, drainage, marsupialization, and packing. A patient with this condition may come in to the office in severe pain, exhausted from several sleepless nights and repeated unsuccessful attempts at spontaneous drainage by means of hot baths. This patient should receive preoperative intravenous medications, including an analgesic such as meperidine, fentanyl or butorphanol and a calming agent such as diazepam or midazolam.

Extreme gentleness must be exercised in anesthetizing the dome and the surrounding tissues of a Bartholin abscess (Fig. 10.1). After a 1-minute delay to allow a full anesthetic effect, an ellipse of skin near the mucocutaneous junction and above the site of maximal fluctuance should be incised with a scalpel blade and the abscess cavity entered along one margin of the incision. The instant relief of pain after drainage is spectacular. Before the

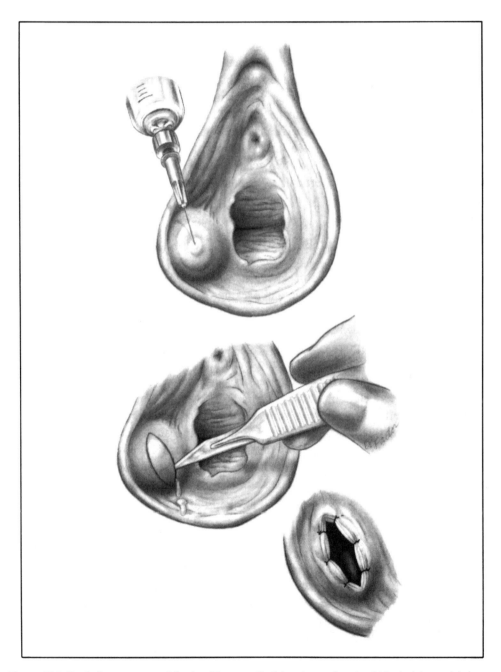

Figure 10.1. Bartholin cyst marsupialization. Top, anesthetizing dome of cyst; middle, incision and drainage; bottom, cyst wall sutured to skin.

landmarks are lost, the ellipse of skin and underlying abscess capsule should be excised. The margins of skin and capsule may be grasped with Allis clamps, and the surgeon's fingertip should be gently inserted to explore the cavity and break down any septa within. Four to six fine polyglycolate sutures are placed about the perimeter to stitch capsule to skin, and the cavity is packed with iodoform gauze. After 1 hour's rest, the patient returns home and takes nightly sitz baths. After 1 week, she returns to the office, and the packing is replaced with a smaller drain that is left in place for another 3 to 5 days. Further packing is usually unnecessary because sufficient healing has occurred to prevent agglutination of the incisional edges.

If these precautions are not taken, abscesses are likely to roof over prematurely and require secondary drainage. The patient is allowed to perform her normal activities (with the exception of sexual intercourse) while the pack is in place, and she will experience only a fraction of the discomfort present before the operation.

A highly satisfactory alternative to marsupialization is the introduction of a Word catheter that is left in place for 10 to 14 days during which time spontaneous re-epithelialization of the drainage tract takes place.

PLASTIC SURGERY OF THE VULVA, VAGINA, OR PERINEUM

Once the skills of operating under local anesthesia are learned, a remarkable number of plastic surgery operations may be easily performed in an office setting.

Excision of Redundant Tissue of Labia Minora

Not infrequently, hypertrophy of either or both minor labia may occur, and this redundant tissue may develop into a constant source of discomfort to the patient. Because these tissues are extremely vascular and composed of loose skin and frequent infoldings, great care must be taken in preoperative skin cleansing and disinfection. The enveloping skin must be stretched out by an assistant as local anesthetic solution is injected proximal to the proposed line of excision. The surgeon must be careful to excise the redundant tag along natural skin lines to minimize scarring during healing. He or she must also be cautious not to excise too much tissue, which may result in scarring, stricture, and resultant dyspareunia. Large tags must be cut away in small steps after proximal clamping to reduce the possibility of postoperative bleeding from the highly vascular stroma. Deep hemostatic mattress sutures may be placed in areas of brisk oozing, and the skin may be closed with fine polyglycolate sutures. The patient should be able to leave the office within 1 hour of surgery, and she will probably benefit from the application of ice packs for 1 hour upon her return home.

Incision of an Imperforate Hymen

The bulge of a distended hymen in an amenorrheic young woman is diagnostic, and a second bulge into the anterior rectal wall felt by the examining finger is further evidence of cryptomenorrhea. An associated uterine enlargement from a hematometra may also be present. After a povidone-iodine wash, anesthetic solution may be injected with extreme gentleness into the hymen and bordering tissue through a 30-gauge hypodermic needle. Central puncture and cruciate incisions will release the dark chocolate blood, and spontaneous evacuation of the hematometra will occur.

Incision of a Tight or Rigid Hymen

In the United States, where most teenage girls routinely insert menstrual tampons, few complain of intact hymens. For the woman who has never used intravaginal protection and who has never had sexual intercourse, it is appropriate to recommend that she stretch her own hymen every evening in the bath for 1 month, first with one finger, then with two, each time to the point of causing some discomfort. She should be advised that this maneuver is likely to result in a small amount of bleeding. Hymeneal dilatations are recommended either to facilitate pelvic examination or to prepare her for intercourse. Occasionally, if a woman refuses to stretch her own hymen or in the rather rare presence of a thick rigid hymen, cruciate incisions may be made readily under local anesthesia. In these cases, 5% Xylocaine jelly is of little benefit; any anesthetic effect produced is too superficial. What is required is the very gentle, meticulous, radial injection of the local anesthetic such as 0.5% lidocaine with 1:200,000 epinephrine to the lateral margins of the hymen by means of a 30-gauge hypodermic needle. Bleeding caused by the incisions is rarely troublesome. Clamping and suturing small arterial bleeders with fine polyglycolate or catgut suture may be necessary.

Reverse Perineorrhaphy

Some women complain of dyspareunia caused by a band of scar tissue across the posterior fourchette, or the entire introitus may have been artificially narrowed by an overly constrictive midline episiotomy repair. Complaints from these conditions may be made within a few weeks after delivery or may not surface until after the menopause, when the narrowing is more pronounced as the result of hypoestrogenic atrophy.

The older woman may obtain sufficient relief by the use of estrogen vaginal cream. The younger woman may cure her dyspareunia with graduated dilators. In either case, preliminary investigations and management of possible psychosexual problems must be undertaken before any attempt at surgical correction. If it is concluded that surgery is necessary, a vertical incision under local anesthesia through the scarred area, as with an episiotomy, followed by a transverse closure of the opening results in an enlarged introital diameter.

Excision of Vaginal Septum

Anterior-posterior vaginal septa of varying thicknesses are frequently seen. They may first be suspected by young women because of difficulty in inserting or removing tampons. With narrow septa, local anesthetic solution is injected into each end. Then an incision is made through the narrowest portion of the septal column, followed by tying off and excising the remaining tags. Larger septa that create a partial or complete double vagina should be excised under general or conduction anesthesia, because surgical correction in these cases requires much more extensive dissection and suturing.

SUTURE LIGATION OF CERVICAL OR VAGINAL BLEEDERS

Occasionally, the cervix will bleed heavily either right after or even many days after a biopsy or laceration from a sharp tenaculum. Provided the patient is sufficiently relaxed so that the area can be adequately exposed and sponged, a deep well-placed mattress or figure-of-eight suture should control the bleeding promptly. Usually no anesthetic is required for this procedure, but on occasion a paracervical block is helpful.

Immediate or delayed hemorrhage may also occur from vaginal biopsy sites or from lacerations caused by traumatic intercourse. After the area is exposed and cleansed, local anesthetic infiltration is usually necessary before repair because the vaginal wall is abundantly supplied with sensory nerve endings.

Occasionally, it is necessary to suture a vaginal cuff bleeder after hysterectomy. The use of local anesthetic infiltration facilitates this procedure in an office or outpatient setting. The patient should rest quietly in the surgical suite for at least 2 hours after such a repair to rule out either recurrent bleeding or the development of a "concealed" pelvic hematoma.

CONIZATION OF CERVIX

All scalpel conizations I performed were in the hospital operating room because they were quite generous, extending as close as possible to the internal os. My indications included severe exudative cervicitis refractory to antibiotics or cryosurgery, persistent cervical dysplasia, and the need to rule out cervical carcinoma. Endocervical and endometrial curettings are also obtained. After excision of the cone, I customarily draw the rim of cervical mucosa down over the raw cervical bed by means of Sturmdorf sutures. A large cone biopsy may be accompanied by heavy bleeding and is therefore more comfortably accomplished under general anesthesia; considerable manipulation and suturing may be required.

Smaller cone biopsies, however, with or without Sturmdorf suturing, are easily performed under local anesthesia in an office setting (1). A paracervical block should be carried out, and deep lateral cervical sutures for hemostasis and traction, as before larger cone biopsies, are wise precautions. They also serve to stabilize the cervix and bring it down closer to the surgeon to facilitate the conization procedure.

To further prevent excess bleeding with cervical conization or with loop electrical excision procedure (LEEP) (see next paragraph), vasopressin 4 units may be mixed with the local anesthetic solution instead of epinephrine (2).

LOOP ELECTRICAL EXCISION PROCEDURE

In recent years, LEEP, as popularized in the United States by Ralph Richart, MD, has largely replaced the need for sharp conization. This procedure was originally introduced in Great Britain by Prendiville (3), who referred to it as large loop excision of the transformation zone.

After anesthetic infiltration of the cervical periphery, a fine semicircular wire loop supplied by a high frequency power source can be used to excise by rapid vaporization a shallow cone of cervix, suitable for histologic study. A smaller loop is used to obtain an endocervical specimen.

INTRAUTERINE DEVICE INSERTION AND REMOVAL

Intrauterine device (IUD) insertion or removal may occasionally require a paracervical block, particularly in the anxious nulligravida patient with an infantile cervix. Even though such a patient is theoretically a poor candidate for IUD insertion, she may refuse an alternative method of birth control. Unfortunately, she may also experience severe postinsertional uterine spasm requiring prompt removal of the device. Most other patients require no anesthesia for IUD insertion.

Whether a local anesthetic is given for IUD insertion or removal, vasovagal reactions occur in about 5% of these patients. About 1% experience transient syncope and convulsions. I have occasionally witnessed convulsions even after paracervical block alone. If the patient gives a history of easy fainting or previous reactions, she should receive preoperative atropine sulfate, 0.4 mg intravenously.

All IUDs in common use in the United States are fitted with a transcervical tail that facilitates their removal. This tail may retract into the uterine cavity and remain there even during a period. In such a case, and in all patients with a tailless IUD, it may be necessary to dilate the cervix up to 6 mm and insert a buttonhook or narrow forceps into the cavity to retrieve the device. These extra maneuvers may require the administration of an intravenous analgesic and a paracervical block.

CULDOSCOPY AND COLPOTOMY (CULDOTOMY)

Although culdoscopy has been largely superseded by laparoscopy in most parts of the world, in Jamaica it continues to flourish in the skilled hands of Wynter (4) of the University of the West Indies in Kingston. He reported on 1,138 personal cases performed under local anesthetic infiltration of the posterior fornix for the purpose of sterilization. Patients received 75 to 100 mg intravenous meperidine 5 to 10 minutes before the procedure. They were placed in the knee-chest position, and the cul-de-sac tissues were injected with about 3 mL 1% lidocaine. A small trocar was inserted into the cul-de-sac and removed from its sleeve. The culdoscope was then passed through the trocar sleeve. Provided no extensive adhesions prevented mobilization of the pelvic organs, one tube was grasped under culdoscopic vision by means of a double-angled clamp that was slipped in alongside the culdoscope. The culdoscope was then removed, the tube delivered and ligated, the scope replaced, and the second tube grasped and delivered into the vagina for ligation as before. The fornix defect was sutured.

The average operating time in these cases was 11 minutes, which is a tribute to the skill and precision of Dr. Wynter. He has been promoting this method throughout the West Indies as a method of permanent birth control. He cites the advantages of absence of an abdominal scar and prompt discharge of the patient from the operating facility. The method is unlikely to gain much in popularity, however, principally because laparoscopy provides far better visualization of the pelvic and the abdominal structures and pelvic adhesions are more readily circumvented by the laparoscopic approach.

Dr. Wynter's approach requires a small colpotomy incision. A somewhat larger incision is required for the companion operation of vaginal tubal ligation still favored by some surgeons. Keith and Berger (5) prefer to label this incision by the more specific term culdotomy, meaning "an incision through the posterior vaginal fornix into the cul-de-sac or pouch of Douglas." Most gynecologists would agree with their statement that "general or conduction anesthesia provide(s) optimal relaxation and pain relief." However, if great gentleness is exercised in mobilizing and delivering the oviducts, sufficient pain relief can be obtained by infiltration of the posterior fornix tissues with a local anesthetic solution. Brown and Schanzer (6) of San Antonio, Texas wrote the definitive text on culdotomy for female sterilization.

BREAST CYST ASPIRATION

Although gynecologists in many communities leave the management of breast cysts to the general surgeons, fine needle aspiration (FNA) has been introduced successfully into the outpatient clinic or office setting. A 1986 report from the Mayo Clinic (7) showed that in 100 patients, concurrent FNA and excisional biopsies of breast nodules showed an accuracy of 94% and no false-positive results. The authors stated, "FNA may add a measure of confidence in the diagnosis of benign breast lesion, provides a safeguard for preventing misdiagnosis of malignant lesions, and might expedite and reduce the cost of managing both primary and recurrent breast cancer."

SECOND TRIMESTER ABORTION

Fewer than 5% of abortions in the United States are performed during the second trimester; 95% of these are dilatation and evacuation, usually after initial insertion of laminaria or Dilapan (2).

The usual indications for second trimester abortions are for management of fetal anomalies or fetal death. Sonographic guidance of the procedure is considered essential by most gynecologists (see Chapter 11).

For further details of this highly specialized procedure, the reader is referred to Hern (8) and Shulman et al. (9).

SKIN LESIONS BETWEEN THE UMBILICUS AND THE KNEE

Martin (1) designated the above territory as being within the particular purview of the gynecologist. Some of his colleagues would raise the boundaries to the neck, whereas claims to the entire area are being made by dermatologists, general surgeons, and plastic surgeons. Certainly, plastic surgeons are usually better qualified for removal and prevention of keloids, and dermatologist may be consulted if the lesion is obscure or threatening in appearance or if it appears to be a manifestation of a systemic disorder.

Most practicing gynecologists, however, require anesthetic solutions, 24- to 30-gauge hypodermic needles, Luer-Lok syringes, scalpels, dissecting scissors, hemostats, needle holders, sutures, and sterile supplies for the prompt and convenient removal of warts, polyps, nevi, and other isolated skin tumors. The skin should be anesthetized circumferentially about the base of the lesion, and no other agent more concentrated than 0.5 % lidocaine with 1:200,000 epinephrine is needed. Long-acting agents such as mepivacaine, although they provide more prolonged pain relief, may also delay the recognition of an enlarging hematoma that may require immediate drainage and possible resuturing. Incisions should be made along natural skin lines, and the tumor should be submitted to the pathologist with an adequate margin of apparently normal skin on all sides.

Nonabsorbable sutures (e.g., silk or nylon) used to close the skin should be removed in 5 to 7 days. Catgut sutures do not require removal but may produce inflammation during the process of enzymatic digestion. Polyglycolate sutures produce little or no inflammation but may take several weeks to undergo hydrolysis. Their continued presence may irritate the skin and require removal after initial healing has occurred.

REFERENCES

1. Martin PL. Ambulatory gynecologic surgery. Littleton, MA: PSG Publishing Company, Inc., 1979.
2. Darney PD, Horbach NS, Korn AP. Protocols for office gynecologic surgery. Cambridge, MA: Blackwell Science, 1996.
3. Prendiville W, Cullimore J, Norman S. Large loop excision of the transformation zone (LLETZ). Br J Obstet Gynaecol 1989;96:1054–1060.

4. Wynter HH. The development of outpatient culdoscopic sterilization in Jamaica. Kingston, Jamaica: University of the West Indies, 1977.
5. Keith LG, Berger GS. Culdotomy. In: vanLith DAF, Keith LG, van Hall EV, eds. New trends in female sterilization. Chicago, IL: Year Book Medical Publishers, Inc., 1983.
6. Brown HP, Schanzer S.N. Female sterilization: an overview with emphasis on the vaginal route and the organization of a sterilization program. Littleton, MA: John Wright, PSG Inc., 1981.
7. Grant CS, Goellner JR, Welch JS, Martin JK. Fine-needle aspirations of the breast. Mayo Clin Proc 1986;61:377–381.
8. Hern WM, Zen C, Ferguson KA, Hart V, Haseman MV. Outpatient abortion for fetal anomaly and fetal death from 15 to 34 menstrual weeks' gestation. Obstet Gynecol 1993;81:301–306.
9. Shulman LP, Ling FW, Meyers CM, Shanklin DR, Simpson JL, Elias S. Dilatation and evacuation for second-trimester pregnancy termination. Obstet Gynecol 1990;75:1037–1040.

11. Office Ultrasound

ILAN E. TIMOR-TRITSCH AND ANA MONTEAGUDO

No recent statistical data are available on the number of obstetric and gynecologic outpatient office practices that operate ultrasound equipment. However, it is our personal observation that the overwhelming majority of such offices have ultrasound machines equipped with transvaginal and/or transabdominal probes.

An increased number of office-based obstetricians and gynecologists are convinced of the cost-effectiveness of performing limited, but meaningful, transvaginal ultrasound examinations as an enhancement of their bimanual pelvic examination. The same can be said about the new generation of obstetric and gynecologic residents who during their residency years are properly exposed to the diagnostic power of transvaginal sonography (TVS). It is appropriate to quote one of our residents word for word, who, after graduating from the residency program, said "it is hard to imagine how an obstetrician gynecologist can practice today without knowing of or, even more, without operating a transvaginal probe."

This transvaginal probe can and probably should be used in almost every pelvic examination to improve and enhance the diagnostic abilities of the bimanual pelvic examination. For many years we said that the modality would be present in every obstetric and gynecologic office. This process is slow, even slower than we anticipated. However, it is unavoidable, and we need this simple and effective imaging modality to be present everywhere that obstetrics and gynecology is practiced, whether in hospitals or in outpatient offices.

Unfortunately, very few books or dedicated issues of journals include TVS as an integral part of office gynecology (1–4). Similarly, even today, courses organized by official bodies directed toward the subject of office gynecology often completely ignore the presentation of ultrasound in general and TVS in particular.

Another fact, at times inappropriate and definitely expensive, is the overuse of sophisticated, complicated, and more expensive imaging modalities such as computed tomography and magnetic resonance imaging without first taking advantage of, or at least trying to use, the simpler, more clear, and user-friendly TVS. A private practitioner from Asheville, North Carolina wrote, "There are too many magnetic resonance images and computer tomographic scans done when a vaginal (ultrasound) probe would solve the problem" (5).

Because office and emergency room use of ultrasound is somewhat different, they are dealt with separately. However, one should understand that although the geographic place of use may be different, the concept of its use is the same: on-site and immediate availability of the imaging modality operated by the examining physician.

OFFICE USE OF ULTRASOUND

This section is directed toward the growing group of obstetricians and gynecologists who understood the importance of having one or more than one ultrasound machine in their offices or intend in the near future to purchase and operate one. Based on a 1991 survey of the known number of ultrasound machines in offices in 1985 and in 1990, it was projected that by the end of 1995, close to 12,000 offices in the United States would operate ultrasound machines. No new numbers are available at this point; however, it seems that far more offices have purchased ultrasound machines (Fig. 11.1) despite the growing problems in reimbursement and the lack of understanding of managed care administrators as to the cost-effectiveness of reimbursement for or even of deploying such an important laboratory tool in the offices of gynecologists and obstetricians. Quality assurance and training issues vital to this almost revolutionary idea are forthcoming.

One can analyze the reasons for which TVS became so popular and well received by the community of obstetricians and gynecologists who are primarily not imaging specialists. Picture quality is mainly dependent on resolution and clarity with which organs or structures are clearly rendered on the monitor. The difference between the quality or clarity of an image on the monitor becomes evident when the same patient is scanned by transabdominal ultrasound and is then immediately scanned using the transvaginal probe. Given the opportunity for the patient to watch the screen, you frequently will hear the patient remark as to how much better and more clear the transvaginal ultrasound picture is. In a more scientifically designed study, Kossoff et al. (6) proved the clarity of TVS beyond any doubt. The basic physical properties of the probe and the application of new electronic processing technologies aided by increasingly powerful computers make the image generated by ultrasound in general, but more so by the transvaginal probes, clearer and clearer as time goes on. It is interesting to see the sonographic picture of a simple sagittal section of the uterus generated 10 years ago and then to see this same example on considerably improved versions. Even if the user does not know or understand much about the physical basis of the "pretty" pictures, such as the two-point discrimination, resolution, transducer frequency, and the different dynamic focusing techniques that make this happen, the user can appreciate the result, which is the clear on-screen picture.

It is not within the scope of this chapter to review the basic physics of machines and transducers. The interested reader is referred to the pertinent chapters in textbooks of TVS (1–4, 7–9). However, it should suffice that the higher the frequencies, the better the high-resolution images are affected in very little magnification. However, what the operator has to know is that this high-quality picture and high resolution of the high-

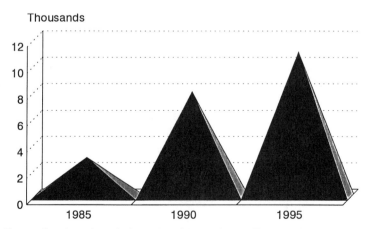

Figure 11.1. The predicted number of obstetric and gynecologic offices equipped with transvaginal ultrasound probes based on estimates from the year 1995. (From Klein Biomedical Consultants 1991 Report.)

frequency probes does not come without paying a price. This "price" comes in terms of a shallow penetration of the sound waves. Because transvaginal ultrasound probes can be placed very close to the target organs, the high-frequency probes such as those of 5 to 9 MHz perform well.

Applying the pertinent physics the higher the frequency, the higher the resolution, whatever the frequency, it is inversely related to penetration. The detection of the embryonic heartbeats at about 4 or 5 days after its "start-up" (at 21 postconception days) when the embryonic pole is only 2 to 4 mm; the detection of the adjacent, thin-walled, 4 mm yolk sac or a small 4- to 5-mm ovarian follicle; or the detection of as little as 5–10 mL of free pelvic fluid are just a few of the clinically important examples of TVS that are appreciated by practicing clinicians.

The next attribute of the transvaginal probe is the possibility of its dynamic use. Because the structures and organs can be gently touched and even pushed by the tip of the probe under constant observation on the monitor, the site of tenderness or overt pain can literally be "seen." By using the bimanual pelvic examination, the palpating finger is able to appreciate and localize pain; however, the transvaginal probe will enhance this task by direct observation of the structure causing the pain. To continue along this line, we should mention that during TVS, the abdominal hand should be used in a similar fashion to that of a simple bimanual pelvic examination. The abdominal hand at the time of the ultrasound examination displaces organs that are "disturbing," such as bowel, and can manipulate and bring structures that have to be examined into "sight." The ovary can at times be localized much faster and better using this well-known "bimanual" technique.

An additional example of the dynamic use of the vaginal probe is to test for free movement and motion of organs in relation to the pelvic wall or to each other. This useful sign was reported by us as the "sliding organs sign" (10). Adhesions between the pelvic organs or absolute immobility of them (frozen pelvis) can be detected by a push-pull motion with the probe and watching the monitor at the same time. One can also create sudden and short tugging movements of small or even large fluid collections and watch the debris or the floating particles drift back and forth and thus reveal its similar content (blood, pus, or clear ascites). It is almost impossible to use these abovementioned dynamic tests using a transabdominal probe. One can definitely use the analogy for the transvaginal probe, which is almost like an observing eye on our pelvic palpating finger.

TVS is extremely valuable to the practicing clinician in two well-known instances, where a thorough bimanual pelvic examination of peculiar patients is almost impossible. The first instance is when an unrevealing bimanual examination is performed in a patient who guards the abdominal wall due to an acute pelvic or abdominal process. In these cases, a gentle examination using the transvaginal probe will furnish more information than both abdominal palpation and a transabdominal ultrasound examination. The same can be said about a patient with thick abdominal walls. Although fatty tissue is present around the pelvic organs, a 5-MHz transvaginal probe will probably result in better and more informative pelvic examinations than the bimanual palpating examination or the transabdominal ultrasound scan.

WHY IS TRANSVAGINAL SONOGRAPHY USEFUL IN THE OFFICE?

First, it can be stated with a great deal of confidence that the technique can be easily mastered by obstetricians and gynecologists, because the vaginal approach to examining the female patient is clear and natural to us from learning to palpate the pelvic organs during a bimanual examination. The obstetrician and gynecologist understands pelvic anatomy and pelvic pathology and can relate the sonographic findings to the history and physical examination of the patient for an "on-sight" integration of the data, resulting in the clinical diagnosis and hence immediate treatment. The ease of operation has another ingredient discussed previously: picture quality and clarity. Of course, previous experience using an abdominal transducer has advantages. However, the speed with which residents in Ob/Gyn and fellows in Maternal Fetal Medicine become reasonably proficient and then even "dependent" on the technique is truly amazing. We deal with the training of the technique later. It can be said that learning to use the transvaginal ultrasound is easy and the technique is operator-friendly.

The next advantage of using the equipment in the office is the immediate availability of the equipment. Even if at this time not all examining rooms in a larger private office can be equipped with a small individual transvaginal ultrasound machine, most smaller machines are portable. They can be wheeled in and out or even hand-carried from one room to another to provide immediate scanning to a patient on the examining table. This issue of portability leads immediately into the main advantage of having an ultrasound unit in the office, and this is the availability of the equipment at the bedside. I usually advise physicians to turn on the machine at the beginning of their office hours and leave it on until they turn off the lights at the end of the day. Experts in handling electronic equipment will tell you that computers and electronic devices such as the ultrasound machine should not be switched on and off constantly. If the ultrasound machine is turned on, it is always ready for the input of the patient's demographic data, and if a scan is needed, it is ready for use right then and there. The immediate availability of the transvaginal probe enables the user to confirm or rule out the most commonly encountered diagnoses. Most problems surfacing through a morning or an afternoon office session are really simple ones: an early pregnancy with a questionable embryonic or fetal heartbeat present or absent? Is the pregnancy in the uterus? Is it a singleton or a twin pregnancy? Can a membrane be discerned between two fetuses? How does the ovary look and what is its size? Does it have a follicle? Is there a cyst in the adnexa? Is the cervix dilated, wedged, shortened, ballooned? Is there a forelying or placenta previa present? How does the adnexa look? And finally, is there an ectopic pregnancy (EP) that at times may be obvious and easy to diagnose? All these commonly occurring questions can be easily answered by using TVS immediately after the bimanual examination. The sonographic images of the abovementioned and many other entities become clear and obvious. We use some commonly seen pictures in the section on clinical cases.

HOW TO INCORPORATE TRANSVAGINAL SONOGRAPHY INTO THE GYNECOLOGIC BIMANUAL EXAMINATION

Patients usually present in the physician's office for a routine yearly examination, for follow-up, for a previously detected problem, or as a medical emergency. The more emergent the problem, the more likely it is that the transvaginal ultrasound will provide valuable information toward making the diagnosis. After the proper history of the patient, a thorough abdominal and bimanual pelvic examination are performed. Most offices offer simple blood and urine tests at the completion of this short process, and attention can be directed toward a narrow range of possible pathologic entities. At this point, sonographic imaging of the pelvis would be indicated and in most cases will focus on the specific problem presented by the patient and is likely to enhance the correct diagnostic process. If instant on-site ultrasound examination is not available, the patient is usually referred to an imaging laboratory and may need to be transferred to another location. Valuable time may be wasted. If the proper equipment is present in the office and the gynecologist is proficient in performing the transvaginal scans, additional objective and evaluation of the pelvis can be affected within minutes. This instant access to real-time pictures of the pelvis and its possible pathologies not only saves time but will be highly appreciated by a receptive patient who will now understand the nature of comprehensive gynecologic care. In most cases, adequate treatment can be offered at the time of the examination (9, 11–16).

Even if it does not pertain strictly to the office use of TVS, a study by Frederick et al. (17) should be mentioned. In this study, preoperative evaluation of gynecologic patients by residents and attendings in obstetrics and gynecology was evaluated. The article states that TVS was quickly mastered by the residents and attendings and that the diagnostic capabilities of this imaging modality before scheduled surgical cases was indeed superior to those of the bimanual pelvic examination. It thus increased the accuracy of preoperative diagnosis in gynecologic patients scheduled for surgery. Such preoperative evaluation can also be done in an office setting by the provider.

Here are some good reasons why the use of TVS in the office setting can be incorporated into the examination of the patient. First, the scan is quickly performed and may add only 5 minutes to the overall examination time. However, more time can be gained by avoiding a second visit and/or unnecessary phone calls. Second, the diagnosis can be established at the time of the first contact with the patient. Third, rescheduling of the patient for an additional diagnostic procedure can be avoided; an example would be a bleeding patient with a thick endometrium in which TVS made the diagnosis of an intracavitary fibroid or polyp; thus, a *diagnostic* hysteroscopy can be dispensed with and one could proceed right away to treatment (i.e., an *operative* hysteroscopy). Fourth, referrals to an outside imaging laboratory may be unnecessary. Fifth, universally, patient acceptance is high, and patient involvement in their own diagnostic process and treatment is rewarding both to the patient and the provider. Finally, the on-site thorough examination combined with sonography will result in fewer misdiagnoses than with a bimanual examination. Therefore, contrary to popular belief, liability is reduced.

More and more obstetricians and gynecologists, including ourselves, believe that there is a clear distinction between the formal and traditional ultrasound examination, usually performed by imaging specialists in dedicated ultrasound laboratories and those performed by examining gynecologists and obstetricians, using mostly or only TVS, as part of the overall pelvic examination. The latter is performed in the office or the emergency room. The first kind is considered "imaging," and the second is what is usually called "office use" of TVS (9–13). The semantics may be of some importance; however, in both cases, in dedicated imaging laboratories, in the office of the practicing obstetrician and gynecologist, and in the emergency room, the use of this powerful tool has to be preceded by adequate training.

OFFICE-BASED ULTRASOUND SCREENING FOR OVARIAN CANCER

The office use of TVS is always the subject of questions as to whether it can be used for a first-line screening for ovarian cancer. An increasing number of articles are devoted to the morphologic description of ovarian and/or adnexal masses by transvaginal gray-scale sonography (18–25). However, good studies using the transvaginal probe as a screening tool in early detection of ovarian cancer have yet to be published. The articles are mainly devoted to finding and describing adnexal masses and trying to distinguish between benign and malignant histologic types. These studies are performed in selected populations of women in pre- or postmenopause who have been referred for scanning or who are part of a study that includes only patients who are at high risk for ovarian cancer. Since the introduction of color Doppler imaging, the measurements of resistance-to-flow and the peak systolic velocities within the suspected adnexal lesion are considered to be diagnostic for ovarian cancer (26–35). Because these measurements require a more elaborate and more expensive color ultrasound machine and because they are seldom available in an office setting, we defer from expanding on this subject. Studies including the screening of an entire population of women at this point would present an insurmountable task for which the medical community is not yet ready and would present an expense that may not be realistic at this point (36–39).

Despite the abovementioned, the combination of a yearly bimanual palpating examination followed by thorough TVS scan in the office will necessarily enhance the odds of detecting an early ovarian cancer. This we speculate will come at the expense of a large number of false-positive findings. These findings, however, can be triaged and diagnosed thanks to our increasing understanding and the use of the different scoring systems. These office-based examinations would not be prohibitive as far as their cost is concerned. As our understanding and experience increases and the equipment improves, the screening for ovarian cancer in the general population will begin in the office of the Ob/Gyn practitioner.

TRAINING

Those who oppose the introduction of TVS in the office often vocalize their concern of its misuse in the hands of the untrained physician. If this would happen, it could present the most powerful argument against the honest and professional users of TVS.

It is easy to master the technique of TVS because of the unusually clear and good resolution pictures. The best time to learn to use this scanning technique is during residency. More and more chairpersons and Ob/Gyn residency program directors become aware of the importance of formally teaching ultrasound in general and TVS in particular.

After graduating from residency, TVS has to be learned on an individual basis by taking courses and spending some time in a recognized ultrasound laboratory offering hands-on training. The importance of reading dedicated textbooks and journals has to be stressed. There are very few excuses not to learn TVS.

HOW TO USE TVS: CLINICAL ASPECTS

Cervix

Patients should be asked, usually after an initial transabdominal scan, to empty their bladders; however, a minimal amount of urine in the bladder is helpful to mark the approximate position of the internal os. We usually advise that the bladder be examined at the time of the probe insertion or at the completion of the transvaginal scan. At the end of a scanning session, the bladder accumulates some urine to make its examination easier.

The cervix is usually examined in the sagittal (median) plane. In an anteverted uterus,

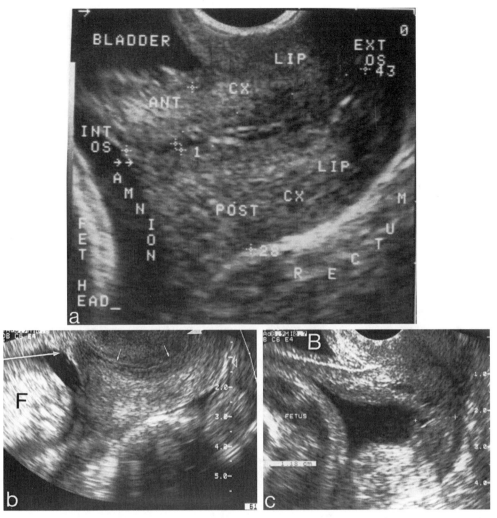

Figure 11.2. The cervix in pregnancy. **a.** Sonographic anatomy of the cervix depicting all the important structures. **b.** Normal-appearing cervix. The two small arrows point to the cervical canal, which has a normal length. The long arrow points to the internal os, and the short one to the external os. F, fetus. **c.** An incompetent cervix at 24 postmenstrual weeks measuring 1.18 cm. B, bladder.

the footprint of the probe will touch the anterior lip of the cervix, and in a retroverted uterus, the posterior lip of the cervix. To achieve a clear picture, the probe should be extracted to assume a position about 1 cm away from the anterior lip. In a pregnant patient, the normal competent cervix should measure about 4 cm (40–44) and the entire length of the cervical canal should be seen (Fig. 11.2a). The shape of a normal internal os in pregnancy should be that of a capital letter T lying on its side. At times, a ballooning or wedge-shaped cervix may indicate an impending premature labor or a cervix that is incompetent (Figs. 11.2c and 11.3, a and b). Contractions may modulate the shape of the internal os and the cervical length. Any cervix measuring less than 3 cm should alert the practitioner to a possible problem and warrants follow-up (45–52). A significant wedge and a short cervix (1.35 cm) at 27 weeks gestation is shown in Figure 11.4.

One concern that is often raised in the office of the Ob/Gyn practitioner is the

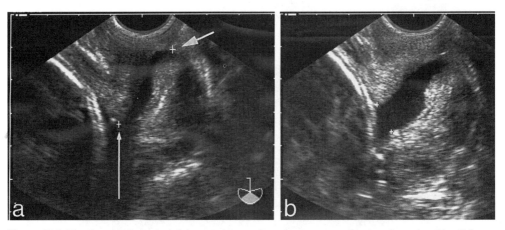

Figure 11.3. The dynamic behavior of the cervix over time due to contractions. **a.** A cervix with a 3.2-mm length with no dilatation or wedging shown. **b.** The same cervix after several minutes and during the peak of a contraction felt by the patient shows a dilatation at wedging of the internal os to 1 cm and a slightly dilated external os. The long arrow points to the internal os, and the short arrow to the external os.

possibility of placenta previa in a patient who is bleeding and seeks emergent advise. It is extremely easy to image the area of the internal os, as demonstrated earlier, and if the placenta is overlying the os, this will be evident immediately (Fig. 11.5). There should be no fear in performing this scan vaginally because the probe cannot penetrate the cervical canal because of the differences in the angle of their longitudinal axis (Fig. 11.6) (53).

There are several other uses of TVS for the evaluation of the cervix, including cervical fibroids, small subchorionic bleeding at the level of the internal os with a live fetus and firmly attached placenta, the follow-up of patients with cervical sutures (54–56), and the rare event of a cervical pregnancy. Remember that a positive heartbeat has to be demonstrated in the cervically located chorionic sac containing the embryo/fetus (57).

Uterus

First, one should determine its position in the pelvis. If the bladder and fundus appear on the same side (e.g., on the left side of the picture), the uterus is anteverted (Fig. 11.7).

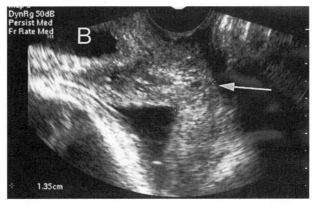

Figure 11.4. A short 1.35-cm cervix showing a significant wedge at 27 postmenstrual weeks. *B*, bladder. The arrow points to the external os.

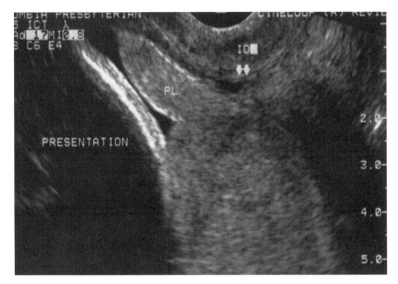

Figure 11.5. Placenta previa in the third trimester. *IO*, internal os.

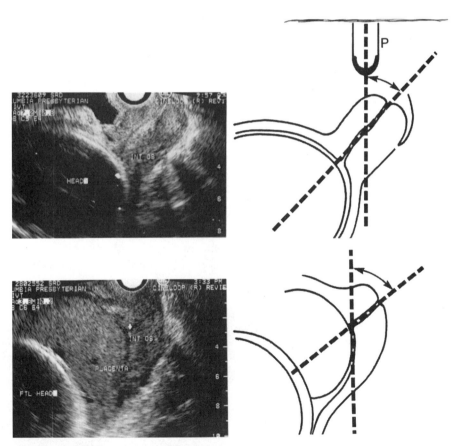

Figure 11.6. These two sonograms with their respective line drawings show the angle between the vaginally placed probe and the axis of the normal cervical canal (the upper pair). The matching lower pair shows a case with placenta previa. These images and the line drawings illustrate that it is practically impossible to penetrate the cervical canal with the vaginal probe due to the angle difference between them. (From Timor-Tritsch IE, Yunis AR. Confirming the safety of transvaginal sonography in patients suspected of placenta previa. Obstet Gynecol 1993;81:742; with permission from Elsevier.)

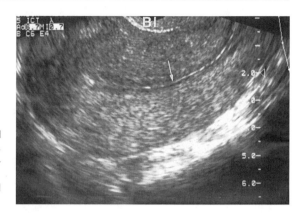

Figure 11.7. An anteverted normal-sized uterus is shown. Endometrial thickness is approximately 8 mm, demonstrating the distinct feature of a midcycle endometrium (i.e., the cavity line; *small arrow*). The contracted empty bladder walls are marked (*Bl*).

If the bladder and the uterine fundus are on opposite sides, the uterus is retroverted (Fig. 11.8). The size and shape of the uterus and the echogenicity of the myometrium should be evaluated on the median section and on a coronal section (Fig. 11.9*b*). The thickness and the echogenicity of the endometrium is evaluated for an eventual invasion of endometrial cancer into the myometrium or beyond. The cavity may contain an intrauterine device (Fig. 11.9) with its typical appearance and shadowing.

Combining the appearance of the endometrium, the cervical canal, and the size of the dominant follicle, one can sonographically date the menstrual cycle (Fig. 11.10).

At times, patients who miscarry or bleed after a dilatation and curettage procedure are evaluated by TVS; the typical picture of residual placental tissue within the cavity is shown on Figure 11.11. At other times, a "polyp-like" structure with significant blood supply develops with almost indistinguishable sonographic properties from those of a true endometrial polyp. Because of this similarity, the term "placental polyp" is used for these cases (Fig. 11.11*e*).

During the last several years, an extremely simple and useful procedure to evaluate the uterine cavity was developed by Parson and Lense (58) and Syrop and Sahakian (59). The procedure consists of saline instillation into the uterine cavity under continuous transvaginal sonographic control. The sonolucent fluid slowly distends the cavity, outlining its contours and/or any intracavitary pathology such as fibroids and polyps (60, 61).

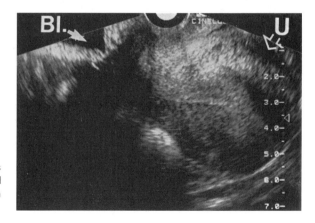

Figure 11.8. A retroverted uterus is shown. The fundus of the uterus labeled with an open arrow and the letter *U* is on the opposite side of the bladder (*Bl*).

CHAPTER 11 / OFFICE ULTRASOUND

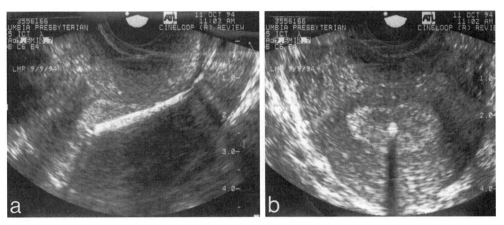

Figure 11.9. An intrauterine device (IUD) in place. **a.** The sagittal image shows the shaft of the IUD. **b.** The cross-section of the IUD casting a shadow. Note that the endometrium is in the late secretory phase.

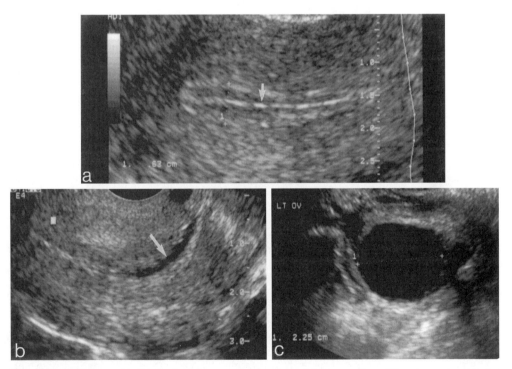

Figure 11.10. Sonographic "dating" of the menstrual cycle. **a.** Median section of the uterus showing the cavity line (*small arrow*). **b.** The sonolucent mucus in the cervix (*arrow*). **c.** The dominant follicle measuring 2.25 cm is shown in the left ovary. This combination places this woman to be at, or very close to, midcycle (i.e., ovulation day).

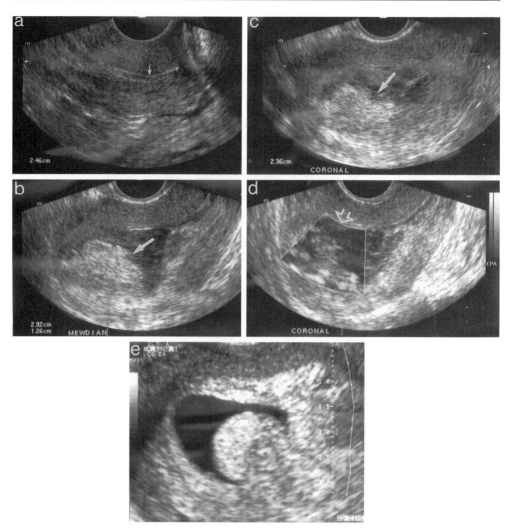

Figure 11.11. Sonographic workup of a patient who is still bleeding 11 days after dilatation and evacuation after a miscarriage at 18 weeks. This is a typical sonographic appearance of residual placental tissue. **a.** The cervix is 2.46 cm long and appears to be closed (*small arrow*). **b.** The median section of the body shows a hypoechoic structure measuring 2.9 × 1.2 cm (*arrow*) above which a more sonolucent content is shown (*arrow*). **c** and **d.** Shown are coronal sections of the hyperechoic placental polyp (*arrow*) and the clot above it as well as the active blood flow (open) to the placental polyp. **e.** The sonogram of different patient with a placental polyp surrounded by sonolucent fluid (blood).

The procedure called saline infusion sonohysterography (SIS) is simple and can be performed in the office or the emergency room, enabling an instant diagnosis and the appropriate triage of the patient as far as management is concerned. It always should be preceded by a pelvic bimanual examination. The necessary instruments are a speculum, antiseptic solution, a large cotton swab or a sponge forceps with a cotton ball, any insemination catheter (several are marketed), at times a special catheter with an inflatable balloon is used to prevent fluid loss in the case of a patulous cervix, 20–30 mL saline, a syringe, and, rarely, a tenaculum to hold the cervix.

At first, the necessity of performing the SIS is established by a careful vaginal scan.

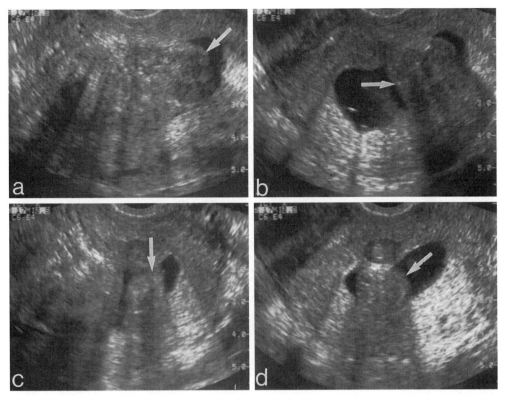

Figure 11.12. Saline infusion sonohysterography. This uterus has the typical sonographic appearance of fibroids casting multiple and parallel shadows. **a.** Before a saline infusion sonohysterography was performed, the center of the uterus shows a questionable structure within the cavity (*arrow*). **b.** Saline is infused in the cavity; the intracavitary structure is revealed (*arrow*). **c.** The intracavitary structure (*arrow*) casts a shadow. **d.** On the coronal section, further information about the fibroid (*arrow*) in the cavity is gained.

The cervix is then cleaned through the open speculum. The 20-mL syringe is filled with saline and the catheter attached. The air should be carefully expelled to avoid the creation of air bubble artifacts. After removal of the speculum (without dislodging the catheter), the vaginal probe is reinserted. Under continuous scanning, saline is instilled. A careful sweep from "side to side" in the sagittal plane as well as "up and down" in the coronal plane has to be performed and is imperative to detect any pathology. Videotaping the procedure is important. This sonographic procedure has a short learning curve and should be used by all office-based gynecologists and the more sophisticated imaging laboratories.

The most prevalent clinical situations in which SIS are useful are irregular uterine bleeding, in which case the findings may be fibroids (Fig. 11.12) or an intracavitary polyp (Fig. 11.13, *a–c*). Sonohysterography is used in the basic infertility workup and lately in the workup of postmenopausal patients and in patients receiving tamoxifen treatment for breast cancer (62–72). In the latter case, SIS can shed light on the actual thickness of the endometrium, regardless of the typical central tiny multicystic structure produced by the tamoxifen. This central structure, which is in the proximal myometrium (and is *not* part of the endometrium), may at times be incorporated into a true polyp, but most of the time is mistakenly measured and expressed as "endometrial thickening." It is now clear that only the actual endometrial thickness after SIS should be measured separately on

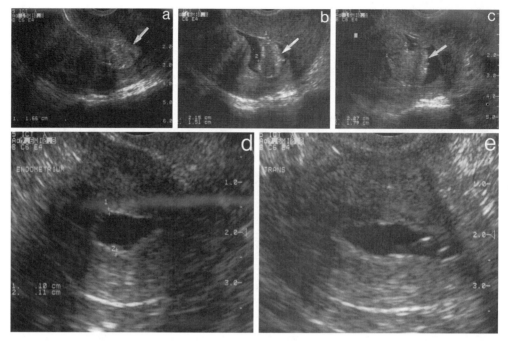

Figure 11.13. An intracavitary polyp. **a–c.** Different stages of the saline infusion sonohysterography (SIS) highlighting the real dimensions of the uterine polyp (*arrows*). **d.** A study using SIS demonstrating the thin endometrium measured separately as 0.1 and 0.11 cm. Total thickness is therefore 0.21 cm. This median section of the uterus in a patient with tamoxifen has normal endometrial thickness. **e.** The cross-section of the same uterus.

both sides of the distended cavity and then added up to represent the customary endometrial thickness (Fig. 11.13, *c* and *d*).

Ovaries

After some experience is gained, it will be relatively easy to detect the normal ovaries. In the reproductive years, they will be above and slightly medial to the large hypogastric vein, in close proximity to the lateral uterine wall (Fig. 11.14).

Their volume rarely exceeds 8–10 cm^3 and they have several sonolucent follicles of different sizes. These are their sonographic markers by which they can be recognized and found.

In menopause it may be somewhat harder to find the ovaries because of the lack of folliculogenesis, which are typical sonographic markers. Therefore, more experience and patience is needed to locate them. Usually, the postmenopausal ovaries are smaller and slightly more sonolucent than the surrounding tissues, the bowel, and the uterus. Bowel peristalsis will help to differentiate between "everything that moves" in the pelvis and the static somewhat sonolucent oval ovary, which will "quietly stand out" (7).

It is important to know when in the menstrual cycle the patient is being scanned. At midcycle, the ovary becomes larger due to the easily seen dominant follicle of about 2.0 cm in diameter. After ovulation, the corpus luteum (CL) may help in the identification process.

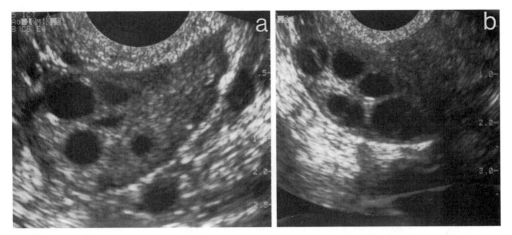

Figure 11.14. The normal-appearing and normal-sized left and right ovary with numerous follicles typical of the reproductive age. **a.** Right ovary; **b.** left ovary.

The CL is far from being a static structure. Sonographically, it presents with an endless variation of pictures depending on the days from ovulation and reflecting the process of bleeding (at times into the pelvis) clot formation, clot lysis, and clot retraction (Fig. 11.15). Finally it disappears, leaving behind a slightly hyperechoic area for several days.

The picture depicted by TVS of a fresh CL at times does not lend itself to easy detection because blood replaces the enrolled sonolucent clear follicular fluid. If color flow (or lately, color power angio) capabilities exist on the ultrasound machine, it is helpful to activate them because a clear ring of extensive and impressive vascular mesh will surround the structure (Fig. 11.15, *c* and *d*).

If flow velocity measurements are performed on the feeding vessel around the CL arising from the ovarian artery, these may show low impedance to flow (low resistance index or low pulsatile index) and a relatively high peak systolic velocity. The bizarre sonographic picture of the CL with its typical blood flow patterns carry a warning for the novice and at times even for the experienced sonographer. In the presence of a CL or in the time window from ovulation until the menses occurs, one should avoid drawing conclusions as far as the differential diagnosis of ovarian cancer or EP is concerned. The resistance index and the pulsatility index for ovarian cancer, inflammatory processes and ectopic tubal gestations, are similarly low and therefore nondiscriminatory. In the case of an equivocal adnexal finding by TVS, good clinical judgement will help to make the emergent and important diagnosis of ectopic gestation. The occasional patient in whom one has to rule out benign or malignant adnexal mass should be rescheduled for a repeated scan immediately after the next menstrual period to minimize or avoid the confusion caused by a normal process of ovulation. In a patient who had a previous hysterectomy, the rescan has to be done within 2 or 6 weeks after the initial scan that revealed the suspicious structure.

The Ob/Gyn practitioner will undoubtedly encounter the sonographic picture of a peculiar kind of an ovary. This slightly larger (>10 cm^3) ovary has a hyperechogenic and prominent capsule around which small equal-sized follicles are crowded beneath its surface. These follicles, measuring 3–5 mm, render this ovary the "beads-on-a-string" or "pearls-on-a-string" appearance (73–75); the polycystic ovary was just described (Fig.

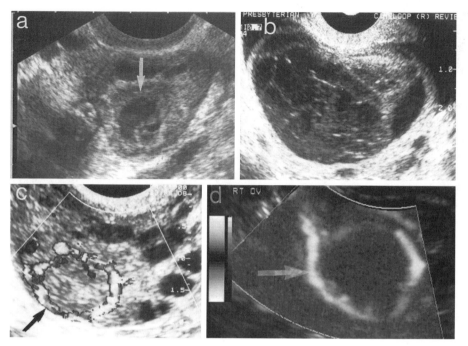

Figure 11.15. Different kinds of CL are shown. **a.** A fresh CL having a thicker wall (*arrow*) contained by a normal ovary. **b.** All of several days shows that the wall of the CL is much thinner and contains a bizarre web-like structure rendered by the clotting blood, which started to undergo lysis. **c.** Color flow (shown here in black and white) reveals the vascular ring around the otherwise undetectable CL (*arrow*). **d.** Power angio image of a CL (*arrow*).

11.16). One has to bear in mind that this picture alone does not constitute the diagnosis of the well-known syndrome of polycystic ovary syndrome. It merely describes an appearance of the ovary that may be found in fertile women with no other apparent hormonal dysfunction.

After recognizing normal ovaries and their changes as a function of the menstrual cycle and menopause, the transvaginal sonographic images of ovarian pathologies should

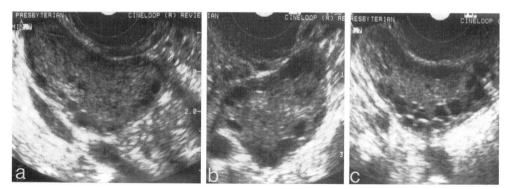

Figure 11.16. Three sections of a polycystic appearing ovary. All three images show a hyperechoic and prominent hilus and a string of small 3- to 4-mm follicles, rendering this picture the "beads-on-a-string" appearance.

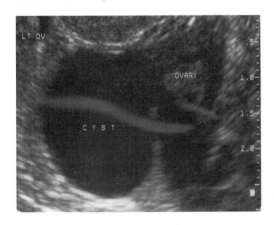

Figure 11.17. A typical ovarian cyst of the left ovary that has the sonographic attributes of a simple cyst: thin smooth walls, no papillations, no septations, and a sonolucent content.

be described. Some, such as the simple-appearing cysts, teratomas, or benign cystadenomas, may be quite common. Others, such as the overt cancers, are rarely encountered. Both, however, have to be recognized and further elucidated to arrive at the correct diagnosis.

The practitioner will most commonly encounter simple functional cysts. These are usually less than 6 cm in size, have thin smooth walls, and are completely sonolucent (Fig. 11.17). The normal ovarian tissue is found to be in very close proximity to these cysts or even "embrace" part of the cyst by gradually "thinning out" over the sides of it.

Figure 11.18 demonstrates neoplastic pathologies of the ovary. The cystadenoma usually is characterized by a multilocular septated lesion containing sonolucent (the serous types) or low level echogenic (the mucinous types) content, at times coexisting side by side. The cystadenoma may contain or be adjacent to other areas of mixed echogenicity (Fig. 11.18*a*). The endometrioma usually has atypical sonographic appearance: smooth walls, at times septations, and always a low level echo-filled content (ground glass appearance; Fig. 11.18*b*). The cystic teratomas are quite common findings and may, at times, be as small as 1–1.5 cm, barely enlarging a normal size ovary. They may also reach larger sizes. In one fifth of the cases, they may be bilateral. Their sonographic appearances vary from cystic with low-level echogenic content, which have a somewhat echogenic round structure casting a typical shadow (Fig. 11.18*c*), to those that are multiseptated, exhibiting bizarre appearances.

Malignant ovarian lesions come in different sizes with or without septations, thick walls, and echogenic solid components; however, if an ovarian lesion reveals inner and outer mural papillations or excrescences, it should immediately trigger the high suspicion of cancer (Figs. 11.18*d* and 11.19).

Several scoring systems have been developed to distinguish between benign and malignant ovarian lesions (18, 20–22, 24, 25, 33, 35). The most quoted was devised by Sassone et al. (18) and later modified by Lerner et al. (21). All are based on the morphologic properties of the ovarian lesions (e.g., wall structure, thickness, septae, loculations, solid components, and papillations). Some take size into consideration. Lately, the physiologic attributes such as the resistance to flow and the peak systolic velocity of the feeding vessel were also added to enhance the statistical power of this discrimination. The main goal is to detect the relatively small ovarian tumors, possibly in stage I, to enhance the 5-year survival rate and possibly even cure the disease (28).

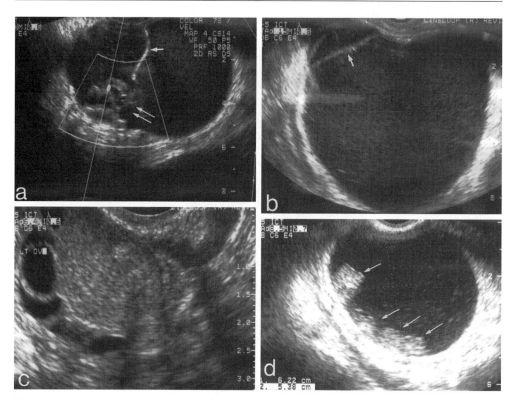

Figure 11.18. Four commonly appearing ovarian masses. **a.** A benign cystadenoma showing a septation (*small arrow*) is filled with low-level echoes and shows an area of mixed echogenicity (two *small arrows*). **b.** An endometrioma with a septation (*arrow*) demonstrating the low-level echoes filling the cyst. **c.** The small dermoid contained within an almost normal-sized left ovary. One or two shadows typical of cystic teratomas of the ovary are seen (*small arrows*). **d.** Ovarian tumor with papillary protrusions into the cavity (*small arrows*). These papillations render the ovary high risk for malignancy.

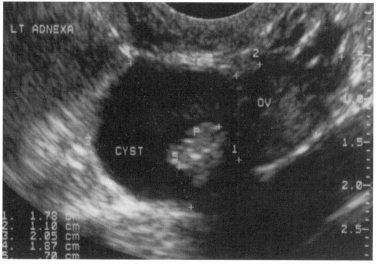

Figure 11.19. A small stage I ovarian carcinoma measuring 2.05 × 1.87 × 2.3 cm. It has mixed echogenicity, but, more significantly, it has a 0.7-cm papilla.

The wide discussion of screening for ovarian cancer is beyond the scope of this chapter. However, it should be clear to all engaging in office gynecology combined with TVS that what the practitioner does day in and day out at the time of a palpating bimanual examination of the female pelvis is also a sort of "screening" for pathology. Using TVS, this ineffective and low yield palpating examination becomes a more powerful tool to detect adnexal pathology often missed by even the best bimanual examination. If such a pathology is found, the first steps have been taken toward a more accurate workup to pinpoint the diagnosis. Routine use of TVS in the office will undoubtedly detect more pelvic pathology than the yearly pelvic examination using the fingers only. Among the pathologies will be an occasional ovarian cancer that possibly will be small and in its early stages.

Fallopian Tubes

The normal tubes can be followed only for about 1–3 cm as they leave their cornual junction with the uterus. Only pathologic tubes can be detected by TVS unless a normal tube is surrounded by fluid outlining its boundaries (76).

The foremost and important pathology of the tubes is EP. Because an ectopic gestation involving the tube can be intact or ruptured, bleeding (tubal abortion) or live, small or large, containing a clot or even a molar gestation, it is clear that the anatomic and the clinical presentation is different in each case (76–81). It should be clear that an inconclusive ultrasound scan in the case of a suspected EP is an unacceptable endpoint.

As far as a practical classification, we suggest that developed by Rottem et al. (82), which enables the clinician to reach a fast and reliable management plan. A live EP with positive heartbeats within an intact tube without bleeding in the pelvis is type I (Fig. 11.20).

Usually, at least in 80% of the cases, the ectopic gestation is on the side of the CL. The differential diagnosis between the two is easier than thought. Both are donut shaped; however, the tubal ring (due to the trophoblastic placental tissue) is almost always more echogenic than the CL. If one of them contains a beating heart within the fetal pole, the diagnosis becomes easy.

If such a live tubal EP is not diagnosed, the next task of the operator is to find or to rule out pelvic bleeding. This is of utmost importance because together with a positive

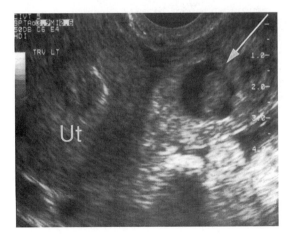

Figure 11.20. Left unruptured live tubal ectopic pregnancy at 8 weeks and 2 days. *U,* uterus.

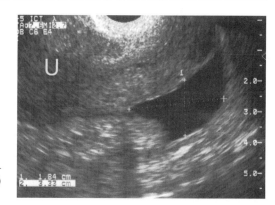

Figure 11.21. Sagittal image of the cul-de-sac containing a 3.3 × 1.8-cm free fluid collection (*arrow*) below the uterus (*U*).

beta human chorionic gonadotropin (β-hCG) test and clinical signs and symptoms, it will determine whether the patient needs immediate surgical attention or can follow a more conservative management plan. If the probe is pointed posteriorly toward the rectum in a sagittal or a coronal plan, one can scrutinize the cul-de-sac. A minimum of 10–15 mL of free fluid is easily detectable (Fig. 11.21). An approximate estimation of the amount in milliliters is possible using the formula A × B × C × 0.523, where A and B are the size of the largest pocket in the coronal plane and C the depth of the fluid pocket in the sagittal plane.

Any fluid collection in excess of 10–20 mL in the cul-de-sac (Fig. 11.22) should trigger the careful scanning of the space between the right kidney and the liver—called Morrison's pouch—along the anterior axillary line just below the ribs (Fig. 11.23). If free fluid is seen in this space, its amount is probably more than 400–500 mL.

If an actively bleeding tubal abortion or ruptured tubal EP is diagnosed using TVS, this would constitute type III in the abovementioned classification.

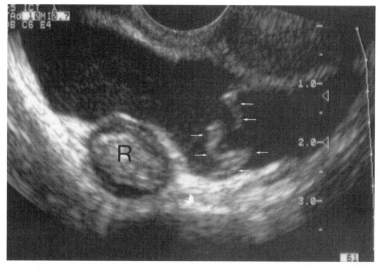

Figure 11.22. Coronal image of the cul-de-sac containing fluid with low level echoes and two undulating slightly hyperechoic structures (*small arrows* above the cross-section of the rectum [*R*]). This is the result of a ruptured bleeding tubal ectopic pregnancy.

CHAPTER 11 / OFFICE ULTRASOUND 217

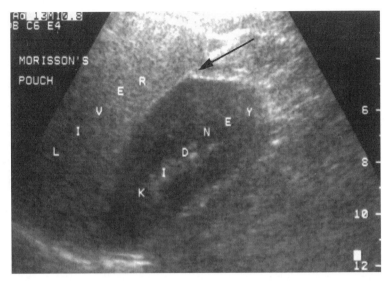

Figure 11.23. Morrison's pouch (*arrow*) can be imaged by holding the transducer along the right anterior axillary line below the ribs. The lower edge of the liver and the kidney are included in this image. This picture shows normal anatomy; no fluid is seen between the liver and the kidney.

Type II EP is diagnosed if no intrauterine pregnancy is present in the presence of a positive β-hCG and there is no or only extremely small amounts of free pelvic fluid; however, a complex adnexal mass is seen alongside the ovary. The management of these cases depends on the symptomatology, the trend of the β-hCG, and other clinically important variables (83–89).

At times, relatively rarely, an EP treated in the cornual area or the cervix is encountered. These ectopic gestations are harder to diagnose; however, if they are suspected, they should undergo a thorough evaluation. Their diagnoses and treatment is widely discussed in the literature (57, 90–95).

The second most important entity that deserves attention as far as its sonographic pictures are concerned is the continuum of the inflammatory processes of the fallopian tubes. These processes usually start out on one side only and frequently at the time of or shortly after ovulation occurs. After a brief period of days, the process may spread to the contralateral side. This is the reason that at times the two adnexa show a delay or an "out-of-phase" picture as far as the stage of the disease is concerned. The sonographic pictures of these tubal inflammatory processes are the hydro- or pyosalpinx, which can be acute or chronic. As far as the acute process is concerned, they can involve the ovaries. In this latter case, the process can progress from a tubo-ovarian complex to a full-blown tubo-ovarian abscess (76).

Acute Phase

The walls of the fluid-filled tube are thick (Fig. 11.24). On cross-section, they may show one or several loops and the sonolucent fluid within the thick tube and its edematous endosalpingeal folds form a typical picture called "cogwheel sign" (see reference 82) seen on Figure 11.24. If the adnexa containing the inflamed tube is touched by the vaginal probe, the typical motion tenderness can be elicited. If the ovaries become involved in

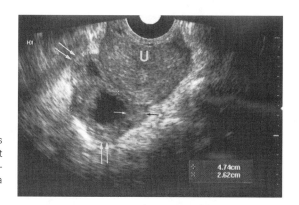

Figure 11.24. Cross-section through two loops of an acute salpingitis. Below and to the right of the uterus (*U*), the thick walls are seen (arrows). Some fluid fills the cumen, rendering a "cogwheel" appearance in the tube.

the inflammatory process, a tubo-ovarian complex develops (Fig. 11.25). The thick-walled, fluid-filled tube "embracing" the ovary can still be recognized as such. If the process continues, the anatomic structures of the ovary and tube "break down" and become sonographically unrecognizable. A complex mass with fluid-filled compartments and bizarre tissue formations are seen above the rectum in the cul-de-sac and the adnexa. This now constitutes the full-blown picture of tubo-ovarian abscess (Fig. 11.26). This distinction is made because management may require different approaches (e.g., intravenous antibiotics versus surgical drainage).

Chronic Phase

The tubes are usually much more distended than in the acute phase. The walls of the hydrosalpinx are thin and usually show a retort shape with an incomplete septum (Fig. 11.27*a*). On cross-section, the thin wall is lined with hyperechoic mural nodules that are the fibrous remnants of the endosalpingeal folds. This is the "beads-on-a-string sign" (Fig. 11.27*b*). The hydrosalpinx is not tender if touched and tugged by the vaginal probe. It is important to differentiate between this structure and the papillary formations inside an ovarian cyst; the latter may be due to ovarian malignancy. Therefore, the normal ovary has to be imaged at the side of a hydrosalpinx.

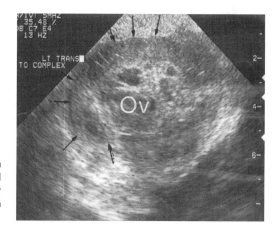

Figure 11.25. Typical picture of a tubo-ovarian complex, where the ovary (*Ov*) is embraced and surrounded by a thickened tube highlighted by several small arrows. This is not yet a tubo-ovarian abscess.

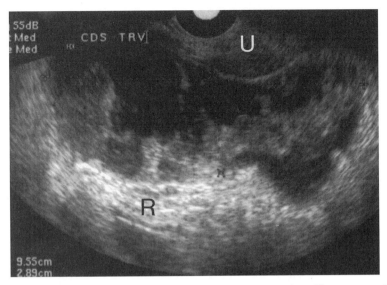

Figure 11.26. This is a typical pelvic/cul-de-sac abscess on a transverse view. The structures in the pelvis cannot be recognized anymore. *R*, rectum; *U*, uterus.

Early Pregnancy

A normal as well as an abnormal early intrauterine pregnancy will be seen at first by the gynecologist even if he or she does not take care of advanced pregnancies. It is therefore important to recognize the various pictures of the different developmental stages of an early gestation as seen with TVS. Detailed discussions on these two topics are available elsewhere (96, 97).

The earliest diagnosis of an intrauterine pregnancy using a 5- to 7.5-MHz vaginal probe can be made at 4.5 postmenstrual weeks (Fig. 11.28). At this time, the small chorionic sac, measuring only several millimeters, is clearly seen embedded on one side of the cavity line into the thick hyperechoic endometrium. Only 1 week later, the yolk

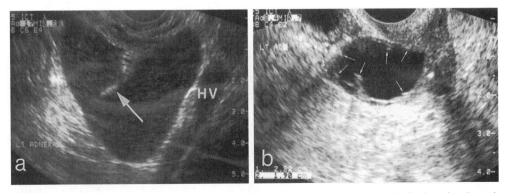

Figure 11.27. A typical thin-walled chronic hydrosalpinx in the left adnexa. **a.** Longitudinal section through the retort-shaped distended fluid-filled tube with an incomplete septum (*arrow*). **b.** Cross-section of the tube demonstrating the "beads-on-a-string" sign (i.e., the remnants of fibroid endosalingeal folds; *small arrows*).

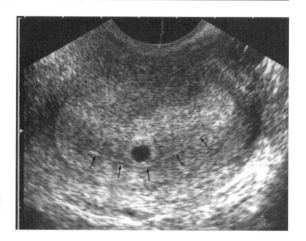

Figure 11.28. An early (4 weeks and 3 days) intrauterine pregnancy is shown implanted into the interior endometrial wall on one side of the cavity line marked by small arrows.

sac can be demonstrated in the growing chorionic sac (Fig. 11.29). The chorionic sac grows with a rate of about 1 mm/day. Close to end of the sixth week (at or after 5 postmenstrual weeks and 5–6 days), the fetal heartbeats appear even before a clear embryonic pole can be seen. The embryo can be discerned at around 6 weeks and 1–2 days measuring 3–4 mm. It then assumes a growth rate of about 1 mm/day. Using an M-mode cursor, now provided even in the inexpensive ultrasound machines, the heart rate can be counted and documented on a hard copy picture (Fig. 11.30) The development of an embryo is best followed by TVS. It is extremely rare that one should use the serum β-hCG titers in the follow-up.

At times, multifetal pregnancies are seen. The first trimester presents the best opportunity to assess chorionicity and amnionicity. Later management depends on this crucially important information that may not be available at later scans (98). Based on a study by Monteagudo et al. (98), at 5 postmenstrual weeks, the number of chorionic sacs and hence chorionicity can be determined. At 6–7 postmenstrual weeks, the number of embryos can be counted on the basis of the number of beating hearts. At 8–9 postmenstrual weeks, the amnionicity (mono- or diamniotic) can reliably be detected (Fig. 11.31).

The woman with a pathologic early intrauterine pregnancy presenting with vaginal bleeding belongs also to the patient population attending the office-based Ob/Gyn prac-

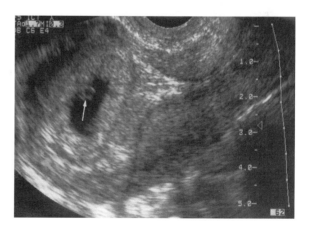

Figure 11.29. A 5.5-week normal intrauterine pregnancy shown with the yolk sac (*small arrow*). At this time, the fetal pole and heartbeats cannot yet be seen.

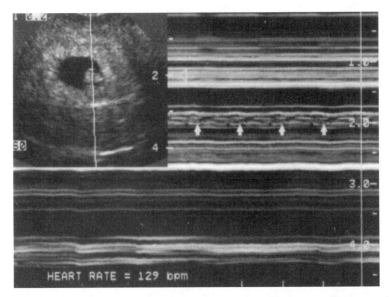

Figure 11.30. An early detection of fetal heartbeats using the M-mode cursor crossing over the tiny fetal heart at 6 weeks and 3 days. The heartbeats are marked by arrows on the M-mode display. The heart rate is 129 beats/min.

titioner. Using TVS, it is easy to determine whether the pregnancy is still progressing normally or if there is any pathology present. During the first trimester or even beyond, the reason for vaginal bleeding is a variable-sized subchorionic hemorrhage. Its location becomes clear seconds after the introduction of the vaginal probe. If the subchorionic bleed does not detach the placenta (which can also be located), the prognosis of the pregnancy may be good (Fig. 11.32a). The patient can be counseled according to the size and location of the hematoma (Fig. 11.32b).

If a fetus is scanned between 9 and 12 weeks, one should concentrate on the posterior contours of the neck and upper spine. At times, a more prominent and obvious nuchal translucency is seen. Lately it has become evident that a fetal nuchal translucency larger than 3 mm measured on a sagittal picture (Fig. 11.33) is associated with an increased risk for chromosomal aneuploidies (99). This measurement should optimally be made between

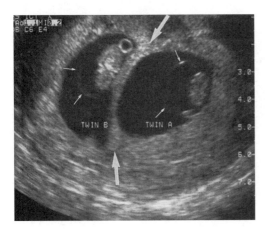

Figure 11.31. Intrauterine dichorionic-diamniotic twins at 9 weeks and 3 days. The amnions are marked by small arrows. The delta-shaped origin of the chorions is marked by two larger arrows, one on each side.

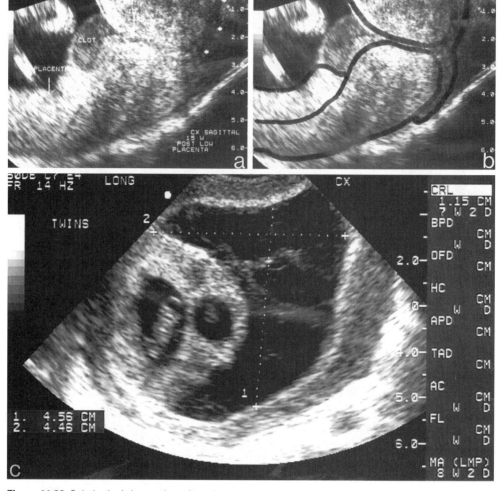

Figure 11.32. Subchorionic hemorrhage in early pregnancy. **a.** At 15 weeks, the area of the internal os reveals a small 1.5 × 2-cm subchorionic clot. The placenta is firmly attached. For easier orientation on this sagittal image, the right picture **b.** highlights the anatomy. **c.** Subchorionic bleeding. An early (8 weeks and 2 days) twin pregnancy in a patient who was bleeding reveals a large 4.5 × 4.4-cm subchorionic bleed. The cervix points to the upper right of this median section. The detachment of the entire gestational sac with the two embryos continued and the pregnancy was lost.

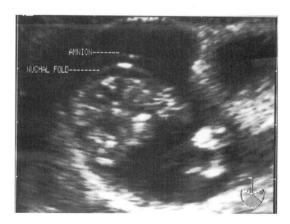

Figure 11.33. An intrauterine pregnancy at 9 weeks. An approximately 4-mm-thick nuchal translucency or nuchal fold is evident and can be differentiated from the amnion above it.

CHAPTER 11 / OFFICE ULTRASOUND

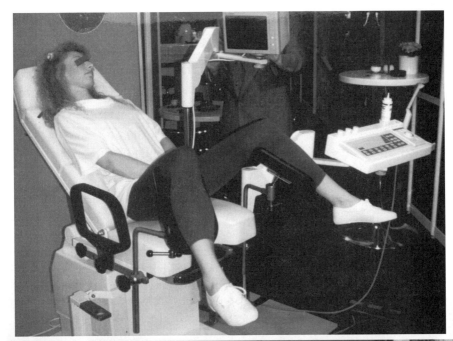

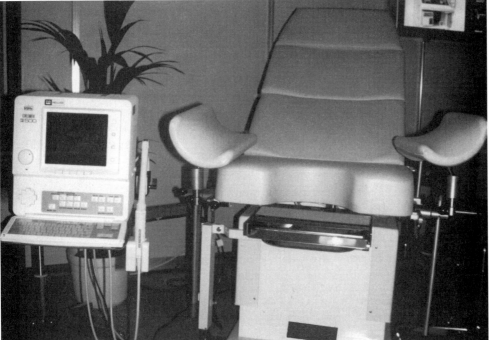

Figure 11.34. Ultrasound equipment setup for the office. **a.** The monitor and the keyboard, on swinging arms, are easy to move. The monitor screen monitor is at the eye level of the patient and doctor. **b.** A different setup that includes the entire unit placed on a swinging platform just as some of the colposcopes are mounted to the examination table. (Reprinted with permission from Timor-Tritsch IE. Transvaginal sonographic gynecologic office practice. Curr Opin Obstet Gynecol 1992;4:919.)

postmenstrual weeks 9 and 11. Because this translucency tends to disappear later during the next 4–8 weeks—at times even in cases of chromosomally affected fetuses—it becomes important to take advantage of this narrow gestation age "window" and routinely assess each and every fetus for the presence or the absence of this easily detectable transient marker of anomaly (Fig. 11.34).

CONCLUSIONS

Office-based TVS should be differentiated from that of a "formal" imaging study of an obstetric or gynecologic patient performed in a dedicated ultrasound department or laboratory. In the office of the Ob/Gyn practitioner, the ultrasound enhancement of the bimanual examination has immense importance and power to help make a diagnosis more accurately on the spot. Management can be started immediately, many times without requiring additional tests or sending the patient to an imaging laboratory. It will save time for the patient and the doctor, alleviating anxieties on both sides.

The unique opportunity to have ultrasound in the office now being presented to gynecologists and obstetricians needs to be grabbed with both hands (100). Such an opportunity, at the introduction of transabdominal real-time ultrasonography, was overlooked and missed in the late 1970s. Let us not repeat this mistake now when TVS is available.

REFERENCES

1. Heine MW. Office gynecology. Curr Opin Obstet Gynecol 1992;4:875–914.
2. Timor-Tritsch IE. Office and emergency room use of transvaginal sonography. In: Timor-Tritsch IE, Rottem S, eds. Transvaginal sonography. 2nd ed. New York: Chapman and Hall, 1991:493–506.
3. Goldstein SR. Beyond the ultrasound-enhanced bimanual examination. In: Goldstein SR, Timor-Tritsch IE, eds. Ultrasound in gynecology. New York: Churchill-Livingston, 1996:271–282.
4. Timor-Tritsch IE, Goldstein SR. Gynecologic ultrasound in the emergency room. In: Goldstein SR, Timor-Tritsch IE, eds. Ultrasound in Gynecology. New York: Churchill-Livingston, 1996:283–288.
5. Sanridge DA. Office vaginal sonogram may obviate CT or MRI referral. Obstet Gynecol News 1991; 26:5.
6. Kossoff G, Griffith KA, Dixon CE. Is the quality of transvaginal images superior to transabdominal ones under matched conditions? Ultrasound Obstet Gynecol 1991;1:29–35.
7. Peisner DB. Transvaginal sonography: equipment. In: Timor-Tritsch IE, Rottem S, eds. Transvaginal sonography. 2nd ed. New York: Chapman and Hall, 1991:29–60.
8. Peisner DB. Applied physics: how do the "gray-scale" and "color" work. In: Goldstein SR, Timor-Tritsch IE, eds. Ultrasound and gynecology. New York: Churchill-Livingston, 1995:5–31.
9. Timor-Tritsch IE. Transvaginal sonography in gynecologic office practice. Curr Opin Obstet Gynecol 1992;4:914–920.
10. Timor-Tritsch IE, Bar-Yam Y, Elgali S, Rottem S. The technique of transvaginal sonography with the use of a 6.5 MHz probe. Am J Obstet Gynecol 1988;158:1019–1024.
11. Goldstein SR. Incorporating endovaginal ultrasonography into the overall gynecologic examination. Am J Obstet Gynecol 1990;162:625–633.
12. Timor-Tritsch IE. Is office use of vaginal sonography feasible. Am J Obstet Gynecol 1990;162:983–985.
13. Goldstein SR. How ultrasound enhances the bimanual exam. Contemp Obstet Gynecol 1992;37:102–119.
14. Davis RO, Brumfield CG. The use of real-time ultrasound in the management of obstetric emergencies. Clin Obstet Gynecol 1984;27:68–77.
15. Stabile I, Campbell S, Gruszinskas JG. Can ultrasound reliably diagnose ectopic pregnancy? Br J Obstet Gynaecol 1988;95:1247–1252.

16. Cilotti A, Weiss C, Bagnolesi P, et al. Echography in gynecologic emergencies. Radol Med Torino 1992;34:488–495.
17. Frederick JL, Paulson RJ, Sauer MV. Routine ultrasound in the preoperative evaluation of gynecologic patients. An adjunct to resident education. J Reprod Med 1991;36:779–782.
18. Sassone AM, Timor-Tritsch IE, Artner A, et al. Transvaginal sonographic characterization of ovarian disease: evaluation of a new scoring system to predict ovarian malignancy. Obstet Gynecol 1991; 78:70–77.
19. Granberg S, Wikland M. Endovaginal ultrasound in the diagnosis of unilocular ovarian cysts in postmenopausal women. Ultrasound Q 1992;10:1–13.
20. Granberg S, Wikland M, Jansson I. Macroscopic characterization of ovarian tumors and the relation to the histological diagnosis: criteria to be used for ultrasound evaluation. Gynecol Oncol 1989; 35:139–144.
21. Lerner JP, Timor-Tritsch IE, Federman A, Abramovich G. Transvaginal sonographic characterization of ovarian masses using an improved weighted scoring system. Am J Obstet Gynecol 1994;170:81–85.
22. Van Nagell JR Jr, DePriest PD, Puls LE, et al. Ovarian cancer screening in asymptomatic postmenopausal women by transvaginal sonography. Cancer 1991;68:458–462.
23. Van Nagell JR Jr, DePriest PD, Gallion HH, Pavlik EJ. Ovarian cancer screening. Cancer 1993; 71(Suppl):1523–1528.
24. Bourne TH, Campbell S, Whitehead MI, Collins WP. Ultrasound screening for sporadic and familial early ovarian cancer. J Ultrasound Med 1991:10:S43.
25. Rottem S, Levit N, Thaler I, et al. Classification of ovarian lesions by high frequency transvaginal sonography. JCU 1990;18:359–363.
26. Bourne T, Campbell S, Steer C, Whitehead MI, Collins WP. Transvaginal color flow imaging: a possible new screening technique for ovarian cancer. BMJ 1989;299:1367.
27. Kurjak A, Zalud I, Alfirevic A. Evaluation of adnexal masses with transvaginal color ultrasound. J Ultrasound Med 1991;10:295–297.
28. Kurjak A, Shalan H, Matjevic R, et al. Stage I ovarian cancer by transvaginal color Doppler sonography: a report of 18 cases. Ultrasound Obstet Gynecol 1993;3:195–198.
29. Weiner Z, Thaler I, Beck D, et al. Differentiating malignant from benign ovarian tumors with transvaginal color flow imaging. Obstet Gynecol 1992;79:159–162.
30. Kawai M, Kano T, Kikkawa F, et al. Transvaginal Doppler ultrasound with color flow imaging in the diagnosis of ovarian cancer. Obstet Gynecol 1992:79;163–167.
31. Hata K, Makihara K, Hata T, et al. Transvaginal color Doppler imaging for hemodynamic assessment of reproductive tract tumors. Int J Gynecol Obstet 1991;36:301–308.
32. Tekay A, Jouppila P. Validity or pulsatile and resistance indices in classification of adnexal tumor with transvaginal color Doppler ultrasound. Ultrasound Obstet Gynecol 1992;2:338–344.
33. Timor-Tritsch IE, Lerner JP, Monteagudo A, Santos R. Transvaginal sonographic characterization of ovarian masses using color flow directed Doppler measurements and a morphologic scoring system. Am J Obstet Gynecol 1993;168:909–913.
34. Fleischer AC, Rogers WH, Rao BK, et al. Transvaginal color Doppler sonography of ovarian masses with pathological correlation. Ultrasound Obstet Gynecol 1991;1:275–278.
35. Kurjak A, Predanic M. New scoring system for prediction of ovarian malignancy based on transvaginal color Doppler. J Ultrasound Med 1993;11:631–638.
36. Westhoff C, Randall MC. Ovarian cancer screening: potential effect on mortality. Am J Obstet Gynecol 1991;165:502–505.
37. Karlan BY, Raffel LJ, Crvenkovic G, et al. A multidisciplinary approach to the early detection of ovarian carcinoma: rationale, protocol design, and early results. Am J Obstet Gynecol 1993;169:494–501.
38. Droegemuller W. Screening for ovarian carcinoma: hopeful and wishful thinking. Am J Obstet Gynecol 1994;170:1095–1098.
39. Herbst AL. The epidemiology of ovarian carcinoma and current status of tumor markers to detect disease. Am J Obstet Gynecol 1994;170:1099–1107.
40. Kushnir O, Vigil DA, Izquierdo L, et al. Vaginal sonographic assessment of cervical length changes during normal pregnancy. Am J Obstet Gynecol 1990;162:991–993.

41. Anderson HF. Transabdominal and transvaginal sonography of the uterine cervix during pregnancy. J Clin Ultrasound 1991;19:77–82.
42. Murakawa H, Utumi T, Hasegawa I, et al. Evaluation of threatened preterm delivery by transvaginal ultrasonographic measurement of cervical length. Obstet Gynecol 1993;82:829–832.
43. Smith CV, Anderson JC, Matamoros A, Rayburn WF. Transvaginal sonography of cervical width and length during pregnancy. J Ultrasound Med 1992;11:465–467.
44. Soneck JD, Iams JD, Blumenfeld M, et al. Measurement of cervical length in pregnancy: comparison between vaginal ultrasonography and digital examination. Obstet Gynecol 1990;76:172–175.
45. Andersen HF, Nugent CE, Wanty SD, et al. Prediction of risk for preterm delivery by ultrasonographic measurement of cervical length. Am J Obstet Gynecol 1990;163:589–593.
46. Stubbs TM, Van Dorsten P, Miller MC. The preterm cervix and preterm labor: relative risk, predicative values and change over time. Am J Obstet Gynecol 1986;155:829–834.
47. Papiernik E, Bonyer J, Collin D, et al. Precocious cervical ripening and preterm labor. Obstet Gynecol 1986;238–242.
48. Okitsu O, Mimura X, Nakayama T, Aono T. Early prediction of preterm delivery by transvaginal ultrasonography. Ultrasound Obstet Gynecol 1992;2:402–409.
49. Gomez R, Galasso M, Romero R, et al. Sonographic examination of the uterine cervix is a better predictor of the likelihood of preterm delivery than digital examination of the cervix in preterm labor with intact membranes. Am J Obstet Gynecol 1994;170:296.
50. Guzman ER, Rosenberg JC, Houlihan C, et al. A new method using vaginal ultrasound and transfundal pressure to evaluate the asymptomatic incompetent cervix. Obstet Gynecol 1994;83:248–252.
51. Romero R, Gomez R, Sepulveda W. The uterine cervix, ultrasound and prematurity [editorial]. Ultrasound Obstet Gynecol 1992;2:385–388.
52. Timor-Tritsch IE, Boozarjomehri F, Masakowski MY, Monteagudo A, Chao CR. Can a "snapshot" sagittal view of the cervix by transvaginal sonography predict active preterm labor? Am J Obstet Gynecol 1996;174:990–995.
53. Timor-Tritsch IE, Yunis AR. Confirming the safety of transvaginal sonography in patients suspected of placenta previa. Obstet Gynecol 1993;81:742–744.
54. Raner J, Davis Harrigan JT. Improving the outcome of cerclage by sonographic follow-up. J Ultrasound Med 1990;9:275–278.
55. Quinn MJ. Vaginal ultrasound and cervical cerclage: a prospective study. Ultrasound Obstet Gynecol 1992;9:410–416.
56. Brown JE, Thiema GA, Shah DM, et al. Transabdominal and transvaginal endosonography: evaluation of the cervix and lower uterine segment in pregnancy. Am J Obstet Gynecol 1986;155:721–726.
57. Timor-Tritsch IE, Monteagudo A, Mandeville EO, et al. Successful management of viable cervical pregnancy by local injection of methotrexate guided by transvaginal sonography. Am J Obstet Gynecol 1994;170:737–739.
58. Parson AK, Lense JJ. Sonohysterography for endometrial abnormalities: preliminary results. J Clin Ultrasound 1993;21:87–95.
59. Syrop C, Sahakian V. Transvaginal sonographic detection of endometrial polyps with fluid contrast augmentation. Obstet Gynecol 1992;79:1041–1043.
60. Goldstein SR. Postmenopausal endometrial fluid collections revisited: look at the doughnut not at the hole. Obstet Gynecol 1994;83:738–740.
61. Goldstein SR. Use of ultrasonohysterography for triage of perimenopausal patients with unexplained uterine bleeding. Am J Obstet Gynecol 1994;170:565–570.
62. Hardell L. Tamoxifen as risk factor for carcinoma of corpus uteri [letter]. Lancet 1988;2:563.
63. Stewart HJ, Knight GM. Tamoxifen and the uterus and endometrium [letter]. Lancet 1989;1:375–376.
64. Neven P, De Muyleder X, Van Belle Y, et al. Tamoxifen and the uterus and endometrium [letter]. Lancet 1989;1:375.
65. Mathew A, Chabon AB, Kabakow B, et al. Endometrial carcinoma in five patients with breast cancer on tamoxifen therapy. NY J Med 1990;90:207–208.
66. Atlanta G, Pozzi M, Vincenzoni C, et al. Four case reports presenting new acquisitions on the association between breast and endometrial carcinoma. Gynecol Oncol 1990;37:378–380.

67. Fornander T, Cedermark B, Mattsson A, et al. Adjuvant tamoxifen in early breast cancer: occurrence of new primary cancers. Lancet 1989;1:117–120.
68. Neven P, DeMuylder X, Van Belle Y, et al. Hysteroscopic follow-up during tamoxifen treatment. Eur J Obstet Reprod Biol 1990;35:235–238.
69. Gal D, Kopel S, Bashevkin M, et al. Oncogenic potential of tamoxifen on endometria of postmenopausal women with breast cancer-preliminary report. Gynecol Oncol 1991;42:120–123.
70. Gusberg SB. Tamoxifen for breast cancer: associated endometrial cancer [editorial]. Cancer 1990; 65:1463–1464.
71. Goldstein SR. Unusual ultrasonographic appearance of the uterus in patients receiving tamoxifen. Am J Obstet Gynecol 1994;170:447–451.
72. Perrot N, Guyot B, Antoine M, Uzan S. The effects of tamoxifen on the endometrium. Ultrasound Obstet Gynecol 1994;4:83–84.
73. Orsini LF, Venturoli S, Lorusso R, et al. Ultrasonic findings in polycystic ovarian disease. Fertil Steril 1985;43:709–714.
74. Yeh H-C, Futterwert W, Thornton JC. Polycystic ovarian disease: US features in 104 patients. Radiology 1987;163:111–116.
75. Takahashi K, Nishigaki A, Eda Y, et al. Transvaginal ultrasound is an effective method for screening in polycystic ovarian disease: preliminary study. Gynecol Obstet Invest 1990;30:34–36.
76. Timor-Tritsch IE, Rottem S. Transvaginal sonographic study of the fallopian tube. Gynecol Obstet 1987;70:424–428.
77. de Crespigny IC. Demonstration of ectopic pregnancy by transvaginal ultrasound. Br J Obstet Gynaecol 1988;95:1253–1256.
78. Timor-Tritsch IE, Yeh MN, Peisner DB, et al. The use of transvaginal ultrasonography in the diagnosis of ectopic pregnancy. Am J Obstet Gynecol 1989;161:157–161.
79. Cacciatore B, Stenman U-H, Ylostalo P. Comparison of abdominal and vaginal sonography in suspected ectopic pregnancy. Obstet Gynecol 1989;73:770–774.
80. Stiller RJ, de Regt RH, Blair E. Transvaginal ultrasonography in patients at risk for ectopic pregnancy. Am J Obstet Gynecol 1989;161:930–933.
81. Fleischer AC, Pennell RG, McKee MS, et al. Ectopic pregnancy: features at transvaginal sonography. Radiology 1990;174:375–378.
82. Rottem S, Thaler I, Timor-Tritsch IE. Classification of tubal gestation by transvaginal sonography. Ultrasound Obstet Gynecol 1991;1:197.
83. Carson SA, Buster JE. Ectopic pregnancy. N Engl J Med 1993;329:1174–1181.
84. Sauer MV, Gorrill M, Rodi IA, et al. Nonsurgical management of unruptured ectopic pregnancy: an extended clinical trial. Fertil Steril 1987;48:752–755.
85. Stovall TG, Ling FW, Buster JE. Outpatient chemotherapy of unruptured ectopic pregnancy. Fertil Steril 1981;51:453–458.
86. Stovall T, Ling FW, Buster JE. Reproductive performance after methotrexate treatment of ectopic pregnancy. Am J Obstet Gynecol 1990;162:1620–1624.
87. Brown DL, Felker RE, Stovall TG, et al. Serial endovaginal sonography of ectopic pregnancies treated with methotrexate. Obstet Gynecol 1991;77:406–409.
88. Stovall TG, Ling FW, Gray LA, et al. Methotrexate treatment of unruptured ectopic pregnancy: a report of 100 cases. Obstet Gynecol 1991;77:749–753.
89. Stovall TG, Ling FW, Gray LA. Single-dose methotrexate for treatment of ectopic pregnancy. Obstet Gynecol 1991;77:754–757.
90. Sherer DM, Allen T, Singh GS, Wods JR Jr. Transvaginal sonographic diagnosis of an unruptured interstitial pregnancy. J Clin Ultrasound 1990;18:582–585.
91. Timor-Tritsch IE, Monteagudo A, Matera C, Veit CR. Sonographic evaluation of cornual pregnancies treated without surgery. Obstet Gynecol 1992;79:1044–1049.
92. Fernandez H, Baton C, Leelaider C, et al. Conservative management of ectopic pregnancy: prospective randomized clinical trial of methotrexate versus prostaglandin sulpostone by combined transvaginal and systemic administration. Fertil Steril 1991;55:756.
93. Oelsner GF, Admon D, Shalev, et al. A new approach for the treatment of interstitial pregnancy. Fertil Steril 1993;59:924–925.

94. Zalel Y, Caspi B, Insler V. Expectant management of interstitial pregnancy. Ultrasound Obstet Gynecol 1994;4:238–240.
95. Timor-Tritsch IE, Monteagudo A, Lerner JP. A "potentially safer" route for puncture and injection of cornual ectopic pregnancies. Ultrasound Obstet Gynecol 1996;7:313–315.
96. Goldstein SR, Timor-Tritsch IE, eds. Early pregnancy. In: Ultrasound in gynecology. New York: Churchill-Livingston, 1996:139–154.
97. Goldstein SR. Pregnancy failure. In: Goldstein SR, Timor-Tritsch IE, eds.Ultrasound in gynecology. New York: Churchill-Livingston, 1966:155–168.
98. Monteagudo A, Timor-Tritsch IE, Sharma S. Early and simple determination or chorionic and amniotic type in multifetal gestations in the first 14 weeks by high frequency transvaginal ultrasound. Am J Obstet Gynecol 1994;170:824–829.
99. Suijders RJM, Nicoleides KH, eds. Ultrasound markers for fetal chromosomal defects. London: Parthenon, 1996.
100. Timor-Tritsch IE. Office use of transvaginal ultrasound: ostriches in the sand? Ultrasound Obstet Gynecol 1993;3:157–159.

12. Transvaginal Sonographic Puncture Procedures

ANA MONTEAGUDO, JODI P. LERNER, AND ILAN E. TIMOR-TRITSCH

The aim of this chapter is to present the office-based obstetrician and gynecologist with the various puncture procedures performed with the guidance of the transvaginal probe. Not everyone will choose this as a diagnostic or therapeutic tool; however, their description may provide additional alternatives to be considered.

During its short existence, transvaginal sonography (TVS) has been found to be important in imaging and in various invasive diagnostic and therapeutic procedures. Most gynecologists and obstetricians in the world learned about TVS from in vitro fertilization/embryo transfer programs. The reason to use ultrasound-guided punctures is to save the patient from a more complicated surgical procedure and render the patient good clinical care. Punctures are used as diagnostic and therapeutic tools. Their advantages are that the needle placement is accurate, there is almost no injury to the neighboring organs, it is easy to master, it is portable, and, finally, it has a relatively low cost and minimal risks.

One engaging in transvaginally directed puncture procedures should be familiar with the term *slice thickness*. Obviously, and due to its physical properties, there is a third dimension to the ultrasound "slice." Although this thickness is negligible and decreases with increased frequency, it still has to be taken into account. The scanning display (which, as has been stated, has a third dimension) shows the picture only in two dimensions, "collapsing" the information of the slice thickness into this two-dimensional picture. This is the reason that at times, despite the fact that the tip of the needle is seen within the desired structure, in reality it may be in front or behind it.

Another important aspect is the "free-hand" approach to puncture procedures. Transabdominally, it is easy to use the free-hand approach, which is dependent on the operator's eye–hand coordination. It is easy to readjust the needle or its direction tip under sonographic control. However, using transvaginal punctures, there is extremely limited mobility of the probe and the needle. It is therefore much easier to "force" the entire length of the needle into the scanning plane, where it can readily be seen, by using a needle guide and thus have perfect control over the exact placement of the tip of the needle.

In this chapter, we reference an automated spring-loaded puncture device (Labotect, Gottingen, Germany) that is mated to the vaginal probe, pictured in Figure 12.1*b*. This automated puncture device (APD), which was first used in reproductive technologies (1), uses a dotted double line that is displayed on the monitor and is generated by the software program of the machine. The directional line measures depth for accurate needle penetration. The APD is equipped with a depth setting that is then adjusted according to the depth measured on the screen. In addition to its accuracy, the needle penetration is virtually painless due to the high velocity of the needle. Very little or no analgesia is needed. Almost all puncture procedures in our center are performed using this ingenious and highly accurate device (2–7). However, puncture needle guides are available for every

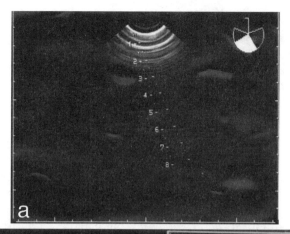
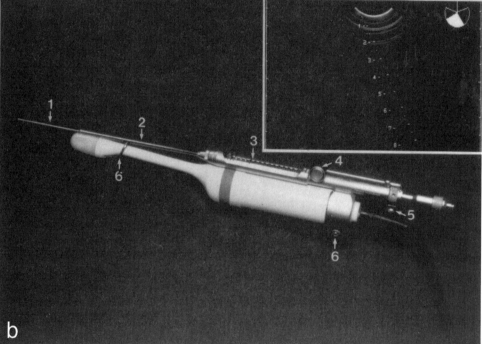

Figure 12.1. Software-generated directional in-depth markers and the puncture device. **a.** The on-screen direction and depth is marked by two lines, dots, and numbers representing centimeters. **b.** The automated puncture device is mated to the shaft of the transvaginal ultrasound probe.

transvaginal ultrasound probe. These should be used during every single transvaginal ultrasound-guided puncture procedure. Most transvaginal puncture procedures can be performed in the office or any emergency suite.

TECHNIQUE

Generally, the punctures are performed after the patient is informed about the specific procedure and is asked to sign a consent form. For special puncture procedures that involve an unusual puncture or research, a specially worded consent form approved by an Institutional Review Board should be used.

The puncture device or any needle guide is mated to the shaft of the probe. Needles ranging from gauge 21 to gauge 14 are used. The thinnest possible needle is used.

Procedures are usually documented by still images and/or by video tape recordings. It is important to watch the pelvic structures and the cul-de-sac after the withdrawal of the needle. Patients are rescanned after 2–3 hours for possible complications.

PUNCTURE PROCEDURES

Transvaginal Puncture and Catheterization Procedures in Reproductive Endocrinology

As mentioned before, the first transvaginal puncture procedure was egg aspiration. Initially, ovum aspiration was performed using transabdominal ultrasound (8). Later, however, transvaginal needle puncture proved to be faster, safer, and much more accurate (9). There is a large body of literature regarding ovum pickup; therefore, we defer from expanding on this subject here. An attempt to use transvaginal probes in embryo transfer proved to be impractical (10). Tubal catheterization or embryo transfer was attempted, but soon this technique was abandoned in favor of transabdominally directed procedures (11).

Puncture of Ovarian Cysts

Despite this being a simple procedure, its use is involved in one of the biggest controversies regarding puncture procedures. Technically, puncturing ovarian cysts is simple and consists of keeping the tip of the needle in the center of the sonolucency representing the fluid, throughout the entire time of the aspiration (Fig. 12.2). One should attempt to estimate the volume of the structure to be punctured and at the completion of the procedure to evaluate whether the obtained amount of fluid matches the estimated one. The problem of ovarian cyst puncture is the concern of spilling potentially malignant ovarian cells into the abdominal cavity. Opposing views are expressed in the literature, their concern based on the fact that a potentially present ovarian cancer can be spread after the puncture procedure (12, 13).

Several articles deal with the puncture of benign-appearing cystic pelvic lesions (14–18). Recently, the ultrasound-guided puncture was used in combination with cytologic examination of the aspirates as a means of preventing or at least limiting surgical intervention (19). The different ovarian scoring systems can be used to classify sonographically defined ovarian cysts, and if they show a low score, the puncture can be attempted (19, 20). Other articles deal with the possibility of puncturing and aspirating endometriotic cysts. However, these definitely lack the enthusiasm of most centers in which follicular aspiration or puncture of ovarian cysts is performed within their infertility programs (21, 22).

The most important question, of course, is whether it is clinically beneficial to puncture ovarian cysts or, to be more precise, cysts with simple architecture. Every time puncture of ovarian cysts is undertaken, one should consider the fact that very little is known about the natural history of simple-appearing ovarian cysts. There are two articles in the literature dealing with this question; the nature and the long-term follow-up of simple-

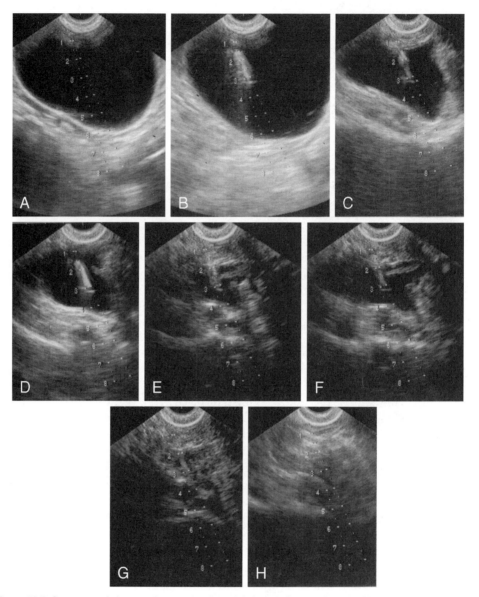

Figure 12.2. Sequence of pictures show puncture and drainage of an ovarian cyst. Note that the approximate diameter of the cyst is 6–7 cm and the needle is inserted into its center. As aspiration is in progress, the tip of the needle is always kept in the middle of the largest sonolucent and available fluid collection. The last picture on the lower right shows the result: all the fluid was aspirated.

appearing ovarian cysts in postmenopausal patients is discussed by Levine et al. (23) and by Goldstein (24). They conclude that in postmenopausal women, simple adnexal cysts less than 3 cm with normal Doppler flow studies and normal Ca–125 levels are most likely benign and may be or should be followed-up safely with ultrasonography. These cysts are very unlikely to be malignant, and the patients should be reassured.

The last word on the use of puncture treatment for diagnosis of ovarian cysts has yet to be said. More evidence, research, and clinical experience is needed.

Multifetal Pregnancy Reduction

The increased use of ovulation-inducing drugs and the number of programs performing in vitro fertilization and embryo transfer have resulted in the appearance of a significant number of multifetal pregnancies. It is well known that as the number of fetuses increase, so does the risk of complications during the pregnancy for the mother, the fetuses, and the neonates. The complications of multifetal pregnancies are extensively discussed elsewhere (25–29). The first multifetal pregnancy reductions (MFPRs) were introduced by French physicians who took advantage of the appearance of ultrasonography (30, 31). Ultrasonography at this time is still the tool of choice to direct the puncture needle into the fetus to be reduced. At first, transcervical ultrasound-guided suction procedures were performed. Later, transabdominal techniques were adopted (32–38). With the appearance of TVS, some centers shifted to this technique (4, 39–46). To date, two main techniques remain in practice: the transabdominal and the transvaginal routes.

The technique of MFPR is quite simple. After an informed consent is signed by the patient, the fetuses are mapped for their spacial interrelationships. After the sonographic evaluation of their anatomy to find major structural malformations obvious at this early gestational age, a needle is aimed at the fetus considered to be reduced. Classically, the transabdominal approach selects fetuses that lie in the upper part, and the transvaginal MFPR reduces the lower lying fetuses in the uterus. A low concentration KCl solution is injected in the vicinity of the heart. The cessation of the heartbeat is then watched for several minutes. Figure 12.3 depicts the MFPR of a quadruplet pregnancy to twins. The patients are usually followed-up at later dates. There have been several published series describing the transabdominal approach and the transvaginal technique. In the last few years, a comprehensive registry has been started by Evans in Detroit, the results of which have been published (47, 48). These articles contain an evaluation of over 1,000 and 1,700 MFPRs, respectively, and also a comparison of the transabdominal, transvaginal, and transcervical methods.

There is no question about the necessity of MFPR in pregnancies containing four or more fetuses. There are also no major differences in opinion about the fact that twins should not be reduced to singletons, unless a liberal social approach to this problem is the case. The main dilemma of each and every obstetrician is whether to reduce triplets to twins or singletons. Only a few articles in the literature touch on this problem (49, 50). Articles concerning specific complications of MFPR also appeared. The one of greatest concern was early rupture of the membranes in several cases (51). The scope of this chapter does not permit an in-depth discussion of this specific topic.

It seems important to perform a structural evaluation of the fetuses, as limited as it may be (52), because in the individual experience of each center, several anomalous fetuses have been detected among those present in the uterine cavity.

The ethical aspect of MFPRs has been reviewed in a number of publications, and the consensus is that the procedure should be offered to patients as a way to maintain a viable and planned pregnancy (53–55). Choosing among the modalities, the physician must advise the one resulting in the least harm and most good for both the fetus and the pregnant patient.

In summary, it can be stated that at the time of this writing, the MFPRs are important for women with an unwanted or unplanned multifetal pregnancy. The procedure can be performed transabdominally or transvaginally in the late first and the very early second trimester. Transabdominal and transvaginal approaches carry a risk of losing the entire

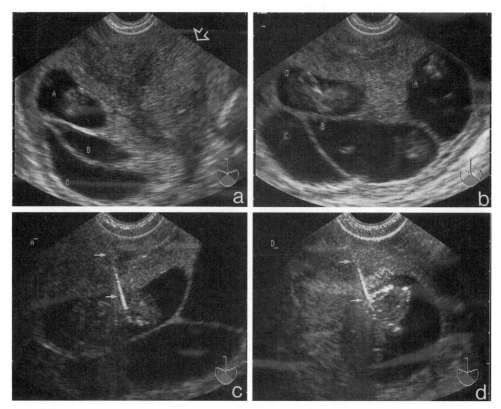

Figure 12.3. Multifetal pregnancy reduction from quadruplet to twins. **a.** Sagittal image. The open arrow indicates that approximate area of the cervix. Only the sacs marked A, B, and C are shown on this section. **b.** Transverse section. All four sacs are clearly demarcated and show separate chorionicity. **c.** The needle marked by small arrows penetrates into the chest area of fetus A. **d.** The needle marked by arrows is reducing fetus D.

pregnancy of about 15% and 12%, respectively. The use of the automated spring-loaded device is useful if the procedure is performed transvaginally. This device may be available in the near future in the United States.

It is our hope that if the number of embryo transfers is limited to three or less and there is tighter control on the administration of ovulation-induction hormonal drugs, the number of MFPRs will shrink to a minimum.

Treatment of Ectopic Pregnancies

Since the introduction of TVS, it is now clear that the entity of "ectopic pregnancy" contains a large number of diseases with different expressions requiring different treatment. The classic approach to ectopic gestation has always been surgical; the diseased tube, ovary, or cornual area was resected. In the case of a cervical pregnancy, hysterectomy was the rule.

The possibility of classifying the different clinical patterns of the disease has enabled the consideration of different therapeutic approaches (56). The introduction of TVS with a high-frequency probe and the knowledgable use of local or systemic administration of methotrexate has opened new possibilities for treatment. It is not by chance that the first puncture procedure treating tubal ectopic pregnancies by injecting methotrexate using the transvaginal probe was developed by a group proficient in technologies of in vitro fertilization. This group used the skills acquired for performing ovum aspiration (55, 56).

Three kinds of ectopic gestations and their puncture treatment are discussed: tubal pregnancies (salpingocentesis), cornual pregnancies, and cervical pregnancies.

Salpingocentesis

We reviewed almost 100 tubal ectopic pregnancies published in the literature treated by transvaginally directed injection of KCl and/or methotrexate (57, 58–67). Before describing the technique, we stress that this procedure should still be considered experimental and requires the signing of an informed consent by the patient.

The technique is similar to the technique of MFPRs. As said before, our group uses the APD, which in the case of injecting different kinds of ectopic gestations is even more useful than in the case of MFPR. The high-velocity delivery of the needle tip into the tubal, cornual, or cervical pregnancy is crucial, because the slowly penetrating needle pushed by hand may displace the target organ before it is penetrated. However, as in any transvaginal puncture, a simple needle guide is attached to the shaft of the probe. The technique is essentially the same as described in the MFPR section (Fig. 12.4).

The complication rates at this time are in the mid to high teens. However, it is hard to compare the success rate because there is no agreed upon basis for comparison. In the literature, different kinds of ectopic pregnancies (nonviable and viable, different gestational ages, different sizes) have been injected. Careful evaluation of the publications reveal that because of the lack of understanding of the natural disease course after the injection, some reported cases do not match the strict definition of a failed treatment. Some authors,

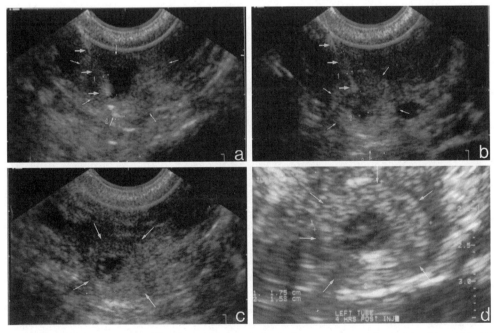

Figure 12.4. Salpingocentesis. A live 6-week, 3-day tubal ectopic pregnancy was treated. In all four pictures, the cross-section of the tubal ring is outlined by small white arrows. **a** and **b**. The needle in place. The length of the needle is marked by three small arrows. **c**. The needle is extracted. No bleeding is evident. **d**. Four hours after the injection, the tube is intact and measures 1.75 × 1.58 cm. This patient was followed until the β-hCG returned to nonpregnant levels. No complications were encountered.

including us, were quick to consider a case a failure and instituted additional treatment because of signs that now are considered the natural disease course after injection (68).

Recently, the clinical course after the puncture treatment has been better understood. There are different clinical pictures. First, a relatively slow decrease of serum beta human chorionic gonadotropin (β-hCG) levels is seen. The difference was also seen if KCl or methotrexate was injected. It is considered that injecting methotrexate causes the β-hCG levels to fall more abruptly. Second, lower abdominal cramping or pain occurs when the decidual cast from the uterine cavity is expelled by the uterine contractions. Third, tubal abortion with various degrees of intraabdominal bleeding should always be kept in mind. If the patient's vital signs and the amount of free fluid (blood in the pelvis) is not significant, the patient may be followed-up conservatively. Finally, the upper limit of the gestational age or tubal size seems to be 8.5 weeks and 2.5–3 cm, respectively.

Cornual Pregnancy

Only about 2–4% of all ectopic gestations are located in the cornual/isthmic area of the uterus. The rupture of a cornual pregnancy brings about severe hemorrhage and exposes the patient to significant risk. The usual procedure of choice is cornual resection. However, at times, hysterectomy is unavoidable.

Our group developed a nonsurgical puncture injection treatment performed using the APD for the treatment of cornual pregnancies less than 12 weeks of gestation (5). To date, five patients have been treated with injection of KCl or methotrexate. It is of importance that nonviable cornual pregnancies with stable or declining β-hCGs be followed-up by TVS, with or without parenteral methotrexate treatment, without injecting them or without taking them to the operating room.

A potentially safer route for the advancing needle into the cornual pregnancy was described by us (69). If the needle avoids the outer thin myometrial mantle surrounding the bulging cornual pregnancy and instead is directed into the chorionic sac and the embryo, traversing the myometrium, a rupture caused by the puncture may be avoided.

Our conclusion is that puncture injection of the very early pregnancy (6–8.5 menstrual weeks gestation) by the guidance of TVS is a valid alternative to a more definitive surgical procedure. More information is desired, but these observations point toward a possibility to treat selected cases of cornual pregnancies.

Cervical Pregnancy

The rare occurrence of cervical pregnancy is in clear contrast with the severity of the complications seen in these cases. Because of underreporting, the true incidence of cervical pregnancy is largely unknown. There is usually severe bleeding and improvised unplanned treatment. These sometimes unorthodox treatment regimens have given rise to a significant body of short communications. However, a general consensus has not yet been developed toward detecting and preventing the sometimes unavoidable hysterectomies (70).

We evaluated the feasibility of transvaginal methotrexate injection of viable cervical pregnancies to avoid complications of the more classic surgical procedures and to preserve fertility (6). The first task of the obstetrician is to rule out the possibility of a nonviable pregnancy in the process of passing through the cervix from the uterine cavity, raising the differential diagnosis of a cervical pregnancy. As in the case of tubal or cornual pregnancies, only viable cervical pregnancies should be considered. In addition, our group suggests new sonographic diagnostic criteria for a cervical pregnancy:

CHAPTER 12 / TRANSVAGINAL SONOGRAPHIC PUNCTURE PROCEDURES

1. The placenta and the entire chorionic sac containing the live fetus should be below the internal os. The level of the internal os on a coronal view is considered to be at the level of the insertion of the uterine arteries (using Doppler or color Doppler sonography).
2. The uterine cavity should be empty.
3. The cervical canal is barrel-shaped and significantly dilated.

We published a study of five viable cervical pregnancies treated by transvaginal injection of methotrexate (Fig. 12.5). In three, the APD was used (6). All five cases were successful. No complications were noted, and the more extensive surgical procedure was

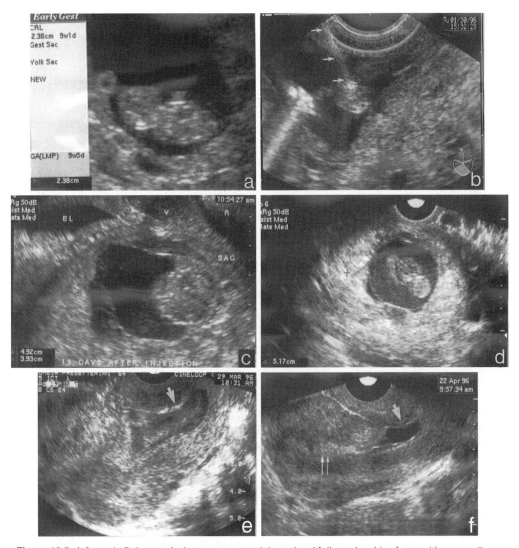

Figure 12.5. A 9-week, 5-day cervical pregnancy was injected and followed. **a.** Live fetus with a crown rump length of 2.38 cm. **b.** The needle (*arrows*) is within the body of the fetus shown in cross-section. **c** and **d.** Sagittal and the transverse section of the cervix 13 days after injection. Initially, the chorionic sac measured 3 cm, however, these pictures show the increase in size to 4.9 × 3.9 × 5.1 cm. *BL*, bladder; *V*, vagina; *R*, rectum. The nonviable fetus (F), the amnion (A), and the extra embryonic coelom (E). **e.** The arrow points to the remnants of the injected cervical pregnancy 8 weeks after the procedure. **f.** The sagittal image of the uterus. The arrow shows the liquefied content of the area of the injection and a double arrow shows the normal-appearing uterine cavity 11.5 weeks after injection.

avoided. Four additional cases of viable cervical pregnancies were also injected by KCl (71). These were also successful, and the highest gestational age was 7 weeks and 1 day. This new treatment modality should be considered when cervical pregnancies are diagnosed early in gestation as an additional therapeutic modality.

A final statement should be made about the gradual decrease of the levels of β-hCG after the puncture and injection of the different kinds of ectopic pregnancies. After an initial rise or sometimes a plateauing of the titers, the values usually decrease, and a return to nonpregnant levels is experienced within 3–13 weeks.

Recently, we treated two heterotopic pregnancies that involved a viable and normal intrauterine and a viable cervical pregnancy each. The cervical pregnancies in both cases were injected using KCl. The follow-up showed various complications such as slow bleeding and invasion of the cervical placenta into the bladder (72). In both cases, the intrauterine fetus was delivered by cesarean section between 32 and 34 weeks. It is our belief that an early, and maybe compulsory, transvaginal sonographic examination of all pregnant patients, but definitely the high-risk population for ectopic pregnancy, is to be considered and scientifically tested to identify and classify ectopic gestations to apply the best and most efficient therapeutic approach, leading to fewer complications and a better distribution of funds.

Drainage Procedures

The drainage procedures were the first ones performed using ultrasonic guidance. As expected, the first drainage procedures were directed by transabdominal sonography (73). Using the same concept of transvaginal sonographic imaging and guidance of a needle along the shaft of the probe, transvaginal drainage procedures were quickly adopted. A word of caution: One should always be reasonably certain about the fact that the structure to be punctured, indeed, is liquefied, and even more so it is loculated in one major or main compartment. Although it is possible to redirect the needle and empty certain loculations behind septations, in those cases an open surgical procedure may be more desirable. For drainage procedures, a slightly larger gauge needle should be used. We developed the insertion of a catheter that was advanced over a lead wire introduced through a 14-gauge needle. Thus, a continuous drainage for several days can be ensured. Two main kinds of fluid collections are considered for transvaginal sonographic drainage. The most frequent kind is the postoperative peritoneal inclusion cyst that is a result of a previous inflammatory process or pelvic surgery (Fig. 12.6). The second is the inflammatory kind, where a collection of purulent material is to be drained. Blood collections resulting from a liquefaction of a postoperative hematoma is probably the wrong procedure because of incomplete liquefaction of the blood, making it very difficult to completely empty the structure (7).

Culdocentesis

Before the advent of sonography, culdocentesis was the "gold standard" diagnostic test to identify a ruptured ectopic pregnancy. More recently, with the increased availability of TVS and its high sensitivity in imaging the cul-de-sac and any fluid that it may contain, the indication to perform a diagnostic culdocentesis has significantly decreased. Culdocentesis is not significantly different from draining pelvic fluid. It is considered as a separate entity because its connotation as a diagnostic process is usually used in the initial

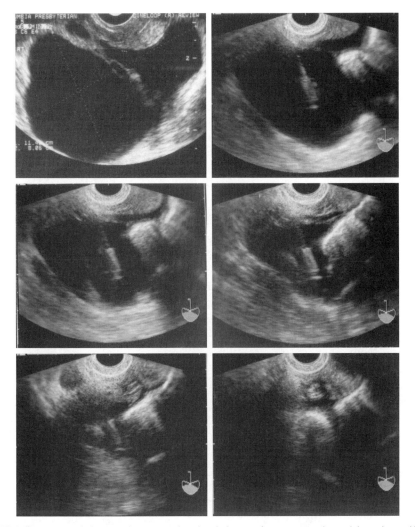

Figure 12.6. Sequence of pictures demonstrating the drainage of a postoperative pelvic peritoneal inclusion cyst. Similar to the ovarian cyst drainage, the needle is kept in the middle of the sonolucent fluid collection. The last picture on the lower right side demonstrates the result.

workup of ectopic pregnancies. The technique is simple and is used in the evaluation of pelvic fluid; it is mostly performed in the emergency room and without proper local anaesthetic for a patient suspected of this disease.

There are several problems in the diagnostic value of culdocentesis for the workup of ectopic pregnancies. In a recent study, Vermesh et al. (74) concluded that culdocentesis is an invasive and painful procedure with very little value in the clinical setting where TVS and rapid pregnancy testing are available. Patients in whom the ectopic gestation could not be ruled out by means of ultrasonographpy and pregnancy testing are probably best managed by laparoscopy rather than culdocentesis. It is easy to understand this statement because TVS can readily detect the smallest amounts of pelvic fluid and even, at times, distinguish between completely sonolucent pelvic content and particulate matter containing fluid in the pelvis. In the right clinical setting, fluid containing particulate matter strongly suggests the presence of blood.

If the need to perform an analysis of the pelvic fluid remains, we strongly suggest the use of directed transvaginal puncture, which enables an accurate needle insertion and avoids dry taps, or inserting the needle into unwanted structures.

Early Amniocentesis

The traditional gestational age at which amniotic fluid is aspirated using the transabdominal route is about 14–18 weeks. Using the transvaginally directed needle, it is possible to aspirate amniotic fluid earlier (75). This can be performed as early as 8–9 weeks gestation (76–78). The only pertinent questions are whether the fluid will yield enough amniocytes for culture and whether the puncture will result in an infectious complication (79).

Early chromosomal analysis of the pregnancy provides the patient information at a time in which the pregnancy is not yet obvious, and at times the termination of this pregnancy is planned. It allows a more simple procedure than later in pregnancy. Transvaginal sonographic needle insertion may be of particular interest and use in obese patients or in patients with lower abdominal or uterine scarring from previous cesarean sections and, of course, in multifetal pregnancies where one of the fetuses can better be approached by the transvaginal route. The literature reflects the research use of early amniocentesis. Several groups have attempted studies to answer the abovementioned questions to introduce this procedure into routine clinical use (79–82).

Transvaginally guided amniocentesis during the late first trimester is feasible. Some techniques using the filtration techniques and recirculating the amniotic fluid may enhance the cell cultures (83–84). However, more information on long-term effects and complication rates of this transvaginal procedure are needed. At the time of this writing, TVS for early amniocentesis is used in several research programs (85–89).

Chorionic Villi Sampling

The initial enthusiasm concerning transvaginal chorionic villi sampling (90, 91) has quieted down quite significantly. In the low number of cases in which chorionic villi sampling by TVS guidance was attempted, they were successful (79, 80). However, as in the previous procedure, this one, also, is in need of further research and larger studies.

SUMMARY

The advantages and disadvantages of transvaginally performed puncture procedures have been described and summarized. It is clear that the transvaginal route provides us with a simple and accurate way of inserting a thin needle into the desired structure. These puncture procedures enable diagnostic and therapeutic procedures. In most cases, abdominal and vaginal surgery can be avoided. There is a very low procedure complication rate, and the simplicity and ease with which it can be performed renders it a desirable outpatient procedure. The use of the APD has to be considered as the most accurate and least painful needle insertion to date.

The experience brought to the reader in this chapter should also raise the possibility of performing some of the more simple transvaginal puncture procedures in the office or emergency room.

REFERENCES

1. Kemeter P, Feichtinger W. Transvaginal oocyte retrieval using a transvaginal sector-scan probe combined with an automated puncture device. Hum Reprod 1986;1:21–24.
2. Timor-Tritsch IE, Baxi L, Peisner DB. Transvaginal salpingocentesis: a new technique for treating ectopic pregnancy. Am J Obstet Gynecol 1989;160:459–461.
3. Timor-Tritsch IE, Peisner DB, Monteagudo A. Puncture procedures utilizing transvaginal ultrasonic guidance. Ultrasound Obstet Gynecol 1991;1:144–150.
4. Timor-Tritsch IE, Peisner DB, Monteagudo A, Lerner JP, Sharma S. Multifetal pregnancy reduction by transvaginal puncture: evaluation of the technique used in 134 cases. Am J Obstet Gynecol 1993;168:799–804.
5. Timor-Tritsch IE, Monteagudo A, Matera C, Veit CR. Sonographic evolution of cornual pregnancies treated without surgery. Obstet Gynecol 1992;79:1044–1049.
6. Timor-Tritsch IE, Monteagudo A, Mandeville EO, Peisner DB, Anaya GP, Pirrone EC. Successful management of viable cervical pregnancy by local injection of methotrexate guided by transvaginal sonography. Am J Obstet Gynecol 1994;170:737–739.
7. Timor-Tritsch IE, Monteagudo A, Peisner DB. Puncture procedures using the transvaginal probe in obstetrics and gynecology. Ultrasound Q 1993;11:41–57.
8. Lenz S, Lauritsen JG. Ultrasonically guided percutaneous aspiration of human follicles under local anesthesia: a new method of collecting oocytes for in-vitro fertilization. Fertil Steril 1983;38:673–677.
9. Dellenbach P, Nisand I, Moreau L, et al. Transvaginal sonographically controlled ovarian follicle puncture for egg retrieval. Lancet 1984;1:1467.
10. Hurley VA, Osborn JC, Leoni MA, Leeton J. Ultrasound-guided embryo transfer: a controlled trial. Fertil Steril 1991;55:559–562.
11. Jansen RPS, Anderson JC. Catheterization of the fallopian tubes from the vagina. Lancet 1987;2:309–310.
12. Trimbos JB, Hacker NF. The case against aspirational ovarian cysts. Cancer 1993;72:828–831.
13. De Crespigny LCH, Robinson HP, Davoren RAM, Fortuen D. The "simple" ovarian cyst: aspirate or operate? Br J Obstet Gynaecol 1989;96:1035–1039.
14. Fornage BD, O'Keeffe F. Ultrasound-guided transvaginal biopsy of malignant cystic pelvic mass. J Ultrasound Med 1990;9:53–55.
15. Granberg S, Crona N, Enk L, et al. Ultrasound-guided puncture of cystic tumors in the lower pelvis of young women. J Clin Ultrasound 1989;17:107.
16. Ron-El H, Herman A, Weinraub Z, et al. Clear ovarian cyst aspiration guided by vaginal ultrasonography. Eur J Obstet Gynecol Reprod Biol 1991;42:43–47.
17. Weinraub Z, Avrech O, Fuchs C, et al. Transvaginal aspiration of ovarian cysts: prognosis based on outcome over a 12-month period. J Ultrasound Med 1994;13:275.
18. Bret PM, Guibaud L, Atri M, Gillette P, Seymour RJ, Senterman MK. Transvaginal US-guided aspiration of ovarian cysts and solid pelvic masses. Radiology 1992;185:377.
19. Yeh H, Greenebaum E, Lerner JP, Heller D, Timor-Tritsch IE. Transvaginal sonographic characterization combined with cytologic evaluation in the diagnosis of ovarian and adnexal cysts. Diagn Cythopathol 1994;10:107–112.
20. Sassone AM, Timor-Tritsch IE, Artner A, Westhoff C, Warren WB. Transvaginal sonographic characterization of ovarian disease: evaluation of a new scoring system to predict ovarian malignancy. Obstet Gynecol 1991;78:70–76.
21. Abu Musa A, Takahashi K, Nagata H, Kitao M. Pregnancy following transvaginal sonographic guided aspiration of endometrioma. Gynecol Obstet Invest 1991;31:90–92.
22. Aboulghar MA, Mansour RT, Serour GI, Rizk B. Ultrasonic transvaginal aspiration of endometriotic cysts. An optional line of treatment in selected cases of endometriosis. Hum Reprod 1991;6:1408–1410.
23. Levine DL, Gosink BB, Wolf SI, Feldesman MR, Pretorius DH. Simple adnexal cysts: the natural history in postmenopausal women. Radiology 1992;18:653–659.
24. Goldstein S. Conservative management of small postmenopausal cystic masses. Clin Obstet Gynecol 1993;36:395–401.

25. Syrop CH, Varner MW. Triplet gestation: maternal and neonatal implication. Acta Genet Med Gemellol (Roma) 1985;34:81–88.
26. Botting BJ, Davies IM, Macfarlane AJ. Recent trends in the incidence of multiple births and associated mortality. Arch Dis Child 1987;62:941–950.
27. McKeown T, Record RG. Observations on foetal growth in multiple pregnancy in man. J Endocrinol 1982;5:387.
28. Levine MI. Grand multiple pregnancies and demand for neonatal intensive care. Lancet 1986;2:347.
29. Gonen R, Heyman E, Asztalos EV, et al. The outcome of triplet, quadruplet and quintuplet pregnancies managed in a perinatal unit. Obstetric, neonatal and follow-up data. AJOG 1990;162:454.
30. Dumez Y, Oury JF. Method for first trimester selective abortion in multiple pregnancy. Contrib Gynecol Obstet 1986;15:50–53.
31. Bessis R, Milanese C, Frydman R. Preventive partial termination in multiple pregnancy. Presented at the Second International Symposium, the Fetus as a Patient-Diagnosis and Therapy, Jerusalem, Israel, 1985.
32. Brandes JM, Itskovits J, Timor-Tritsch IE, Drugan A, Frydman R. Reduction of the number of embryos in multiple pregnancy. Fertil Steril 1987;48:326–327.
33. Berkovitz RL, Lynch L, Chitkara U, Wilkins IA, Mehalek KE, Alvarez E. Selective reduction of multifetal pregnancies in the first trimester. N Engl J Med 1988;318:1042–1047.
34. Evans MI, Fletcher JH, Zador IE, et al. Selective first-trimester termination in octuplet and quadruplet pregnancies: clinical and ethical issue. Obstet Gynecol 1988;71:289–296.
35. Birnholz JC, Dmowski WP, Binor Z, Radwanska E. Selective continuation in gonadotropin-induced multiple pregnancy. Fertil Steril 1987;48:873.
36. Farquharson DF, Wittmann BK, Hansmann M, Ho Yuen B, Bladwin VJ, Lindahl S. Management of quintuplet pregnancy by selective embryocide. Am J Obstet Gynecol 1988;158:413–416.
37. Tabsh KMA. Transabdominal multifetal pregnancy reduction: report of 40 cases. Obstet Gynecol 1990; 74:739–741.
38. Lynch L, Berkowitz RL, Chitkara U, Alvarez M. First trimester transabdominal multifetal pregnancy reduction: a report of 85 cases. Obstet Gynecol 1990;75:735–738.
39. Itskovitz J, Boldes R, Thaler I, Bronstein M, Erlik Y, Brandes JM. Tansvaginal ultrasonography-guided aspiration of gestational sacs for selective abortion in multiple pregnancy. Am J Obstet Gynecol 1989; 160:215–217.
40. Itskovits J, Boldes R, Thaler I, Levron Y, Rottem S, Brandes JM. First trimester selective reduction in multiple pregnancy guided by tansvaginal sonography. J Clin Ultrasound 1990;18:323–327.
41. Shalev E, Frenkel Y, Goldenberg M, Shalev E. Selective reduction in multiple gestations: pregnancy outcome after transvaginal and transabdominal needle-guided procedures. Fertil Steril 1989;52:416–420.
42. Donnor C, McGinnis, Simon P, Rodesch F. Multifetal pregnancy reduction: A Belgian experience. Europ J Obstet Gynecol Repro Biol 1990;38:183–187.
43. Monteagudo A, Timor-Tritsch IE. Transvaginal multifetal pregnancy reduction: Which? When? How many? Ann Med 1993;25:275–278.
44. Timor-Tritsch IE, Peisner DB, Monteagudo A. Puncture procedures utilizing transvaginal ultrasonic guidance. Ultrasound Obstet Gynecol 1991;1:144–150.
45. Itskovitz-Eldor J, Drugan A, Levron J, Thaler I, Brandes JM. Transvaginal embryo aspiration—a safe method for selective reduction in multiple pregnancies. Fertil Steril 1992;58:351–355.
46. Monteagudo A, Timor-Tritsch IE. An approach to multifetal pregnancy reduction in a pregnancy of grand order (12 fetuses). Ultrasound Obstet Gynecol 1994;4:339–341.
47. Evans MI, Dommergues M, Timor-Tritsch IE, et al. Transabdominal versus transcervical and transvaginal multifetal pregnancy reduction. International collaborative experience of more than one thousand cases. Am J Obstet Gynecol 1994;170:902–909.
48. Evans MI, Dommergues M, Wapner RJ, et al. International collaborative experience of 1789 patients having multifetal pregnancy reduction: a plateauing of risks and outcomes. J Soc Gynecol Invest 1996; 3:23–26.
49. Macones GA, Schlemmer G, Pritts E, Weinblat V, Wapner RJ. Multifetal reduction of triplets to twins improves perinatal outcome. Am J Obstet Gynecol 1993;169:982–986.

50. Lipitz S, Reichman B, Ural J, et al. A prospective comparison of the outcome of triplet pregnancies managed expectantly or by multifetal reduction to twins. Am J Obstet Gynecol 1994;170:874–879.
51. Lipitz S, Grisaru D, Achiron R, Lidor A, Mashiach S, Schiff E. Pregnancy outcome after early amniotic fluid leakage after transabdominal multifetal reduction. Fertil Steril 1996;65:1055–1058.
52. Timor-Tritsch IE, Monteagudo A, Peisner DB. High frequency transvaginal sonographic examination for the potential malformation assessment of the 9 to 14 week fetus. J Clin Ultrasound 1992;20:231–238.
53. Berkowitz RL, Lynch L. Selective reduction: an unfortunate misnomer. Obstet Gynecol 1990;75:273–274.
54. Hobbins JC. Selective reduction—a perinatal necessity. N Engl J Med 1988;318:1062–1063.
55. McCormick RA. How brave a new world? Washington DC: Georgetown University Press, 1981:199–200, 443–444.
56. Rottem S, Thaler I, Timor-Tritsch IE. Classification of tubal gestations by transvaginal sonography. Ultrasound Obstet Gynecol 1991;1:197–201.
57. Feichtinger W, Kemeter P. Conservative treatment of ectopic pregnancy by transvaginal aspiration undersonographic control and methotrexate injection. Lancet 1987;1:381.
58. Feichtinger W, Kemeter P. Treatment of unruptured ectopic pregnancy by needling of sac and injection of methotrexate or PGE_2 under transvaginal sonography control: report of 10 cases. Arch Gynecol Obstet 1989;246:85–89.
59. Menard A, Crequat J, Mandelbrot L, Hauuy JP, Madelanat P. Treatment of unruptured tubal pregnancy by local injection of methotrexate under transvaginal sonographic control. Fertil Steril 1990;54:47–50.
60. Jeng CJ, Yang YG, Lan CC. Transvaginal ultrasound guided salpingocentesis with methotrexate injection: a minimally invasive treatment for early ectopic pregnancy. Presented at The Third World Congress on Vaginosonography in Gynecology, San Antonio, Texas, 1990.
61. Fernandez H, Baton C, Lelaidier C, Frydman R. Conservative management of ectopic pregnancy: prospective randomized clinical trial of methotrexate versus prostaglandin sulpostrone by combined transvaginal and systemic administration. Fertil Steril 1991;55:746.
62. Tulandi T, Bret PM, Atri M, Senterman M. Treatment of ectopic pregnancy by transvaginal intratubal methotrexate administration. Obstet Gynecol 1991;77:627–643.
63. Popp LW, Mettler L, Weisner H, Mecke I, Freys I, Semm K. Ectopic pregnancy treatment using pelvicscopic or vaginosonographically guided intrachorionic injection of methotrexate. Ultrasound Obstet Gynecol 1991;1:136–143.
64. Shalev E, Zalel Y, Bustan M, Weiner E. Ectopic pregnancy: sonographically guided transvaginal reduction. Ultrasound Obstet Gynecol 1991;1:127–131.
65. Venezia R, Zangara C, Comparetto G, Cittadini E. Conservative treatment of ectopic pregnancies using a single echo-guided injection of methotrexate into a gestational sac. Ultrasound Obstet Gynecol 1991;1:132–135.
66. Jehng CH, Ng Ky, Jou HJ, Jenh AL, Lien YR. Successful treatment of two viable tubal pregnancies by two-step local injection. J Formos Med Assoc 1992;91:823–827.
67. Caspi B, Barash A, Friedman A, Appelman Z, Pausky M, Borenstein R. Aspiration of ectopic pregnancy under guidance of vaginal ultrasonography. Eur J Obstet Gynecol Reprod Biol 1992;46:51–52.
68. Carson SA, Buster JE. Ectopic pregnancy. N Engl J Med 1993;329:1174–1181.
69. Timor-Tritsch IE, Monteagudo A, Lerner JP. A "potentially safer" route for puncture and injection of cornual ectopic pregnancies. Ultrasound Obstet Gynecol 1996;7:3553–3555.
70. Yanowitz J, Leake J, Huggins G, Gazaway P, Gates E. Cervical ectopic pregnancy: review of the literature and report of a case treated by single-dose methotrexate therapy. Obstet Gynecol Surv 1990;45:405–414.
71. Frate MC, Benson CB, Doubilet PM, DiSalvo DN, Laing FC, Brown DL. The sonographic diagnosis and nonsurgical treatment of cervical ectopic pregnancy. J Ultrasound Med 1994;13(Suppl):S1–S86.
72. Monteagudo A, Tarricone NJ, Timor-Tritsch IE, Lerner JP. Successful transvaginal ultrasound guided puncture and injection of a cervical pregnancy with a simultaneous intrauterine pregnancy in a patient with a history of a previous cervical pregnancy. Ultrasound Obstet Gynecol (in press).
73. McArdle CR, Simon L, Kiejna C. Vaginal drainage of posthysterectomy abscess under direct ultrasonic guidance. Obstet Gynecol 1984;63:908.

74. Vermesh M, Graczykowski JW, Sauer MV. Reevaluation of the role of culdocentesis in the management of ectopic pregnancy. Am J Obstet Gynecol 1990;162:411–413.
75. Shalev E, Dan U, Machiach S, Chaki R, Shalev J, Barkai S, Goldman B. First trimester transvaginal amniocentesis for genetic evaluation of multiple gestation. Prenat Diagn 1990;10:344–345.
76. Byrne D, Azar G, Nicolaides K. Why cell culture is successful after early amniocentesis. Fetal Diagn Ther 1991;6(1–2):84–6.
77. Nelson MM. Amniotic fluid volume in early pregnancy. J Obstet Gynaecol Br Cwlth 1972;70:50–53.
78. Byrne DL, Marks K, Azar G, Nicolaides KH. Randomized study of early amniocentesis versus chorion villus sampling: technical and cytogenetic comparison of 650 patients. Ultrasound Obstet Gynecol 1991;1:235–240.
79. Hanson W, Zorn EM, Tennant FR, Marianos S, Samuels S. Amniocentesis before 15 weeks' gestation: outcome risks and technical problems. Am J Obstet Gynecol 1987;156:1524.
80. Nevin J, Nevin NC, Dornan JC, Sim D, Armstrong MJ. Early amniocentesis: experience of 222 consecutive patients, 1987–1988. Prenat Diagn 1990;10:79–83.
81. Rooney DE, MacLachlan N, Smith J, et al. Early amniocentesis: a cytogenetic evaluation. Br Med J 1989;299:24.
82. Elejalde BR, Elejalde MM, Acuna MJ, Thelen D, Trujillo C, Karrmann M. Prospective study of amniocentesis performed between week 9 and 16 of gestation: its feasability, risks, complications and use in early genetic prenatal diagnosis. Am J Med Genet 1990;35:188–196.
83. Sundberg K, Smidt-Jensen S, Philip J. Amniocentesis with increased cell yield, obtained by filtration and reinjection of the amniotic fluid. Ultrasound Obstet Gynecol 1991;1:91–94.
84. Bryne DL, Marks K, Braude PR, Nicolaides KH. Amnifiltration in the first trimester: feasbility, technical aspects and citological outcome. Ultrasound Obstet Gynecol 1991;1:320–324.
85. Campbell J, Cass P, Wathen N, Stone R, Wald N. First-trimester amniotic fluid and extraembryonic coelomic fluid acetylcholinesterase electrophoresis. Prenat Diagn 1992;12:609–612.
86. Wathen NC, Cass PL, Campbell DJ, Wald N, Chard T. Alpha-fetoprotein levels and yolk sac size in the first trimester of pregnancy. Prenat Diagn 1992;12:649–652.
87. Campbell J, Mainwaring-Burton R, Wathen N, Cass P, Chard T. Microvillar enzyme activity in amniotic fluid, extraembryonic coelomic fluid and maternal serum in the first trimester of pregnancy. Eur J Obstet Gynecol Reprod Biol 1992;45:169–172.
88. Campbell J, Wathen N, Lewis M, Fingerova H, Chard T. Erythropoietin levels in amniotic fluid and extraembryonic coelomic fluid in the first trimester of pregnancy. Br J Obstet Gynaecol 1992;99:974–976.
89. Campbell J, Wathen N, Macintosh M, Cass P, Chard T, Mainwaring-Burton R. Biochemical composition of amniotic fluid and extraembryonic coelomic fluid in the first trimester of pregnancy. Br J Obstet Gynaecol 1992;99:563–565.
90. Ghirardini G, Popp LW, Camurri L, Stoeckenius M. Vaginosonographic guided chorionic villi biopsy (transvaginal chorionic villi sampling). Eur J Obstet Gynecol Reprod Biol 1986;23:315–319.
91. Popp LW, Girardini A. The role of transvaginal sonography in chorionic villi sampling. J Clin Ultrasound 1990;18:315–322.

13. Accreditation, Risk Management, and Reimbursement

PAUL M. ALLEN

ACCREDITATION

The preceding chapters in this text effectively describe the basics of outpatient gynecologic surgery and provide a solid background for the practicing gynecologist to complete a variety of surgical procedures in an office-based surgical facility or similar setting. Because this aspect of ambulatory surgical health care has continued to shift away from the institutional setting of a hospital or medical center and into the distinctively noninstitutional setting of a physician office, it is important that the practitioner ensure that systems are in place to maximize quality of operations and minimize risk for the patient, staff, and physician. We should be able to assure patients, staff, the general public, and regulatory bodies that continuous improvements are ongoing to meet nationally recognized standards through the accreditation process. Reimbursement to the physician should be adequate yet cost effective to patients and third-party payers to ensure ongoing operational success.

Our traditionally hospital-centric view of health care has assigned these administrative responsibilities to various highly organized departments of medical centers. We firmly believe, and our experience has shown, that the individual physician or small group of physicians can, with the support of a dedicated and committed office staff, develop, implement, and monitor a quality improvement and risk management program that can be validated and recognized through the challenging process of practice accreditation.

Achieving a favorable accreditation decision bestows many benefits on a practice, including the ability to generate a facility fee based on fixed practice costs, which is separate and distinct from professional fees, to provide reimbursement to cover occupancy, personnel, equipment, and accreditation costs incurred in the operation of an office-based surgical facility.

Maximizing Safety in the Office-Based Surgical Facility

A safe surgical environment is equally important to quality patient care as a competent skilled surgeon. Just as a hospital undergoes periodic inspection by various regulatory, accrediting, certifying, and licensing bodies to ensure patient safety and quality of care, the office-based surgical facility must have in place similar or corresponding systems that also ensure a safe setting. An office-based surgical facility can achieve validation and public recognition of a safe operating environment through the process of accreditation.

Practice Accreditation

In this context, we define accreditation as a voluntary process whereby an agency or an association grants public recognition to a school, institute, college, or university or any organization that meets certain established standards, as determined through initial and periodic evaluations (1).

Although the accreditation process has been developed and used most widely in the educational sector of society, it was first introduced to health care in 1915, when the American College of Surgeons established operational standards for hospitals. Evolving from this earlier endeavor, the Joint Commission on Accreditation of Hospitals was established in 1951 and has since changed its name to the Joint Commission on Accreditation of Health Care Organizations (JCAHO). Other health care accrediting bodies include the Accreditation Association for Ambulatory Health Care (AAAHC), the National Committee on Quality Assurance, the Commission on Accreditation of Rehabilitation Facilities, and the Commission on Office Laboratory Accreditation.

In distinguishing the accreditation process from that of certification and/or licensure, an organization or entity rather than an individual is conferred recognition in the accreditation process. In addition to the practicing physician(s), the organization's staff, physical plant, and policies and procedures are reviewed as well in the accreditation survey. In contradistinction to this, the certification process generally grants recognition to an individual professional who has met certain standards of knowledge and performance. This traditional meaning of certification has been somewhat distorted by the Health Care Financing Administration (HCFA) by referring to its member Ambulatory Service Centers (ASCs) as Medicare-certified when meeting Medicare conditions of participation.

Medicare certification, state licensure, and state Certificate of Need reviews are carried out by state government health agencies and their representatives with whom HCFA contracts to conduct Medicare ASC certification reviews. Medicare ASC certification and state ASC licensure reviews may be conducted simultaneously in some states. On the other hand, accreditation surveys are conducted by private agencies, which are usually not for profit organizations.

Accreditation, Certification, Licensure, and Certificate of Need

Whereas requirements necessary to achieve accreditation are nationally uniform, conditions required to be granted Medicare ASC certification, Certificate of Need, and/or state ASC licensure vary widely among different states. Also, accreditation standards tend to be more generic and process oriented in nature than are Medicare ASC certification standards, which are more specific and prescriptive in both structure and tone. On July 23, 1996, as a result of legislation enacted by Congress, HCFA published in the *Federal Register* a long awaited proposal notice to grant deeming authority to both AAAHC and JCAHO for ambulatory surgical centers. The deemed status proposal has been finalized, and this was published by HCFA in the *Federal Register* on December 19, 1996. ASCs will now have the option of obtaining Medicare certification either by becoming accredited or by completing a Medicare certification survey conducted by state agencies that have historically performed this function. In conducting Medicare reviews, both AAAHC and JCAHO will apply certain additional standards beyond the normal accreditation standards, and both agencies have agreed to conduct surveys on an unannounced basis rather than on a normally scheduled and announced basis of accreditation surveys.

Accreditation Association for Ambulatory Health Care

Both AAAHC and now JCAHO will accredit ambulatory surgical centers, including solo physician office surgery centers and practices. As both a AAAHC surveyor and proprietor of an accredited solo physician office surgical facility and practice, I am familiar and experienced both with AAAHC accreditation standards and the survey process. With this in mind, we focus on the accreditation process and standards of AAAHC.

History of AAAHC

Founded in 1979 as a not for profit corporation in Illinois, AAAHC stated as its purpose to organize and operate a peer-based assessment, education, and accreditation program for ambulatory health care organizations as a means of assisting them to provide the highest achievable level of care for recipients in the most efficient and economically sound manner.

The birth of this organization followed a decision by the JCAH in 1978 to dissolve its Accreditation Counsels, including the Accreditation Counsel for Ambulatory Health Care, which was formed in 1975. The six charter members of the AAAHC corporation had either withdrawn from or suspended discussion about cooperative accreditation efforts with JCAH as a result of its reorganization. Each charter member designated AAAHC as its national accrediting body, appointed members to its governing board, and contributed funds to the development and operation of its programs.

Current AAAHC Membership and Programs

There are now 13 member associations of AAAHC, which is governed by a 22-member board of directors, which includes one public member. Fourteen of 22 board members represent surgical associations or specialties. Most AAAHC surveyors are involved in ambulatory surgery. These member organizations include

- American College Health Association;
- Federated Ambulatory Surgery Association;
- Medical Group Management Association;
- National Association of Community Health Centers;
- Outpatient Ophthalmic Surgery Society;
- American Academy of Facial Plastic and Reconstructive Surgery;
- American Society of Outpatient Surgeons;
- American College of Occupational and Environmental Medicine;
- American Academy of Dental Group Practice;
- American Association of Oral and Maxillofacial Surgeons;
- American Academy of Cosmetic Surgery;
- Association of Free Standing Radiation Oncology Centers;
- American Society for Dermatologic Surgery.

Now in its 17th year of operation, AAAHC has accredited more than 500 ambulatory health care organizations, 75–80% of which are ambulatory surgical providers. The continued growth and success of AAAHC reflects increasing acceptance and recognition of its accreditation program by the health care community, state and federal government agencies, third-party payers, managed care organizations, and the general public.

AAAHC has continued its tradition of using physicians, administrators, and other health care professionals who are actively involved in ambulatory health care to conduct its accreditation surveys. There are now more than 200 individuals listed on the active surveyor roster.

In the last 2 years, AAAHC has sponsored and conducted several full-length educational programs in response to an expressed need for more training and education in quality improvement and accreditation standards. These programs have supplemented workshops and presentations provided by AAAHC at other ambulatory health care meetings. In addition to providing Ambulatory Health Care Accreditation Conferences, AAAHC also conducts educational programs for its team of surveyors.

AAAHC Accreditation Policies and Procedures

Dedicated to improving the quality of medical, surgical, and dental care to this nation's patients in various ambulatory venues, AAAHC has played an important role in facilitating cost-effective delivery of high quality health care in the ambulatory setting. In fulfilling its mission, AAAHC has assisted many small health care organizations, including solo surgeon's offices, in both understanding and integrating into operations the basic tenets of quality assurance and quality improvement. AAAHC has noticed a dramatic increase in demand for surveys in the last year because of increasing incentives for ambulatory health care providers to seek public recognition through the accreditation process.

Survey Eligibility Criteria

AAAHC considers all survey applications on an individual basis and determines whether the standards can be applied to the applicant. Several criteria should be met for an organization to be considered for an accreditation survey:

- Ongoing provision of health care services for at least 6 months before the on-site survey;
- Formal organization and legal constitution either as an entity primarily providing health care services or as a subunit providing such services of another entity which may, but need not be, a health care organization;
- Compliance with applicable federal, state, and local laws and regulations;
- Licensure for the organization if required by the state;
- Sharing of facilities, equipment, business management, and records involved in patient care among members of the organization;
- Operation without limitation because of race, creed, sex, or national origin;
- Submission of signed survey application, presurvey questionnaire, and other documents in advance of the survey;
- Payment of application and survey fees.

AAAHC surveys a wide variety of organizations, including college and university health services, community health centers, dental group practices, health maintenance organizations, occupational health services, radiation oncology centers, surgical recovery centers, and urgent/immediate care centers. Of more specific interest to the readers of this text, other accreditable entities include

- Office surgery centers and practices;
- Single specialty group practices;
- Multispecialty group practices;
- Ambulatory surgery centers;
- Birthing centers.

Application of AAAHC Standards

AAAHC has developed standards to reflect characteristics of an accreditable organization striving to attain the highest possible levels of quality patient care. The standards tend to be written in general rather than specific terms where possible to allow an organization to achieve compliance in a manner most consistent with its particular situation. In interpreting the standards, AAAHC is concerned with the intent of the standard first and with the letter of the standard second. A series of core standards applies to all organizations (see below), and another series of adjunct standards are applied as appropriate to services provided by the entity being accredited.

Ambulatory surgery centers and office surgery practices are evaluated for compliance with standards for anesthesia and surgical services and other relevant adjunct standards such as those for pharmaceutical services and pathology and medical laboratory services. AAAHC expects an accreditable organization to demonstrate substantial compliance with the applicable standards, and this is evaluated by review of documented evidence, by answers to detailed questions concerning implementation and/or by on site observations and interviews by surveyors.

AAAHC Survey Process

Details of the survey process are described in the *Accreditation Handbook for Ambulatory Health Care*,[a] which has undergone eight revisions since it was first published in 1979. An organization can evaluate its readiness for accreditation by reviewing the *Accreditation Handbook* and *Self Assessment Manual*. After this assessment is completed, the *Application for Accreditation Survey* may be requested, completed, and then submitted to AAAHC with a nonrefundable survey application fee (currently $375.00).

A *Presurvey Questionnaire* should also be completed and submitted before the survey to enable the AAAHC staff to review the governing structure and health care services provided by the applicant organization.

Accreditation Survey Site Visit

After the appropriate materials are submitted by the applicant organization, AAAHC staff members review the documents and determine the number of surveyors needed, as well as the number of days required for the site survey, and then determines and quotes a survey fee that can range from $2,900.00 for a small surgical office to $7,500.00 for a large ambulatory surgery facility. A survey team and survey date are then selected.

During the site visit, the surveyors first meet with the organization's staff in an orientation session. A tour of the facility follows, and then the survey team reviews a sample of at least 25 clinical records. Interviews with medical and administrative staff members are conducted by the surveyors, who also review quality improvement projects, governance and administrative documents, and materials relevant to patient rights and satisfaction. The surveyors observe a surgical procedure and inspect the facilities and environment, including the anesthesia equipment and operating room.

At the conclusion of this fact-finding visit, the surveyors complete a *Survey Report Form* to evaluate the organization's compliance with the standards and to make recommendations based on observed variances, as well as other consultative comments not necessarily related directly to compliance with the standards. The surveyors findings are then discussed at a summation conference with the organization's staff.

---

[a]AAAHC has published several texts including *Accreditation Handbook for Ambulatory Health Care, Self Assessment Manual, Pre-survey Questionnaire,* and *Physical Environment Checklist for Ambulatory Surgical Centers*. The *Survey Report Form* is used by members of the survey teams to submit a report after a survey site visit.

Figure 13.1. Certificate of Accreditation.

Accreditation Decision

After the AAAHC staff reviews the *Survey Report Form*, this document is then presented to the Accreditation Committee, which meets monthly by telephone conference call and which then renders one of five accreditation decisions.

- Accredited for Three Years. The organization demonstrates substantial compliance with the standards, and the Accreditation Committee has no reservations about the organizations commitment to continue providing high quality care.
- Accredited for One Year. The organization is substantially compliant with the standards, but its commitment to ongoing compliance with the standards is not sufficiently well established to warrant a 3-year accreditation decision.
- Deferred Accreditation Decision. The organization is in less than substantial compliance with one or more standards but demonstrates the commitment and capability to correct the identified deficiencies within 6 months. In such instances, the applicant organization may request another survey site visit without paying an additional application fee, and this request may be made within 6 months of notification of the deferred accreditation decision.
- Denial. The organization is not in substantial compliance with the standards and is therefore not accredited.
- Provisionally Accredited. This recently created category is rendered to certain organizations not in substantial compliance with the standards but expected to verify and document changes to achieve compliance within the ensuing 6 months. These organizations may or may not require a follow-up survey. This new category is necessitated by governmental regulations requiring some form of accreditation, and governmental bodies recognize a provisional accreditation decision. A Certificate of Accreditation is issued to the applicant organization after a favorable accreditation decision is rendered (Fig. 13.1).

AAAHC Standards

The standards used by AAAHC for surveys of surgical facilities are described fully in the *Accreditation Handbook for Ambulatory Health Care,* which is updated and revised biannually. Standards contained in the *1996/1997 Handbook* became effective October 1, 1996. We offer summary comments on the standards in this text.

A series of eight core standards are considered so essential to the provision of quality health care by any facility that they are applied consistently to all organizations surveyed by AAAHC:

1. Rights of patients;
2. Governance;
3. Administration;
4. Quality of care provided;
5. Quality management and improvement;
6. Clinical records;
7. Professional improvement;
8. Facilities and environment.

Standards 1 through 8 apply to all organizations seeking accreditation. Adjunct standards are also appropriate to the services provided by the organization and are as follows:

9. Anesthesia services;
10. Surgical services;
11. Overnight care and services;

12. Dental services;
13. Emergency services;
14. Immediate/urgent care services;
15. Pharmaceutical services;
16. Pathology and medical laboratory services;
17. Diagnostic imaging services;
18. Radiation oncology treatment services;
19. Occupational health services;
20. Other professional technical services;
21. Teaching and publication activities;
22. Research activities.

These adjunct standards are applied in the event that an organization being surveyed provides any of the services referenced in one or more of the adjunct standards. For an ambulatory surgical facility, the 8 core standards would be applied along with standard 9 on anesthesia and standard 10 on surgery. Standard 15 on pharmaceutical services and standard 16 on pathology and medical laboratory services would probably also be applied. We focus on adjunct standards 9, 10, 15, and 16 in this text. The reader is referred to the *1996/1997 Accreditation Handbook for Ambulatory Health Care* for additional information on the adjunct standards we do not comment on here.

Rights of Patients

This standard affirms that basic human rights of patients are recognized by an accreditable entity. This can be validated in part by displaying a Patient Bill of Rights prominently in the facility's reception areas; the survey team will look for this document (Fig. 13.2).

It is important that patients be afforded privacy in dressing and treatment areas and also in business areas of the facility when discussing payment and financial obligations. Examining tables should be positioned to face away from the treatment room/operating room doors. Privacy dressing curtains in treatment rooms further demonstrate commitment to this standard. The organization should demonstrate that patient records are treated confidentially; that patients are provided complete information regarding diagnosis, evaluation, treatment, and prognosis; and that they are given the opportunity to participate in decisions involving their health care unless contraindicated. The survey team reviews marketing and advertising materials, information available to patients on fees for services and payment policies, and methods available to patients to express grievances and suggestions to the organizations. A surveyor may telephone the facility after hours to ensure that care is available at that time.

Governance

An accreditable entity needs a functioning governing body that sets policy and is responsible for the organization. The sole proprietor physician of a solo office surgical facility would function as the governing body in such a setting in lieu of a corporate board of directors.

AAAHC requests documentation that the organization is a legally constituted entity or an organized subunit of such a entity in the state or equivalent jurisdiction in which it is located and provides services. Such documentation could be in the form of a charter, articles of incorporation, partnership or franchise agreement, legislative or executive act,

Patient Bill of Rights

Women's Center for Healthcare is committed to providing comprehensive health care in a manner which acknowledges the uniqueness and dignity of each patient. We encourage patients and families to have clear knowledge of, and to participate in, matters and decisions relating to their medical care.

1. A patient has the right to respectful care given by competent personnel.

2. A patient has the right, upon request, to be given the name of his attending practitioner, the names of all other practitioner directly participating in his care, and the names and functions of other health care persons having direct contact with the patient.

3. A patient has the right to consideration of privacy concerning his own medical care program. Case discussion, consultation, examination and treatment are considered confidential and shall be conducted discreetly.

4. A patient has the right to have records pertaining to his medical care treated as confidential except as otherwise provided by law or third party contractual arrangements.

5. A patient has the right to know what facility rules and regulations apply to his conduct as a patient.

6. The patient has the right to expect emergency procedures to be implemented without unnecessary delay.

7. The patient has the right to good quality care and high professional standards that are continually maintained and reviewed.

8. The patient has the right to full information in layman's terms, concerning diagnosis, treatment and prognosis, including information about alternative treatments and possible complications. When it is not medically advisable to give this information to the patient, the information shall be given on his behalf to the responsible person.

9. Except for emergencies, the practitioner shall obtain the necessary informed consent prior to the start of the procedure.

10. A patient or, if the patient is unable to give informed consent, a responsible person has the right to be advised when a practitioner is considering the patient as a part of a medical care research program or donor program, and the patient or the responsible person, shall give informed consent prior to actual participation in the program. A patient, or responsible person may refuse to continue in a program to which he has previously given informed consent.

11. A patient has the right to refuse drugs or procedures, to the extent permitted by statue, and practitioner shall inform the patient of the medical consequences of the patient's refusal of drugs or procedures.

12. A patient has the right to medical and nursing services without discrimination based upon age, race, color, religion, sex, national origin, handicap, disability or source of payment.

13. The patient who does not speak English shall have access, where possible, to an interpreter.

14. The facility shall provide the patient, or patient designee, upon request, access to the information contained in his medical records, unless access is specifically restricted by the attending practitioner for medical reasons.

15. The patient has the right to expect good management techniques to be implemented within the facility. These techniquesshall make effective use of the time of the patient and avoid the personal discomfort of the patient.

16. When an emergency occurs and a patient is transferred to another facility, the responsible person shall be notified. The institution to which the patient is to be transferred shall be notified prior to the patient's transfer.

17. The patient has the right to expect that the facility will provide information for continuing health care requirements following discharge and the means for meeting them.

18. A patient has the right to expect that the facility will provide information for continuing healthcare requirements following discharge and the means for meeting them.

19. A patient has the right to be informed of his rights at the time of his admission.

Figure 13.2. Patient Bill of Rights.

or notation of function as a sole proprietorship. Full disclosure of ownership is also expected of the governing body by AAAHC.

The governing body is expected to address and assume full responsibility, some of which may be professionally delegated, for the operation and performance of the entity being delegated.

The governing body is responsible for articulating organizational mission, goals, and objectives and corresponding strategic planning. Preparation and posting of a mission statement would document this responsibility, and minutes of the governing body meet-

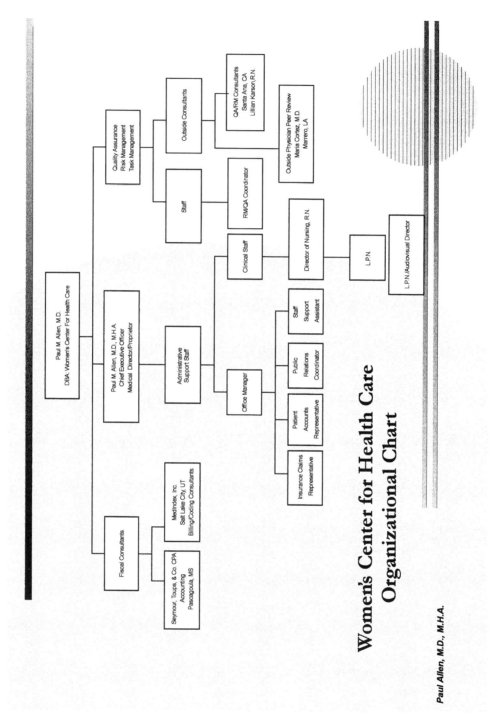

Figure 13.3. Organizational chart.

ings, which should occur at least annually, might reflect formulation of long-range planning.

The governing body is also responsible for establishing an organizational structure, which specifies functional relationships among its various components. Construction of an organizational chart documents compliance with this standard, and the survey team will undoubtedly review such an organizational chart (Fig. 13.3).

The governing body is also responsible for policies and procedures and rules and regulations to ensure the orderly development, management, and conduct of the organization. A manual or book should be maintained by the facility that documents relevant policies and procedures. These policies and procedures should also be validated or archived periodically, perhaps biannually. This manual should be available for surveyor review and should contain policy statements regarding quality of care issues, legal and ethical matters, organizational communication, financial management and accountability, rights of patients, approval of contracts affecting medical/surgical care provided, methods and materials used for marketing and advertising, risk management program, continuing education policies, and mechanisms to ensure compliance with Occupational Safety and Health Administration and Americans with Disabilities Act rules.

A series of criteria to obtain credentials appear with the governance standards that calls for a process to ensure initial appointment, reappointment, and assignment or curtailment of clinical privileges based on professional peer evaluation. A credentials file should be maintained for each physician using the facility and for each allied health care practitioner as well. The organization should have its own independent process to obtain credentials and complete its own primary source verification of credentials. The American Medical Association Physician Profile Service is an excellent resource for such verification and will provide a physician profile of credentials upon request for a minimal fee.

Administration

This standard calls for management of an accreditable facility in a manner that ensures delivery of high quality health services and fulfills the mission, goals, and objectives of the organization.

The policy and procedure manual previously described should document that systematic controls are implemented to enforce policies delegated by the governing board. Administrative policies should demonstrate that qualified personnel are employed, that applicable laws and regulations are recognized, that planning goals are achieved, that the organization's assets are protected, and that fiscal controls have been implemented. Administrative policies should ensure vertical and horizontal communication and delineate lines of authority, accountability, and supervision within the organization. Systems should also be in place to control inventory, control custody of official documents, and secure confidentiality and safety of data on both patients and staff.

The manual should also contain relevant personnel policies, including a listing of job descriptions, performance evaluation methods, procedures for compensation review, and provisions for orientation of newly hired personnel to the facility. A policy should also be articulated to define the status of students and postgraduate trainees when they are present at a facility.

Administrative personnel should ensure that patient satisfaction is assessed, documented, and reported to the governing body (Figs. 13.4 and 13.5).

PATIENT SURVEY QUESTIONNAIRE

Welcome to the office of Dr. Paul M. Allen

It is our desire to provide you with the finest in modern medical care in a courteous and friendly atmosphere. To help us live up to this goal, we ask for your assistance. Your comments are sincerely appreciated and extremely helpful.

<u>**THANK YOU FOR TAKING THE TIME TO COMPLETE THIS QUESTIONNAIRE**</u>

1. Please check: First visit_____ Return visit_____
2. Is the location of this office convenient for you? Yes____ No____
3. How long does it take you to travel to our office? _____
4. How did you get to our office today? Auto____ Bus____ Taxi____ Other____
5. When you called our office, how far in advance was your appointment scheduled? ____Days ____Weeks ____Months. Was this time span satisfactory for you? Yes____ No____
6. When you arrived today, how long did you wait to be seen?_____
7. Do you feel your waiting time was satisfactory? Yes ____ No ____
8. What hours are best for you to schedule an appointment? _____
9. Would childcare be helpful? Yes____ No____
10. Is transportation to the office of concern? Yes____ No____

Please Check

	Excellent	Above Average	Average	Below Average	Poor
The courtesy of our receptionist when you phoned our office?					
The courtesy extended by the doctor?					
The seating in our reception room?					
The selection of reading materials?					
The appearance and neatness of our staff?					
The courteousness of our staff?					
Your general impression of the appearance and cleanliness of our office?					
The doctor's patient and interest in your problem?					
The doctor's explanation of your problem and treatment?					

If you have any suggestions about service in our office, please write them below. Feel welcome to comment on any topic.

_____

_____

_____

Name (optional): _____   Date: ____/____/____

Figure 13.4. Patient Survey Questionnaire.

Quality of Care Provided

The criteria described in this section require provision of high quality health care services in accordance with the principles of professional practice and ethical conduct by an accreditable organization, which should also show concern for the cost of care and for improving the community's health status.

Compliance with this set of standards requires assurance that all health care practitioners have appropriate education and competence to deliver the professional services provided by the organization and that these providers practice in an ethical and legal manner. Support personnel at the facility should also be appropriately trained, qualified, and supervised and should be available in adequate numbers to provide the services offered by the facility.

Other indicators of high quality health care services include education of patients

Women's Center for Health Care

<u>SURGERY SATISFACTION QUESTIONNAIRE</u>

DEAR PATIENT:

We value you as a patient. To help us continue to provide adequate patient care, please complete the following:

Name: _____

Date of Surgery: _____/_____/_____

CATEGORY	Excellent	Above Average	Average	Below Average
COURTESY OF OFFICE STAFF				
CARE GIVEN BY STAFF				
DOCTOR'S EXPLANATION OF YOUR SURGERY				
PRE-OPERATIVE INSTRUCTIONS GIVEN BY STAFF				
POST-OPERATIVE INSTRUCTIONS GIVEN BY STAFF				

COMMENTS:

_____

_____

_____

_____

Figure 13.5. Surgery Satisfaction Questionnaire.

regarding diagnosis and treatment of their conditions, related preventative measures, and access to and use of the health care system. Additionally, documentation should be evident that diagnosis is appropriate, timely, and based on history and physical examination and that treatment is consistent with the clinical impression or working diagnosis. Assurance of appropriate and timely consultation and referral, when indicated, should also be apparent. Other related criteria include absence of clinically unnecessary diagnostic or therapeutic procedures, appropriate and timely follow-up of test results and other findings, and provision of health care services consistent with current professional knowledge. The clinical records should document accurate and complete entries of patient encounters, timely patient contact, follow-up of abnormal findings and significant problems, and transfer of care and information related to care from one health care practitioner to another when needed.

An accreditable organization should demonstrate concern for cost of care issues by avoiding duplicate diagnostic procedures, using the least expensive alternative resources when suitable, providing treatments with appropriate frequency, and using ancillary services that are relevant to and consistent with patient needs.

Provisions should be made for practitioners and staff to communicate with patients in the language primarily used by them. Accessing AT&T Language Line Services gives users quick telephone access to highly trained interpreters in as many as 140 languages, 24 hours a day, 365 days a year.

Quality Management and Improvement

This standard has historically caused the most difficulty for AAAHC organizations and has sometimes been the singular reason for rendering 1-year and deferral accreditation decisions. This standard calls for maintenance of an active, integrated, peer-based program of quality management and improvement that links peer review, quality management activities, and risk management activities in an organized systematic way.

Surveyors look for physician peer involvement in quality management and improvement endeavors. A minimum of two physicians should be involved in quality improvement activities to provide peer-based review, all of which cannot be delegated to the nursing staff. In a solo physician organization such as an office-based surgical facility for a solo practitioner, an outside physician should be involved in the peer review function. Peer review should be conducted on an ongoing regular basis. All peer review activity should be documented, and an example of a physician peer review roster is shown in Figure 13.6. An occurrence screening review worksheet can be used to document physician peer review, and examples of such a worksheet are shown in Figure 13.7.

Because AAAHC standards are generic and process-oriented by design, an accreditable organization may structure its quality improvement program in any manner that best meets its particular situation and needs, as long as it addresses problems and resolves issues. It is not sufficient to merely collect data for ongoing monitoring of care without efforts to improve quality or address problems. AAAHC has traditionally asked a series of questions of a quality assurance program:

- Has an important problem in the care of patients been identified?
- Were the frequency, source, and severity of suspected problems or concerns evaluated?
- Was corrective action taken to solve the problem?
- Was the problem reevaluated to determine whether corrective measures were successful?
- If the problem persisted or recurred after the initial corrective measures were implemented, was alternative corrective action taken?
- Were the results shared with appropriate personnel, the chief executive officer, and the governing body?

Elements of a quality improvement study are shown in Figure 13.8.

A systematized risk management program should be developed and maintained by an accreditable entity to improve the quality of care delivered and to protect the organization's financial, human, and physical assets.

AAAHC criteria call for a person or committee to be responsible for the risk management program. Methods should be in place to refuse care or to dismiss a patient from care. Unpaid accounts should be reviewed before referral to a collection agency with the consideration of factors such as outcome. All incidents reported by employees, visitors, or patients should be reviewed (Fig. 13.9). All litigation involving the organization, its staff, and its health care practitioners should also be reviewed periodically, as should all deaths, trauma, or adverse events. Patient complaints should be addressed. Policies dealing with physician and employee impairment should be developed. Other issues that should be an integral part of the risk management program include communications with professional liability insurance carrier; response to inquiries from governmental agencies, attorneys, consumer advocate groups, and the media; and methods for complying with applicable governmental regulations and contractual agreements. Methods to prevent unauthorized prescribing and to establish and document after-hour coverage should be

WOMEN'S CENTER FOR HEALTHCARE
PASCAGOULA, MS

PHYSICIAN PEER REVIEW ROSTER

PHYSICIAN PEER REVIEW DATE	PATIENT IDENTIFICATION	DESCRIPTION OF VARIATION
May 15, 1993	6530	Unable to complete urodynamic studies because Millar catheters not working.
May 15, 1993	6992	Difficult Norplant cartridge removal.
August 8, 1993	6154	Patient underwent laser vaporization of the cervix for dysplasia December 1990 and has been seen here several times in 1992 and 1993, but pap smears not taken at any of these visits.
December 18, 1993	8382	Severe cervical dysplasia on biopsy. Class I pap smear on cytology.
December 18, 1993	8841	Procedure cancelled after patients arrival because of vasovagal reaction.
January 22, 1994	4701	Urinary retention following urethrocystoscopy with dilatation.
June 19, 1994	7713	Patient with recurrent severe cervical dysplasia, postoperative laser vaporization/conization of cervix and subsequent cold knife cervical conization. Patient seems reluctant to undergo hysterectomy.
May 6, 1995	5316	Review of Class II pap unsatisfactory, limited by obscuring blood. Patient subsequently diagnosed with invasive cervical carcinoma. Pap smear does not reflect diagnosis.
January 13, 1996	8943	Prolonged lower genital tract laser surgical procedure due to inability to reactivate laser beam after procedure was started resulting in 50 minute delay before procedure could be completed.
June 1, 1996	9988	Twenty seven year old female who underwent hysteroscopy May 24, 1996 following difficult laminaria insertion on May 23, 1996 and difficult laminaria removal at the time of hysteroscopy because of cervical stenosis associated with old cervical lacerations and previous cervical cryotherapy. Patient's postoperative course was complicated by endometritis, salpingitis, and hematometra requiring hospitalization one week postoperatively and subsequent dilatation of the cervix with endometrial curetting and drainage of hematometra under general anesthesia.
August 10, 1996	6261	Patient underwent intralesional interferon injection July 30, 1996 for recurrent vulvar condyloma acuminata. Patient returned to office August 1, 1996 with intense local reaction to interferon injection.
August 31, 1996	5156	Forty-five year old female who underwent EMG/electrical stimulation by nursing staff for detrusor instability suffered vulvar burn when EMG probe slipped from vagina.

Figure 13.6. Physician Peer Review Roster.

OCCURRENCE SCREENING REVIEW WORKSHEET

DEPT. *GYN*

RECORD #: *8943*

PHYSICIAN: *PMA*

OCCURRENCE: *Reviewed for prolonged operating time due to inability to reactivate laser beam after procedure was started. There was a 50 minute delay before we could continue and then complete the procedure.*

REVIEWER COMMENTS:

1. Why did this happen? *Technical failure of instruments may happen at any time during a surgical procedure.*

2. How could this have been prevented? *Although preventative maintenance avoids most of the mechanical failures, at times they just occur.*

SIGNIFICANCE SCALE	ACTION TAKEN
0 = No variation (occurrence) 1 = *Variation justified.* 2 = Clinical variation unexpected but acceptable. 3 = Clinical variation unexpected but reasonably avoidable. 4 = Questionable clinical practice. 5 = Highly questionable clinical	*No action at this time* Send letter to M.D. Monitor M.D. for possible trend Refer to Department Refer to Professional Affairs

Physician Reviewer: *M. Cortez, M.D.*   Date Reviewed: *January 13, 1996*

A

Figure 13.7. (**A–C**) Occurrence Screening Review Worksheet.

OCCURRENCE SCREENING REVIEW WORKSHEET

DEPT. *GYN*

RECORD #: *N/A*

PHYSICIAN: *PMA*

OCCURRENCE : *Review and comment on Pap Smear Follow up Surveillance Audit completed by Tracy Dickens in June 1996. Tracy has reviewed 121 patients who are under concurrent pap smear surveillance, and we found ten patients who had been lost to follow up.*

REVIEWER COMMENTS:

1. Why did this happen? *Patients do not respond for various reasons. They move, have follow up elsewhere, etc.*

2. How could this have been prevented? *Cannot prevent certain number of non-responders and non-compliance. A total of only ten out of one hundred and twenty patients is very good.*

SIGNIFICANCE SCALE	ACTION TAKEN
0 = *No variation (occurrence)*	*No action at this time*
1 = *Variation justified.*	*Send letter to M.D.*
2 = *Clinical variation unexpected but acceptable.*	*Monitor M.D. for possible trend*
	Refer to Department
3 = *Clinical variation unexpected but reasonably avoidable.*	*Refer to Professional Affairs*
4 = *Questionable clinical practice.*	
5 = *Highly questionable clinical*	

Physician Reviewer: *Nancy Bryant, M.D.* Date Reviewed: *June 1, 1996*

B

Figure 13.7. *(continued)*

OCCURRENCE SCREENING REVIEW WORKSHEET

DEPT. *GYN*

RECORD #: *9988*

PHYSICIAN: *PMA*

OCCURRENCE : *Twenty seven year old female who underwent hysteroscopy May 24, 1996 following difficult laminaria insertion on May 23, 1996 and difficult laminaria removal at the time of hysteroscopy because of cervical stenosis associated with old cervical lacerations and previous cervical cryotherapy. Patient's postoperative course was complicated by endometritis, salpingitis, and hematometra requiring hospitalization one week postoperatively and subsequent dilatation of the cervix with endometrial curetting and drainage of hematometra under general anesthesia.*

REVIEWER COMMENTS:

1. Why did this happen? *This patient has cervical stenosis.*

2. How could this have been prevented? *Perhaps since this patient presented with cervical stenosis which made it difficult for laminaria insertion and hysteroscopy, she could have been given a full therapeutic antibiotic therapy course for a few days after the procedure was done.*

SIGNIFICANCE SCALE	ACTION TAKEN
0 = No variation (occurrence) 1 = Variation justified. **2 = Clinical variation unexpected but acceptable.** 3 = Clinical variation unexpected but reasonably avoidable. 4 = Questionable clinical practice. 5 = Highly questionable clinical	*No action at this time* Send letter to M.D. Monitor M.D. for possible trend Refer to Department Refer to Professional Affairs *This recommendation was discussed personally with the attending physician.*
Physician Reviewer: *M. Cortez, M.D.*	Date Reviewed: *June 1, 1996*

C

Figure 13.7. *(continued)*

WOMEN'S CENTER FOR HEALTH CARE
Paul M. Allen, M.D.
2812 ANDREW AVENUE • P.O. BOX 1345
PASCAGOULA, MISSISSIPPI 39567
(601) 769-6389 • FAX (601) 769-5073

— Gynecology
— Gynecologic Laser Surgery
— Urogynecology and Urodynamics
— Infertility
— Obstetrics

Diplomate American Board Of Obstetrics And Gynecology
Fellow American College Of
Obstetricians And Gynecologists

QUALITY MANAGEMENT AND IMPROVEMENT STUDY

STANDARD: *Auditor to monitor patients undergoing therapy for lower genital tract neoplasia to be followed up by pap smear surveillance on a semi-annual basis. Note patient follow up over one year to see if compliance with surveillance criteria are being met.*

OBJECTIVES: *To determine if surveillance rate is acceptable.*

ASSESSMENT TOOLS: *Pap smear follow up surveillance variance report.*

SUMMARY OF FINDINGS: *A total of one hundred twenty-one patients were eligible for post treatment pap smear follow up surveillance. Ten patients missed follow up pap smear surveillance or colposcopic evaluation.*

PLAN OF ACTION: *Patients who had been lost to surveillance follow up were contacted immediately upon completion of study to resume surveillance.*

CONCLUSION: *A surveillance variance rate of 8.3% is acceptable.*

FOLLOW UP: *We will repeat this study on an annual basis.*

Prepared by: *Tracy Dickens, R.N.*   Date: *6/13/96*

Title: *Director of Nursing/Quality Assurance Coordinator*

Reviewed by: *Paul M. Allen, M.D.*   Date: *7/17/96*

Title: *Chief Executive Officer/Medical Director*

A Single Specialty Ambulatory Surgical Center
Accredited by **Accreditation Association for Ambulatory Health Care, Inc.**

A

Figure 13.8. (A–C) Quality Improvement Study/Pap Smear Surveillance.

PAP SMEAR FOLLOW UP SURVEILLANCE VARIANCE REPORT

MONTH: *JUNE*   DATE: *1996*

PATIENT NAME	DIAGNOSIS	TREATMENT	DATE OF LAST PAP SMEAR	REASON FOR SURVEILLANCE VARIANCE	ACTION TAKEN
VA	Cervical atypia and condyloma	11/94 - Laser Rx	9/95	Due for pap smear 3/96. On Q 6 month pap smears	Attempted contact 3/96
BT	Condyloma acuminata	9/94 - Laser Rx	6/95	Due for Q 6 month pap smear. Due 12/95	Phone call made, awaiting return call.
CH	Atypical pap smear - cervical dysplasia	6/95 - Laser Rx	5/95	Had 4 month follow up colposcopy 11/95. No follow up since	Dr. Allen dictated letter on 5/21/96
TB	Condyloma acuminata	7/93 - Laser Rx	7/95	No follow up since 7/95. On Q 6 month pap smears	2 letters sent. Attempted to reach by phone x 5.
MC	Cervical atypia	8/94 - Laser Rx	10/95	On Q 6 month pap smears No follow up since 10/95.	Attempted to call 3/96. R.N. called .
DB	Cervical atypia	4/95 - Laser Rx	3/95	Needs 4 month follow up colposcopy 8/95. No follow up since on pap smear or colposcopy.	
ED	Cervical dysplasia	10/94 - Laser Rx	11/94 Laser Rx; 4/95 - Laser Rx.	Due for pap smear 4/96. No follow up noted.	6/96 Message left for patient to call.
KC	Cervical dysplasia	2/95 - Laser Rx	9/95 - Colposcopy done	Due for follow up colposcopy 1/96. Not completed.	Colposcopy recently completed
JM	Cervical dysplasia	2/94 - Laser Rx	6/94 - Colposcopy done	No follow up since 6/94	Dr. Allen dictated letter to patient 5/96
LV	Cervical dysplasia	12/94 - Laser Rx	8/95 - Pap done	No follow up since 8/95. Due for Q 6 month pap smears.	6/96 Message left for patient to call

Total # of patients in surveillance: *121*   Total # of surveillance variances: *10*
Surveillance variance rate: *8.3%*

CRITERIA
1. On an annual basis, nurse auditor will search computer files for all patients with diagnosis 622.1 (cervical dysplasia), 233.1 (cervical carcinoma in situ), 233.3 (vulvar carcinoma in situ), 623.0 (vaginal dysplasia), and search computer files and clinical records if necessary to ensure adequate six month follow up surveillance.
2. Variance report will include patients on whom pap smear surveillance is past due.
3. Nurse auditor will determine date of last pap smear for patients on whom surveillance is past due and will document reason for variance. Nurse will further document follow up action taken in effort to resume pap smear surveillance.
4. This audit will be completed and report submitted annually in the month of June.

REPORT SUBMITTED BY: *Tracy Dickens, R.N*.   DATE: *6/7/96*

REPORT REVIEWED BY: *Paul M. Allen, M.D.*   DATE: *7/13/96*

Figure 13.8. *(continued)*

CHAPTER 13 / ACCREDITATION, RISK MANAGEMENT, AND REIMBURSEMENT

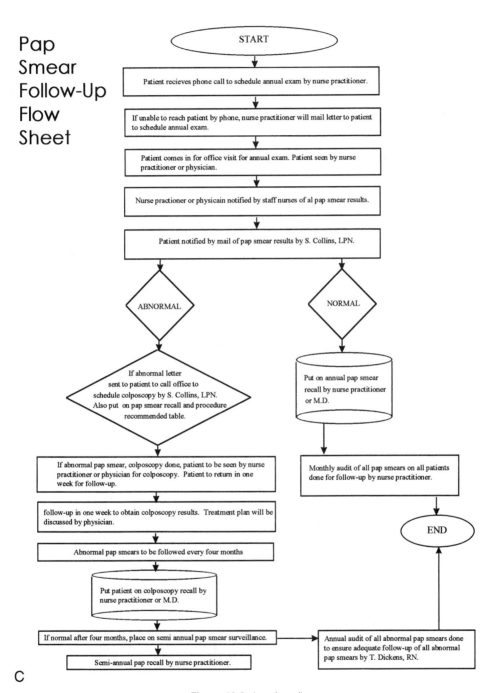

Figure 13.8. *(continued)*

WOMEN'S CENTER FOR HEALTH CARE
Paul M. Allen, M.D.

2812 ANDREW AVENUE • P.O. BOX 1345
PASCAGOULA, MISSISSIPPI 39567
(601) 769-6389 • FAX (601) 769-5073

— Gynecology
— Gynecologic Laser Surgery
— Urogynecology and Urodynamics
— Infertility
— Obstetrics

Diplomate American Board Of Obstetrics And Gynecology
Fellow American College Of
Obstetricians And Gynecologists

QUALITY ASSURANCE PROGRAM FOR WOMEN'S CENTER FOR HEALTH CARE

To effectively monitor quality assurance for Women's Center for Healthcare, the following program will be utilized.

1. QA checklist shall be completed per month including Dedicated Procedure Room Checklist, Exam Room Checklist, Audit Review (Quarterly), Lab Checklist, and QA activity log as monitoring tools to identify problems.

2. All problems identified should be written on the QA Activity Log as well as random problems identified by other staff or physician.

3. After identification of problems, a Quality Assurance study is completed if deemed necessary, and follow up review date is set.

4. Quality Assurance Study is then presented at staff meeting to QA committee (all staff).

5. Study must be signed by QA Coordinator and Physician.

6. Follow up with be completed as set.

 A Single Specialty Ambulatory Surgical Center
Accredited by **Accreditation Association for Ambulatory Health Care, Inc.**

Figure 13.9. (**A** and **B**) Quality Care Control Report.

WOMEN'S CENTER FOR HEALTH CARE

Quality Care Control Report

INSTRUCTION FOR USE
1. This form when completed provides an effective method of reporting occurrences to the practice's Quality Review/Risk Management Department. The reported data is used to monitor and evaluate the quality and safety of services and of the practice environment.
2. What to report? A reportable occurrence is a happening that is not consistent with normal practice operations or patient care.
3. Who should report? The immediate supervisor of the staff member most closely associated with the event is responsible for completing the report or having the most directly involved employee complete it.
4. When to complete the report? The report should be completed as soon after the occurrence as it is practical to do so.
5. Completing the form:
    a. Properly identify patient/individual.
    b. Complete applicable section of the report as it relates to the occurrence.
    c. If the occurrence you are reporting is not listed or additional space is needed, please describe occurrence in Section A below.
    d. Complete additional sections on back side of form as required.

A. BRIEFLY DESCRIBE EVENTS: Give facts: Include injury/damage/loss if any:

B. Occurrence follow-up report:

Completed by_____   _____
               Signature   Date

Reviewed by_____   _____
               Signature   Date

B

Figure 13.9. *(continued)*

evident. Clinical records and clinical record policies should be reviewed periodically. The staff should be educated in risk management activities. We expand our discussion of risk management activities in a office-based surgical facility later in this chapter after concluding remarks concerning accreditation.

Clinical Records

The criteria in this standard require maintenance of a user-friendly clinical records system from which information can be readily retrieved by health care practitioners. Records should be legible, accurate, and timely in documenting patient care.

Any record containing clinical, social, financial, or other data on a patient should be treated as strictly confidential and should be protected from loss, tampering, alteration, destruction, and unauthorized or inadvertent disclosure.

A person should be designated in charge of clinical records to ensure that these protective measures are carried out; to ensure the timely retrieval of records upon request; to provide unique identification of each patient's record; to supervise the collection, processing, maintenance, storage, retrieval, and distribution of records; and to maintain a predetermined organized record format and sequence. Allergies should be consistently declared and displayed in a prominent and uniform location. Reports and notes should be reviewed and filed in a timely manner.

A diagnostic and surgical procedure summary should be maintained to facilitate ongoing provision of rational care when a clinical record is complex and lengthy. Entries for each patient encounter should include date, provider name and professional status, purpose of visit, clinical findings, diagnosis or impression, studies ordered, treatments administered, disposition, recommendations, and instructions given to patients and authentication and verification of contents by the practitioner. Significant medical advice given to the patient by telephone both during and after normal hours of operation should be recorded.

Documentation of the informed consent process should be evident in the clinical record. A Clinical Research Protocol stamp or similar identifying method should distinguish diagnostic or therapeutic research intervention from nonresearch-related care. To ensure continuity of care, summaries or records should be obtained for patients treated elsewhere and conversely a summary forwarded to practitioners when patient care is transferred.

The survey team reviews a minimum of 25 records to ensure compliance with the above criteria.

Professional Improvement

The criteria in this standard call for organizational assurance of efforts to improve the professional competence, skills, and quality of performance of health care practitioners and other professional staff members in an accreditable entity.

A system to ensure orientation of personnel to the policies, procedures, and physical plan of a facility should be evident. Methods should also be in place to monitor continued maintenance of licensure and certification of professional personnel. Policies should be documented that encourage staff members to participate, at the organization's expense, in seminars, workshops, and other educational activities pertinent to the organization's mission, goals, and objectives. Certificates of attendance at such seminars should be placed in the personnel file.

Facilities and Environment

This standard has also caused considerable difficulty for AAAHC organizations striving to achieve compliance. The criteria in this standard call for a functionally safe and sanitary environment for the facility's patients, personnel, and visitors.

The facility must comply with applicable state and local building codes, as well as applicable state and local fire prevention regulations. The NFPA 101 Life Safety Code (both are registered trademarks of the National Fire Protection Association, Inc., Quincy, MA) is a commonly accepted guideline among states and localities. The local fire marshall should inspect the facility at least annually. Fire extinguishers of the proper types should be available to control a limited fire. This equipment should be appropriately positioned and maintained, along with prominently displayed fire instructions and evacuation routing. Personnel should be instructed periodically, perhaps by the fire marshall at the time of annual inspection, in the use of fire extinguishing equipment. Such periodic inspections and instructions should be documented.

Illuminated "exit" signs with emergency power capability should be positioned and readily visible at all exits from each floor or hall. Emergency lighting should be available to allow evacuation of patients and staff in the event of a power failure. All stairwells should be protected by fire doors.

A comprehensive emergency plan including both internal and external emergencies and disasters should be articulated and documented (Fig. 13.10). This should include a

WOMEN'S CENTER FOR HEALTH CARE

INTERNAL DISASTER PLAN

<u>**PURPOSE OF PLAN:**</u> To have guidelines in place to ensure safety of patients and staff in times of emergency/disaster.

<u>After Hour Emergencies</u>: i.e. robberies, flooding (internal or external), hurricanes or other severe damaging weather, fire, and/or power outages.

1. Dr. Allen will be notified after proper authorities have been (i.e. police, fire department, etc.).
2. Notify Executive Director and Director of Nursing.
3. Building will be secured if windows or doors have been damaged before leaving it.
4. Inventory of damage or loss will be taken as soon as possible.
5. Executive Director will submit inventory to insurance company for claims processing.
6. Patients will be notified and rescheduled if the building is deemed unsafe to provide good patient care without endangering them.
7. Safety meeting should be called per Dr. Allen as soon as possible to discuss proper handling of cleanup, changes to regular patient workload, all safety concerns, assisting authorities, etc.
8. Employees will then make every effort to ensure cleanup is done and order restored. This may include contacting necessary outside agencies if available and staff cannot safely complete the cleanup.
9. The Safety Training Coordinator will ensure that proper safety measures are followed by staff and contracted help. OSHA will be contacted if there is a question as to what procedures should be followed.

<u>During Office Disasters</u>: Robberies, or attempted robbery. Refer to Tornado/Inclement Weather Plan for weather emergencies. Refer to Fire Plan for fire emergencies.

1. Dr. Allen and staff are to remain calm.
2. Panic button should be pressed which is easily accessible without alarming intruders/robbers.
3. Staff should keep patients calm and provide for their safety, as well as their own.
4. Staff should cooperate fully with intruders/robbers to ensure safety of others. Under no circumstances should anyone confront the intruders/robbers for this could jeopardize the safety of others.
5. Authorities should be notified as soon as it is safe to do so.
6. The Executive Director should provide police with inventory of missing and damaged items and also insurance company.
7. Staff will cooperate with authorities to ensure that evidence is not tampered with.
8. Patients will be rescheduled if the office is not safe or if they would interfere with police procedures.
9. Refer to transfer and evacuation plans for injuries to personnel and/or staff.
10. Safety meeting should be called by Dr. Allen as soon as possible to discuss further actions and evaluate effectiveness of plan for this or any other internal or external disaster plan.

A

Figure 13.10. (A–D) External and Internal Disaster Policies.

ESCAPE ROUTE POLICY ON FIRES OR EMERGENCIES REQUIRING EVACUATION

In case of need for emergency escape:

<u>From Dr. Allen's office to rear of building:</u>

Emergency escape route shall be to exit down hall to garage in rear of building. Follow exit signs to (R) area of garage through exit door.

<u>From reception waiting to Nursing Office:</u>

Escape route shall be up hallway to front waiting room and out of front door.

In case of emergency, nurses will escort patients to safety via exit route. Office (clerical) personnel shall escort family members, visitor, or vendors to safety via exit route.

All employees, visitors, patients, vendors, shall gather outside in rear of building, and account for all patients, employees, visitors, and vendors. Director of Nursing shall account for all. In her absence, this authority will fall upon Office Manager.

<u>In case of fire:</u>

Person first suspecting fire should announce code red on Intercom#2 and call 911 - if time is available and then follow above instructions.

B

EMERGENCY ACTION PLAN

<u>Weather emergency:</u>

Tornado Warning:

Person first hearing weather alert should announce code blue 2 times on intercom.

Nurses shall gather all patients into hall instructing them to kneel in hall against wall with hands folded over their head.

Clerical staff shall assist visitors and/or vendors to do the same.

Lastly, employees shall take cover as documented above.

Director of Nursing and Office Manager shall listen to weather forecast to establish "all clear" and shall inform all patients, visitors, and vendors to return to previous location.

C

EXTERNAL DISASTER POLICY

In case of external disaster,
the office will be closed until physician deems
the office to be safe to re-open

D

Figure 13.10. *(continued)*

plan to evacuate patients during an internal emergency and provisions for efficient use of the facility and services during an external emergency such as hurricane, tornado, earthquake, or flood. Four fire drills should be conducted annually, and staff participation in these drills should be documented.

It is important that practitioners and staff members achieve and maintain *Advanced Cardiac Life Support Certification* as per the American Heart Association to validate availability of personnel familiar with cardiopulmonary resuscitation and the use of cardiac emergency equipment in the facility during hours of operation. Emergency equipment and supplies should be available and maintained.

Hazards that might result in slipping, falling, electrical shock, burns, poisoning, or other traumas should be eliminated. Smoking should be permitted only in designated areas and prohibited in operating and anesthesia areas where oxygen and other volatile gases are used and stored.

Amenities for patients and visitors such as parking, reception areas, toilets, and telephone should be provided in proportion to patient and visitor volume. Compliance with provisions of the Americans with Disabilities Act should be evident. Handicapped parking, building access, and properly designed bathroom facilities should be available.

Ventilation and lighting should be adequate, and cleaning and maintenance of the facility should also be ensured. Allocation of space for various administrative and clinical functions should be adequate. Infection control procedures should be implemented, including documented surveillance techniques.

Hazardous materials and wastes should be processed in a systematic manner that protects patients, staff, and the environment. This includes identification, management, handling, transport, treatment, and disposal of infectious, radioactive, chemical, and physical hazards.

Periodic testing and proper maintenance of all equipment are criteria in this set of standards, as is availability of an alternate power source, which is adequate for protection of the life and safety of patients and staff. A UPS battery pack or similar alternate power source should provide enough electrical power to complete a surgical procedure in the event of electrical power failure.

Additional Medicare-related standards are applied by AAAHC when an ASC facility requests that its accreditation survey be recognized for Medicare ASC certification. These include presence of a separate recovery room and waiting area and availability of an emergency call system, oxygen, cardiac defibrillator, cardiac monitoring equipment, tracheostomy set, laryngoscopes, endotracheal tubes, and suction equipment.

With few exceptions, Medicare-certified ASCs must also meet the provisions of the 1985 edition of the Life Safety Code of the National Fire Protection Association that apply to ambulatory surgical centers. Complete and accurate information on these regulations can be found in the actual text of the National Fire Protection Association Codes and Standards. AAAHC offers a publication, *Physical Environment Checklist for Ambulatory Surgical Centers*, authored by its consulting architect, William Lindeman, AIA, which assist ASCs in understanding and complying with *NFPA Life Safety Code*. Portions of this document describe highly complex and detailed issues of construction and life safety design, which are best suited for application by architects and/or engineers (Fig. 13.11). Also, each state and locality may have its own fire and building codes and other requirements that must be met. A condensed spot checklist is also published as an appendix in the *1996/1997 Accreditation Handbook for Ambulatory Health Care*. Design features related to exiting, medical gases, and construction/detail are described in that

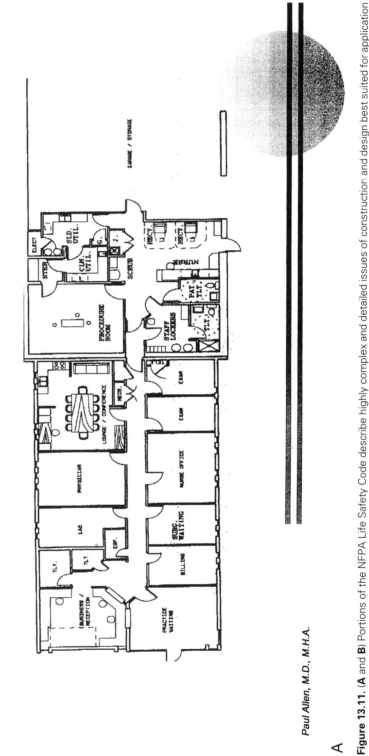

Paul Allen, M.D., M.H.A.

A

Figure 13.11. (A and **B)** Portions of the NFPA Life Safety Code describe highly complex and detailed issues of construction and design best suited for application by architects and/or engineers. AAAHC consulting architect William Lindeman, AIA, reviews surgical suite design documents with the author. These documents were subsequently presented to representatives of the Division of Facilities Licensure and Certification of the Mississippi State Department of Health in Jackson, Mississippi for comments and suggestions.

CHAPTER 13 / ACCREDITATION, RISK MANAGEMENT, AND REIMBURSEMENT 273

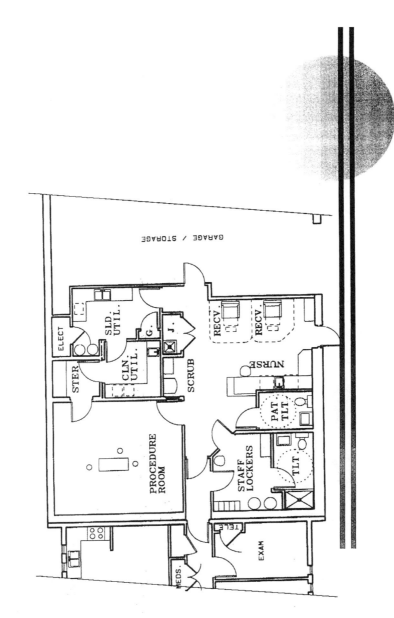

Figure 13.11. *(continued)*

Paul Allen, M.D., M.H.A.

B

appendix. The reader is referred to these referenced publications for more detailed and authoritative information.

Anesthesia Services

The criteria in this standard call for delivery of anesthesia services in a safe and sanitary environment by qualified health care practitioners who have proper credentials and granted privileges by the governing body. This set of standards does not apply when organizations use only unsupplemented local anesthesia and/or inhaled nitrous oxide in low concentrations (not to exceed 50%) that would not result in loss of the patient's life-preserving protective reflexes.

In facilities where conscious sedation is used to supplement local anesthesia or where intravenous block anesthesia techniques are used, the applicable standards require use of techniques approved by the governing body upon the recommendation of qualified professional personnel and supervision of anesthesia services by one or more qualified physicians who are also approved by the governing body upon the recommendation of qualified professional personnel. Policies should be developed addressing the education, training, and supervision of personnel and the responsibilities for both nonphysician anesthetist and supervising physicians.

It is expected that the surgeon or anesthesiologist evaluate the patient immediately before surgery to assess the anesthesia risks relative to the anticipated surgical procedure

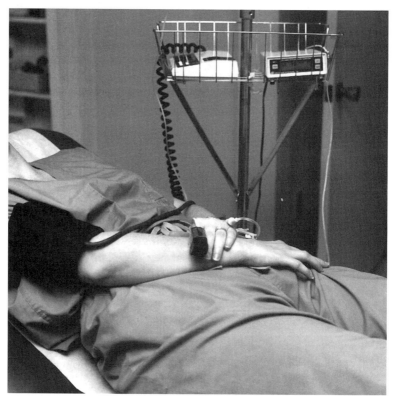

Figure 13.12. Continuous pulse oximetry should be used for intraoperative physiologic monitoring when procedures are completed under conscious sedation.

and that such an assessment be documented in the clinical record. Continuous pulse oximetry monitoring should be used consistently throughout the procedure for intraoperative physiologic monitoring when conscious sedation is used (Fig. 13.12), and a person qualified to administer anesthesia should be available on-site as long as clinically indicated. Furthermore, the operating surgeon or anesthesiologist should personally evaluate the patient for discharge readiness after recovery from anesthesia. Patients should be discharged in the company of a responsible adult. Additional standards apply to organizations using general anesthesia, including the presence or immediate availability of one or more additional health care practitioners in addition to the one performing surgery. End tidal CO_2 monitoring should be used during endotracheal anesthesia. All machinery used for general anesthesia should undergo functional testing at least once annually by technicians with appropriate training, and a log of such testing should be maintained.

Surgical Services

This set of standards recognizes the importance of having appropriately credentialed and licensed practitioners performing surgical procedures in a safe and sanitary environment.

A list of approved surgical procedures should be generated. Appropriate supervisory personnel should be available for management of the surgical suite. Outside physician peer review of surgical procedures is expected in a solo office-based surgical practice. Preoperative history and physical examinations should be documented in the clinical record before surgery. The informed consent process should also be documented in the medical record.

A registered nurse appropriately trained and supervised in surgical techniques should be an integral part of the staff. At least one operating room, adequately designed and equipped, should be available for surgery. A physician trained in resuscitative techniques should be present or immediately available until all patients undergoing surgery that day are discharged. Pathologic tissue examinations should be completed, and a signed pathology report should be part of the clinical record. The surgeon should dictate or write an operative report immediately after completing the surgical procedure, and this report should also be evident in the clinical record.

A series of environmental controls is included in this set of standards to ensure adequate space, equipment, and personnel and to protect the patient from cross-infection. These include use of proper surgical attire, acceptable aseptic techniques, limited access to the surgical suite of authorized persons only, suitable sterilizing equipment, and packaging of sterilized materials and provisions for cleaning the operating room after each procedure followed by a terminal cleaning at the conclusion of the day's surgery schedule. A detailed transfer and evacuation plan should be documented for situations requiring hospitalization of a surgical patient for evaluation and stabilization. Either a written document with a nearby hospital or a stipulation that all surgeons using the facility have admitting and surgical privileges at that hospital provides evidence of continuity of care (Fig. 13.13).

Procedures should be developed to secure blood and blood products on a timely basis as necessary and appropriate for the type of surgery performed.

An emergency power source should be available to ensure completion of a surgical procedure in the event of a power failure. A UPS battery pack may be a cost-effective alternate power source.

Equipment used for surgical procedures should be periodically calibrated and preventatively maintained. Documentation of such preventative maintenance should be evident in the form of a log. Written postoperative self-care instruction protocols should be developed for patient use.

Additional Medicare-related standards also apply for surgical services when an organization requests Medicare ASC certification as part of the accreditation process.

The nearby hospital with which a transfer agreement is executed or at which operating surgeons have admitting and surgical privileges must be a Medicare participating hospital or a nonparticipating hospital that meets the requirements for payment of emergency services under section 405.1011 of Title 42 code of federal regulations.

Additionally, provisions apply regarding exclusivity in the surgical suite. The ambu-

---

TRANSFER AND EVACUATION PLAN FOR DR. PAUL ALLEN'S OFFICE

PURPOSE OF PLAN:

To safely and quickly transfer a patient experiencing complications to the Emergency Room at Singing River Hospital.

If any patient, in the process of having a treatment or procedure done in the office, experiences complications necessitating the need for transfer to Singing River Hospital Emergency Room, the following procedures will be executed:

1. The doctor and a nurse will remain with the patient and appropriate measure implemented to stabilize the patient's condition and reassure the patient.

2. The secretary assigned to the front desk will call 762-4848 or 911 and have an ambulance dispatched to the doctor's office on 2812 Andrew Avenue.

3. The emergency suitcase with resuscitation equipment and emergency drugs will be opened. This emergency equipment is readily available and is located in the dedicated procedure room with a CPR board.

4. The Emergency Room personnel will be notified by the front desk secretary that the patient will be arriving soon. Dr. Allen will call in a brief history and any pertinent orders to the Emergency Room Physician.

5. Vital signs will be monitored and recorded and any medications given will be recorded and time noted. This information will be sent with the patient to the Emergency Room allowing for continuity of care.

6. The ambulance will enter the office through the back garage. The stretcher will be taken to the dedicated room for the patient's transfer to the Emergency Room.

7. Under Dr. Allen's direction, the nurse will notify a family member and offer a brief explanation of the patient's condition.

8. After the patient transfer is completed, the nurse will restock any emergency equipment used and restock any medications used from the suitcase before returning it to its customary storage area.

Figure 13.13. Transfer and Evacuation Plan.

TRANSFER PLAN
PAGE 2

In the non-emergency transfer of a patient, the in-office wheelchair will be used to transport the patient from the dedicated room to a private vehicle. When patients receive a pudendal block as part of their procedure, the patient's relative will bring their vehicle to the back garage, and the nurse will assist the patient in getting from the wheelchair into the car. This will eliminate any apprehension by other patients in the office and protect everyone's privacy.

_____   Date: _____/_____/_____
Paul M. Allen, MD, CEO/Medical Director
Women's Center for Healthcare, Pascagoula

_____   Date: _____/_____/_____
Jamie Swanner, RN, Director of Nursing
Women's Center for Healthcare, Pascagoula

_____   Date: _____/_____/_____
Peggy Guess, RN, Associate Administrator
Singing River Hospital, Pascagoula

Figure 13.13. (continued)

latory surgical center must be a distinct entity, operating exclusively for the provision of surgical services, using an area that is dedicated in time and space exclusively for ambulatory surgery or directly related activities. The ASC may be housed in the same building as a physician's office or clinic, but it must be separated physically from nonsurgical patient care areas by at least semipermanent walls and doors. Furthermore, surgical and nonsurgical functions and operations cannot be mixed during concurrent or overlapping hours of operation. Ambulatory surgery centers staffing and record keeping must also be separate and exclusive.

The Medicare Peer Review Organization program reviews samples of Medicare cases from ASCs. The adequacy of histories and physical examinations is assessed as an element of the generic quality screening criteria. Regardless of the type of anesthesia used, if any, for the surgical procedure, the history should include documentation of indicators or symptoms for surgical practices, a list of current medications and dosages, any known allergies, and any existing comorbid conditions.

The extent of documentation required in the physical examination is related to the anesthesia planned. For procedures requiring either no anesthesia or topical, local, or regional block, an assessment of mental status and an examination specific to the anticipated procedure and any comorbid conditions is expected. For procedures completed under conscious sedation, auscultation of the heart and lungs should also be described. For procedures completed under general, spinal, or epidural anesthesia, an assessment of the patient's general condition should also be written.

A physician, operating practitioner, or individual qualified to administer anesthesia is expected to complete a note before the surgical procedure, evaluating the patient's current status for surgery. An anesthesia history should also be part of such a preprocedure note when general or spinal anesthesia is used. Laboratory, electrocardiogram, and x-ray studies necessary and relevant to the patient's health status should be completed and reports available at the time of surgery. Abnormal results of such studies should be assessed or resolved, or the record should explain why they are unresolved.

Vital signs including blood pressure, pulse, respirations, and temperature should be taken and recorded on the day of surgery before administering preoperative medications or sedation.

Pharmaceutical Standards

The criteria in this set of standards call for provision or availability of pharmaceutical services by an accreditable organization in accordance with ethical and professional practices and legal requirements to meet the needs of patients.

Staff should demonstrate knowledge of applicable state pharmaceutical laws, maintain records and security to ensure control and safe dispensing of drugs in compliance with federal and state laws, and inform patients concerning safe and effective use of medications.

Provision of pharmaceutical services should be supervised by a licensed pharmacist or, when appropriate, by a physician who is qualified to assume responsibility for the quality of the services provided. If the organization owns or operates a pharmacy, supervision by a licensed pharmacist is required. Patients should not be required to use a pharmacy owned or operated by the organization.

Additional Medicare-related standards apply to an ambulatory surgical center requesting recognition of its survey for purposes of Medicare ASC certification.

Adverse reactions to medications should be reported to the physician and documented in the clinical record. Either a physician or registered nurse should administer blood or blood products. Oral orders given for drugs and biologicals should be followed by a written order, signed by prescribing physician.

Pathology and Medical Laboratory Services

AAAHC expects provision or availability of pathology and medical laboratory services by an accreditable entity to meet the needs of patients in accordance with ethical and professional practices and legal requirements.

An organization requiring laboratory services should either meet the requirements of the Clinical Laboratory Improvement Act (CLIA) (part 493 of Title 42 of the code of federal regulation) if it provides its own laboratory services or have procedures in place to obtain routine and emergency laboratory services from a CLIA-certified laboratory if it does not provide its own such services.

Tests should be performed in a timely manner, and test results should be distributed within 24 hours of completion of study. A copy of the results should be maintained in the laboratory, and dated reports of all examinations performed should be part of the patient's clinical record. Appropriate quality assurance procedures should be performed and documented, including periodic calibration of equipment and use of standardized control specimens to validate test results.

A pathologist or other qualified physician should be responsible for directing these services. A sufficient complement of adequately trained supervisory personnel should be available to conduct the work of the laboratory.

Established procedures should be followed in obtaining, identifying, storing, and transporting specimens. For each test procedure performed in the laboratory, a complete description of technique should be available, including sources of reagents, standards, and calibration procedures, and information should be available on the determined normal ranges of reported results. Space, equipment, and supplies should be sufficient to perform the volume of work with accuracy, precision, efficiency, and safety.

RISK MANAGEMENT

The purpose for developing and implementing a risk management program in a physician's practice is twofold: to improve the quality of care delivered and to protect the organizations assets in today's highly litigious climate. Fortunately, as we strive to accomplish the first goal, the latter goal can also be realized if one follows an organized approach to managing the daily requirements of the practice.

Born of a marriage between management and insurance concepts, risk management has as its goal the protection of an organization's financial, human, and physical assets. The opportunities to apply good risk management techniques run through a medical practice's entire operation, from the physical plant to the standards for patient care. This summary concentrates on the medical aspects of risk management in a private practice.

Long before the current embracing of total quality management or continuous quality improvement, the proponents of sound risk management programs emphasized the importance of documenting procedures and then improving them. This aspect of risk management is applicable to all organizations but is especially critical in a complex medical practice where many patient encounters do not occur with the physician but with the staff, acting on his or her behalf. Therefore, the physician must create a system where all procedures are planned in advance and properly documented so the staff members can consistently deliver the proper elements of patient care.

Components of a Risk Management Program

In our practice we have developed a program that follows a basic 5-step approach to risk management and practice management:

1. *Identify* the key processes in the practice that have the potential for creating the greatest element of risk:
   a. Office-based surgical procedures;
   b. High risk patients with noncompliant behavior;
   c. Nursing triage calls;
   d. Patients with complaints about treatments/outcomes;
   e. On-call and/or referral patients with limited contact;
   f. Patients requiring follow-up care.
2. *Develop* the standard procedure(s) to be followed and train all staff members in the procedure(s).
3. *Audit* the practice documentation on a regular basis to ensure that the procedures are being followed.
4. *Document* all patient encounters with standardized forms.
5. *Review and revise* procedures on a regular basis with the staff.

Identify Key Processes and Procedures

Risk management activities include many operational components of a practice and should include administrative, financial, patient communications, treatments, examination procedures, laboratory procedures, patient notification and follow-up, charting, and so on. We identify clinical key processes and procedures as clinical audits pertaining to the medical record, procedure room surgical case review, mammogram audit, and pap smear audit. A methodology for staff development should be articulated including a mission statement, documentation of orientation to all employees to the risk management program, a statement of confidentiality of patient information for employees and contractuals, employee performance appraisals, and personnel chart checklist. A task orientation checklist and skill assessment report for new employees is significant as well as monthly performance profiles to list critical incidents and assist staff in improving performance. Preventative maintenance on equipment and machinery is also recognized as a key procedure. Patient profile determination assists the practice in identifying and directing special attention to difficult or "red flag" patients. Infection control practices are also identified as key procedures and are developed to ensure compliance with standards promulgated by the Occupational Safety and Health Administration. These would include Hazard Communication Plan, Infection Control Plan, Medical Waste Management Plan, and Chemical Hygiene Plan. Informed consent protocol is also identified as a key process in the risk management program. Vehicles and instruments to ensure patient advocacy, including questionnaires and complaint forms, should be developed, and these issues should be assigned to the staff meeting agenda.

Key procedures and policies are also identified for financial management. These include methods to optimize compliance from prospective new patients, detailed methodology for scheduling surgery, and procedures to verify insurance policy benefits for all insured patients. It is also important to provide patients with estimate of fees, particularly for surgical services (Fig. 13.14). Methods to optimize collection opportunities are also identified as a key process. It is also important that job descriptions be fully developed for all staff. Follow-up on the no-show patients is also identified as a key process. Marketing and advertising methods to optimize practice growth, including patient information brochures and newsletters, are also identified as significant procedures to enhance financial management of the practice. Inventory control is also identified as a key process. Methods to enhance revenue recovery, including accurate billing, coding, and reimbursement procedures and UCR data and procedure room pricing analysis, are recognized.

Develop Standard Procedures

These procedures must be well thought out in advance and written up in a standard fashion for all aspects of the practice. In this manner, each staff member, new or old, can quickly use the procedure document as a resource when either training or refreshing their memory. The use of these procedures should lead to better delivery of care in the office. As a byproduct, having the standards of care well-defined can serve as a strong deterrent in the event of litigation. Plaintiff attorneys use the absence of written procedures and charted results to create the impression that proper care was not given.

Procedures can be developed and standardized by using standard spreadsheets with clearly stated criteria for all aspects of various procedures. These spreadsheets state methods to ensure a systematic approach to patient care.

PAUL M. ALLEN, M.D.
2812 ANDREW AVENUE - P. O. BOX 1345
PASCAGOULA, MISSISSIPPI 39567
(601) 769-6389 • FAX (601) 769-5073

- Gynecology
- Gynecologic Laser Surgery
- Urogynecology and Urodynamics
- Infertility
- Obstetrics

Diplomate American Board of Obstetrics and Gynecology
Fellow American College of
Obstetricians and Gynecologists

ESTIMATE OF FEES

Patient's Name: _____

1). Estimated Professional Fee _____

2). Estimated Non-Professional Fee (Supplies, Injections, and related variable procedure costs)
_____

3). Accredited Single Specialty Ambulatory Surgical Center Facility Fee _____

Anticipated Surgical Procedure(s): _____

I understand that the fees quoted above are estimates of minimal charges only. I also understand that additional charges may be generated depending on surgical/obstetrical conditions. I also understand that any tissue collected or removed will be submitted for pathologic examination and that I will be billed separately by pathologist/facility who performs this exam. I understand that pathologic examination of specimens collected or removed in surgery is not performed by Dr. Allen and that again I will be billed separately for pathologic examination of any specimens collected or removed during this procedure. I also understand that charges for anesthesia services at Singing River Hospital, Ocean Springs Hospital, or J. F. Turner Outpatient Surgical Center will be generated separately by the anesthesiologist or anesthesia personnel who will be participating in my care and that I will be billed separately and additionally for anesthesia services. Anesthesiologists, pathologists, radiologists, or other consulting services are not included in this fee estimate. I understand that laparoscopy is a diagnostic procedure and that additional charges will be generated if therapeutic (laser) procedures are also performed. I will receive a multiple surgery adjustment on my balance as soon as insurance benefits are received. I understand after a six week period I will being making monthly payments if a balance remains.

I understand that a facility fee will be generated based on fixed costs per procedure hour for use of the procedure, operating, and recovery room in Dr. Allen's Accredited Single Specialty Ambulatory Surgical Center. I also understand that additional charges will be generated for injections and supply items which represent variable procedure costs.

FOR SERVICES PROVIDED BY DR. ALLEN AND FOR FEES GENERATED FOR THE USE OF HIS PROCEDURE, OPERATING, AND RECOVERY ROOM. THIS CAP DOES NOT INCLUDE CHARGES GENERATED BY ANY OTHER PHYSICIAN AND/OR HOSPITAL FACILITY.

MAXIMUM FEE FOR THIS PROCEDURE WOULD BE : _____

Above conditions explained verbally to patient by:
_____ on _____ (date).

Figure 13.14. Estimate of Fees.

Audit the Practice Documentation

The existing data of a practice can be reviewed by using the patient appointment log, patient charts, telephone log, staffing patterns, patient questionnaires, staff interviews, and so on. By reviewing this data, the auditor (physician, manager, or outside consultant) can readily identify areas that need more emphasis with the staff or could benefit from process improvement.

Acceptable levels of compliance can be stated, and compliance with the criteria outlined in the audits can be precisely determined. The compliance levels for the various criteria can be communicated to the physician and staff at the regularly scheduled staff meetings and through performance profiles. This will assist the staff in improving performance and optimizing compliance with the various standards and criteria associated with the audits. Special attention can be directed to activities identified by the audit in need of improvement or revision.

Document All Patient Encounters With Standards

The most fertile area for plaintiff attorneys to develop cases against a private practitioner is in the area of patient charting and the lack of documentation of delivered care. To protect against this inevitable day, one must develop a complete system for recording all patient encounters. To make this feasible, time should be spent to develop standard forms that simply require a check, time entry, initial, fill-in, or other similarly easy method of entry. This documentation is required at all levels of the practice, including telephone log for the receptionist, post-treatment instructions, routine physical and laboratory entries, vital signs, and so on. Another important aspect of documentation is patient acknowledgment by obtaining a signature on an original document and retain a copy. Once again, the documentation should be established for the purpose of ensuring that the best level of care is given. A byproduct of good documentation is the probability of a good defense case if and when it is necessary.

Review and Revise Procedures

Beyond the personal skills and dedication of the physician, the biggest determinant of good outcomes and good quality of care is the quality and involvement of the staff. To keep the staff involved in both providing good care and in improving the procedures that are in place, the physician should conduct regular staff meetings for the specific purpose of improving the delivery of care. The outcome from those meetings will be suggestions for process improvements and a team commitment to delivering quality health care.

These meetings allow optimal communication between physician and staff on clinical and administrative matters. Concerns and problems can be clearly articulated at these meetings, and attention can thus be directed to resolution of problems and improvement of various procedures. Problems with patient compliance, patient concerns, and patient advocacy can be thoroughly discussed and either resolved or referred for consultation in certain complex or difficult situations. Agenda items at the regularly scheduled staff meetings include review of minutes of previous meeting, reports relating to patient visits, recall activity, patient no-show, patient satisfaction survey questionnaires, and requests for medical records from outside sources.

Administrative reports can also be reviewed and discussed. These include collection activity reports, reports on insurance claim submission and follow-up, public relations report, accounts payable, and inventory control log. These meetings also provide an opportunity to discuss results of the monthly clinical and administrative audits.

In our practice, we found that three key elements enable us to establish this basic process and keep the energy for continued improvement alive and well. First, each staff member is responsible for certain elements of the practice and maintains records for that aspect of patient care or administrative function. Second, we have a clinic manual that is the focal point for developing and documenting the patient care processes to which we are all committed. Finally, we use the services of an outside risk management consultant to audit our program on a regular basis. The consultant helps the staff members identify improvements in their particular assignments and keeps them involved in the procedure changes that document the improvements. Each staff member is provided monetary incentives to manage his or her portion of the practice at a level of excellence so they are motivated to both improve processes and improve the actual care delivered.

Although physicians may believe that a certain threshold of professional liability claims activity is inevitable to a practice, we firmly believe that claims activity can be reduced and even abated with the development of a well-defined and formal risk management program. Although considerable effort and dedication at all organizational levels are necessary for an effective and successful risk management program, these efforts can result in a higher standard of care as demanded by society, a safer medical environment as expected by the community, and a significant decrease in professional liability claims activity.

REIMBURSEMENT

Commercial insurance carriers and managed care plans generally allow additional reimbursement, separate and distinct from reimbursement for professional fees, to an accredited facility in payment of benefits for facility fee charges, which are based on fixed practice costs related to delivery of surgical services. Fiscal agents and intermediaries for the Medicare and Medicaid programs provide similar reimbursement if the organization achieves Medicare ASC certification as well.

The facility fee is based on fixed practice costs per procedure hour and can be determined using standard cost accounting methods, which we describe. Fixed costs are related to occupancy, personnel, equipment, and accreditation expenses. For an office-based surgical facility, only a portion of practice operating (overhead) expenses are allocated for surgical procedures. Such a facility has a relatively small infrastructure with proportionally few indirect costs centers requiring support. For these reasons and because of the relative lack of cost shifting in such a venue, facility fees generated in single specialty ambulatory surgical centers and office-based surgical facilities compare favorably with facility fees set by larger institutions such as free-standing ambulatory surgical centers and hospitals.

Operating and Recovery Room Pricing Analysis

The pricing analysis begins with a computation of annual fixed costs (Fig. 13.15). Only a portion of employed and contractual personnel costs are allocated to the surgical suite. This may be determined by allocating proportions of practice personnel working time dedicated to surgical procedures or proportions of total practice revenues generated from surgical procedures completed on site. An example is cited.

In a similar fashion, a portion of occupancy costs, including rent or depreciation, maintenance and repairs, telephone and utilities, taxes and licenses, and building and contents insurance costs, are allocated to the surgical suite, and this allocation is on a square footage basis as exhibited. As cited in the pricing analysis exhibited, costs associated with remodeling or reconfiguration of existing office space to achieve accreditation and/or Medicare ASC certification can also be considered as part of the occupancy costs, and these remodeling expenses can be prorated or depreciated over an optional period of 3–15 years.

Equipment costs are also considered in the computation of annual fixed costs. For equipment related to surgical procedures that is leased, the lease payments are totaled.

PROCEDURE/OPERATING AND RECOVERY ROOM PRICING ANALYSIS
MARCH 1, 1996

I. **COMPUTATION OF ANNUAL FIXED COSTS**

   A. Personnel Costs

   Only a portion of employed and contractual personnel costs were allocated to the surgical suite. This allocation was based on 25% of personnel activity dedicated to the surgical suite and surgical procedures.

   1. Employed Personnel Salaries
      - .25 Executive Director FTE
      - .25 Insurance Claim Representative FTE
      - .25 Receptionist FTE
      - .25 RN FTE
      - .25 LPN 2.5 FTE

   2. Contractual Personnel Costs
      - .25 Transcriptionist FTE
      - .25 QA/RM Consultant
      - .25 Billing/Collection Representative
      - .25 CPA

   3. *Total Annual Employed and Contractual Personnel Costs*   *$66,846.81*

   B. Occupancy Costs

   Only a portion of the occupancy costs including rent, maintenance and repairs, telephone and utilities, and taxes and licenses, as well as building and contents insurance costs were allocated to the surgical suite. This allocation was on a square footage basis.

A1

Figure 13.15. (A1–A4) Procedure/Operating and Recovery Room Pricing Analysis. **(B)** Memorandum to insurance carriers.

PROCEDURE/OPERATING AND RECOVERY ROOM PRICING ANALYSIS
PAGE 2

1. Procedure and Recovery Room Square Footage = 576 square feet.
   Total Office/Facility Square Footage = 4,292 square feet.
   Percentage of total equals 576 ÷ 4,292 = 13.4%

• Total annual occupancy costs	$13,355.00
• Building Rent	$48,000.00
• Telephone Expenses	$21,402.41
• Taxes and Licenses	$ 1,445.28
• Building Maintenance and Repairs	$13,626.48
• Utilities	$10,892.28
• Building and Contents Insurance	$ 4,298.00

   Subtotal Occupancy Costs **$99,664.47 x 13.4% = $13,355.00**

2. Medicare ASC Certificate Remodeling Costs allocated for one year
   $27,333.00

   Total Annual Occupancy Costs   *$40,688.00*

C. Equipment Costs

   1. Procedure Room Equipment Leases $60,055.63

      - Zeiss Operating Microscope with Floor Stand
      - Midmark Procedure Table
      - Surgitek UDS 1000 Urodynamic System
      - Coherent CO2 Surgical Laser System
      - Hysteroscope with Biopsy Forceps
      - ATL Ultramark4+ Ultrasound System
      - .25 Systems Plus Medical Manager Computer

   2. Procedure Room Equipment Service Contacts and Repairs $13,626.48

   3. Purchased Procedure Room Equipment Depreciation $3,460.00

      - UPS Battery Pack Alternate Power Source
      - Locked Wall Cabinet for Controlled Substances
      - Handicapped Toilet Facilities for Procedure Room
      - Defibrillator

Figure 13.15. *(continued)*

PROCEDURE/OPERATING AND RECOVERY ROOM PRICING ANALYSIS
PAGE 3

        Depreciation for these purchased procedure room items was calculated on a five year straight line basis.

        Total annual equipment cost $77,142.11

  D. ASC Accreditation Fee $2,054.58

        Fee generated for three year Certificate of Accreditation, issued by Accreditation Association for Ambulatory Health Care, allocated over one year.

E. *Summary of total annual fixed costs ASC accreditation cost.*

    1. *Total annual personnel costs* $66,846.81

    2. *Total annual occupancy costs* $40,688.00

    3. *Total annual equipment costs* $77,142.11

    4. *Total annual ASC Accreditation Fee* $2,054.58

    Total annual fixed costs   *$196,731.50*

II. **COMPUTATION OF FIXED COST PER PROCEDURE HOUR**

Procedure Mix	1995 Procedures	Hours of Utilization
½ hour (minor) = 54%	120	60
1 hour (minor) = 21%	46	46
2 hours (major) = 25%	58	116
TOTAL 1995 PROCEDURE HOURS		222

    <u>Fixed Costs Per Hour of Procedure</u>

    1995 Volumes $196,731.51 ÷ 222 hours = $ 886.00 per procedure hour

Figure 13.15. *(continued)*

PROCEDURE/OPERATING AND RECOVERY ROOM PRICING ANALYSIS
PAGE 4

III. FEE COMPARISON

Facility fee at J. F. Turner Outpatient Surgical Center in Pascagoula includes operating and recovery room supplies and equipment but are not inclusive of general anesthesia costs.

Procedure Description	J. F. Turner ASC Facility Fee (1995)
MINOR PROCEDURE - Dilatation and Curettage of the uterus Laser Conization of the cervix	$1,750.00 $2,000.00
MAJOR PROCEDURE - Laser vaporization of vulva/vagina/anus	$3,500.00

A4

Figure 13.15. *(continued)*

For purchased equipment, depreciation is totaled and may be based on elected or preferred accounting methods.

The *straight line (time) method* is most commonly used for financial reporting, wherein the costs of the asset (equipment) less any estimated salvage value is divided by the number of years of the equipments expected useful life: Annual depreciation = Cost less estimated salvage value ÷ Estimated service life in years.

Accelerated depreciation methods can alternatively be used for equipment that provides more and better service in the earlier years of its useful life. The *declining balance method* is one accelerated depreciation method in which depreciation charge results from multiplying the net book value of the equipment (costs less accumulated depreciation but without subtracting salvage value) at the start of each period (year) by a fixed rate. In using the *double declining balance method* of accelerated depreciation, an organization could depreciate an asset with an estimated 5-year life at a rate of 40% per year of book value at the start of the year and then switch to straight line depreciation after 3 years.

Another accelerated depreciation method is the *sum-of-the-years'-digits method,* in which depreciation charge results from applying a diminishing fraction to the cost of the equipment less its estimated salvage value. The numerator of the fraction is the number of the years of remaining life at the beginning of the year of depreciation calculation, and the denominator is the sum of all such numbers, one for each year of estimated service life (Fig. 13.16).

Fees for service contracts and repair expenses for all equipment used for surgical procedures are also considered in the computation of equipment costs. Accreditation costs including application and survey fees are then considered and allocated for 1 year. Personnel, occupancy, equipment, and accreditation costs are then totaled for an aggregate sum of annual fixed costs. Computation of fixed costs per procedure hour is then completed by determining the major and minor procedure mix and then totaling the hours

WOMEN'S CENTER FOR HEALTH CARE
Paul M. Allen, M.D.

2812 ANDREW AVENUE • P.O. BOX 1345
PASCAGOULA, MISSISSIPPI 39567
(601) 769-6389 • FAX (601) 769-5073

— Gynecology
— Gynecologic Laser Surgery
— Urogynecology and Urodynamics
— Infertility
— Obstetrics

Diplomate American Board Of Obstetrics And Gynecology
Fellow American College Of
Obstetricians And Gynecologists

MEMORANDUM

DATE: MARCH 1, 1996

TO: ALL INSURANCE CARRIERS

FROM: PAUL M. ALLEN, M.D., M.H.A. CHIEF EXECUTIVE OFFICER AND MEDICAL DIRECTOR, WOMEN'S CENTER FOR HEALTH CARE

RE: PROCEDURE/OPERATING AND RECOVERY ROOM PRICING ANALYSIS/ FACILITY FEE

We are enclosing an updated procedure/operating and recovery room pricing analysis which shows how we calculate our facility fee. We are fully accredited by the Accreditation Association for Ambulatory Health Care as a single specialty ambulatory surgical center and a copy of our Certificate of Accreditation is attached. We use standard cost accounting methods to calculate our facility fee, and our facility fee computation is based on annual fixed costs per procedure hour. These annual fixed costs are based on the following items.

- A portion of annual personnel costs for both employed and contractual personnel as described.

- A portion of occupancy costs allocated on a square footage basis.

- Expenses related to reconstruction and remodeling required to achieve our Medicare ASC Certificate.

- Equipment costs including procedure room equipment leases, procedure room equipment service contracts and repairs, and depreciation of purchased procedure room equipment as per the attached schedule.

- ASC Accreditation Fee as generated by the Accreditation Association for Ambulatory Health Care allocated for one year,

Please note that our charges for facility fee fixed cost as well as variable costs for surgical tray and supply items are considerably less than charges generated by our local free-standing ambulatory surgical center.

A Single Specialty Ambulatory Surgical Center

Accredited by **Accreditation Association for Ambulatory Health Care, Inc.**

B

Figure 13.15. *(continued)*

SUM-OF-THE-YEARS'-DIGITS DEPRECIATION SCHEDULE

Asset with 5 - Year Life, $5,000 Cost, and $200 Estimated Salvage Value

YEAR	ACQUISITION COST LESS SALVAGE VALUE (1)	REMAINING LIFE IN YEARS (2)	FRACTION = (2)/15 (3)	DEPRECIATION CHARGE FOR THE YEAR = (3) x (1) (4)
1	$4,800.00	5	5/15	$1,600.00
2	$4,800.00	4	4/15	$1,280.00
3	$4,800.00	3	3/15	$960.00
4	$4,800.00	2	2/15	$640.00
5	$4,800.00	1	1/15	$320.00
				$4,800.00

Figure 13.16. Sum-of-the-Years'-Digits Depreciation Schedule.

of use on an annual basis as exhibited. A fee comparison completes the pricing analysis. This data may be collected by telephone survey of free-standing ambulatory surgical centers in the same geographic area.

A memorandum may be styled, which can be submitted to insurance carriers describing the procedure and operating and recovery room pricing analysis, and such a memorandum is also exhibited.

Insurance Claim Processing

Facility fee charges are submitted to commercial and government carriers on either an HCFA 1500 or a UB–92 claim form, depending on the carrier's specification or stated reference. CPT code 99070, which is a supply code descriptor, is used to report facility fee charges on an HCFA 1500 claim form (Fig. 13.17). Use of an ASC Facility Fee stamp assists claims processors in identifying the exact nature of the charge. A copy of the Certificate of Accreditation issued by the accrediting agency can also be attached to the HCFA 1500 claim form as exhibited.

Less familiar to a physician's practice is the uniform bill known as the UB–92, also called the HCFA–1450, which was developed and approved for use in 1992, replacing the UB–82 claim form (Fig. 13.18). The UB–92 is not used for billing the professional components of physician services. It contains 86 data elements called form locators (FL), is printed in red ink for scanning, and is designed to be typed or computer printed. The UB–92 is also formatted for processing claims electronically.

FL 42 calls for a revenue code. Revenue code 490 is a descriptor generally used for ambulatory surgical care as exhibited.

Whereas fixed costs are reflected in the generation of a facility fee, variable costs related to surgical procedures, such as supplies, injections, and surgical trays, are reported separately using HCPCS A or J codes as descriptors. Examples of typical surgical tray itemizations and supply and injection items used frequently in an office-based surgical facility are displayed (Fig. 13.19).

Figure 13.17. HCFA 1500 Insurance Claim Form.

CHAPTER 13 / ACCREDITATION, RISK MANAGEMENT, AND REIMBURSEMENT

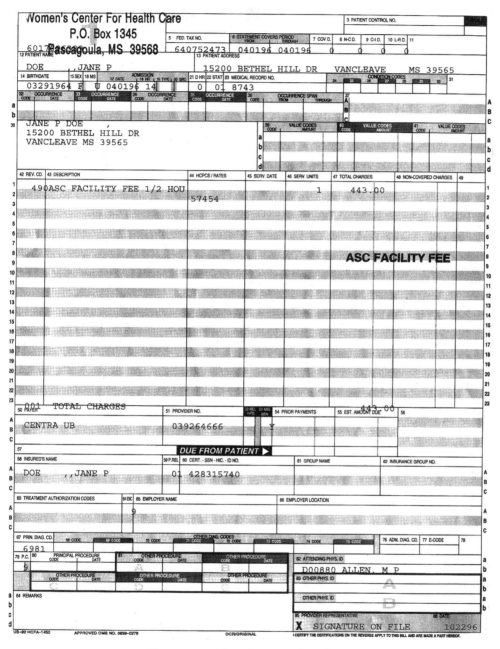

Figure 13.18. UB-92 Insurance Claim Form.

PROCEDURE ROOM COSTS AND INCIDENTALS
PROCEDURE-RELATED EXPENSES

SURGICAL TRAY LIST (A4550)

LOWER GENITAL TRACT LASER SURGERY:

Description

Feminine Pad x 1
4 x 4 x 20
Gloves x 22
Hibiclens
Hurricane
Laser Masks x 4
Needles, 22 G 1 1/2" x 3
Needles 18 G x 10
Needles 25 G x 3
Needles 27 G x 1
Pudendal Tray
Q-Tip x 1
Scopettes x 20
Smoke Evacuator Filter
Smoke Evacuator Tubing
Syringes - 3 cc x10
Syringes - 5 cc x 4
Tape, Surgical - 50 cm.
Tongue Depressor x 1
Underpads x 4
Vaseline Gauze
Vinegar

HYSTEROSCOPY/ENDOMETRIAL CURETTAGE:

Description

4 x 4 x 20
Gloves x 22
Needles, 18G x 5
Needles, 22 G x 1 1/2 in. x 3
Scopettes x 10
Surgical Tape - 50 cm
Syringes, 3 cc x 10
Syringe, 5 cc x 1
Table Paper x 2 m.
Telfa x 1
Tissue Trap
Underpads x 4
Hibiclens
Computer Paper

A

Figure 13.19. (**A** and **B**) Surgical Tray Lists. (**C**) J code injection list and A code supply list.

PROCEDURE ROOM COSTS AND INCIDENTALS
PROCEDURE-RELATED EXPENSES

SURGICAL TRAY LIST (A4550)

Urodynamic Evaluation/Cystourethroscopy with Dilatation:

Description

Alcohol Swabs x 4
Feminine Pads (Kotex) x 1
4 x 4 x 20
Gloves x 22
Hibiclens
Hurricane
Infusion Tube - One set
Needles, 18 G x 1 in. x 10
Needles, 25 G x 1 1/2 in. x 3
Scopettes x 5
Spinal Needle
Sterile Water
Suction Tubing, Small, Sterile
Syringe Tuberculin
Syringes, 3 cc x 10
Syringe, 10 cc x 1
Table Paper
Tape - 100 cm
Underpads x 4
Urodynamic connection tubing
EMG Patches
Computer paper
Surgical Tape 100 cm
Q-Tip x 1

B

Figure 13.19. *(continued)*

INJECTIONS AND SUPPLY ITEMS

Injections:		Supply items:	
Rocephin 250 mg	J0696	Non-emergency taxi transport	A0100
Claforan 1 gm	J0698	Surgicel absorptive dressing	A4204
DMSO (Rimso)	J0970	Sterile Needle	A4215
Interferon 3 mil IU	J9214	Catheter without bag	A4311
Kenalog 10	J1870	Catheter, indwelling with bag	A4338
Kenalog 40	J1880	Surgical tray	A4550
Toradol 60 mg	J1885	Xylocaine ointment	A4735
Demerol 50-100 mg	J2175	Connecting Tubing	A4750
Nesacaine	J2400		
Vistaril 25 mg	J3410		
B&O Suppository	J3490		
Stadol 1-2 mg	J3490		
Normal Saline	J7050		
D5 lactated ringers	J7120		
Effudex Cream	J9190		

C

Figure 13.19. *(continued)*

SUMMARY

In this chapter we describe the merits of achieving public recognition through the process of practice accreditation in an office-based surgical facility and/or single specialty ambulatory surgical center. Descriptive comments on both core and adjunct standards applicable by AAAHC to ambulatory surgical facilities are stated. Quality improvement and risk management endeavors are also described. Methods to optimize reimbursement including generation of facility fee charges for the use of an office-based surgical facility are discussed, including the cost accounting methods used to determine an appropriate facility fee based on fixed practice costs per procedure hour. Additional information is also provided on descriptors and methods used to complete and submit both HCFA–1500 and UB–92 claim forms to report facility fee charges.

Acknowledgment. The author acknowledges Lillian P. Karson, R.N., DASHRM, who coauthored the section on risk management, and Christopher Damon, J.D., AAAHC Executive Director, who provided valuable insight in the preparation of the section relating to accreditation. The interpretive remarks and comments regarding the accreditation process are those of the author and are not the official views of AAAHC.

Appendix
Facility Regulations and Standards for Ambulatory Surgical Centers
A Primer

WILLIAM E. LINDEMAN

A common theme of accreditation, licensure, and certification is recognition that a facility meets or exceeds the reviewing authority's standards. Although the jurisdictions and requirements of these authorities varies widely—between voluntary/private accreditation, State-mandated accreditation,[b] State-required licensure, and Federally directed Medicare Certification—their fundamental premise remains the same: to ensure the "safe and appropriate" delivery of patient care. They also share emphasis within the standards themselves, focusing on the operational makeup of the facility (policies and procedures) and the design and construction (physical environment).

What distinguishes the requirements of various authorities is the degree to which they each mandate literal conformance with standards and the relative importance they place on operational issues compared with facility issues. Traditionally, accreditation for ASCs has emphasized the operational aspects appropriate for the specific patient group and procedure list. Conversely, regulatory bodies tend to place greater importance on a standardized physical environment and relatively little on the clinical aspects of facility operation. Until recently, these circumstances have resulted in a system requiring accreditation as well as licensure and/or certification to fully demonstrate a facility's adherence to the highest operational and physical environment standards.

As noted in this chapter, there is a revolution underway in the regulatory approval process for ASCs desiring to qualify for Medicare Part "B"(facility fee) reimbursement. As this goes to press, it is likely the nation's two largest health care accrediting bodies have been granted "deemed status" for Medicare Certification (2). What this does in effect is to replace the survey portion of the traditional Medicare Certification process with that done by the Accrediting bodies. In their pursuit of deemed status, the accrediting bodies have been required to adopt several standards previously outside their review agenda but fundamental to Medicare Certification, most significantly Life Safety / Physical Environment standards. As a result, it will soon be possible to have a single "authority" evaluating all aspects of operational and physical environment, resulting in a new higher level of recognition/accreditation.

Many have heralded the achievement of Deemed Status as the end to the inequitable variation of Medicare Certification standards from state to state. Although that may eventually prove to be the case, it is not at the onset and may never be. Medicare is a federal

---

[b]California Assembly Bill "AB595," signed and enacted into law September 30, 1996, effectively mandates accreditation, licensure, or Medicare certification of any facility in which patients undergo outpatient surgical procedures involving levels of anesthesia that reduce the patient's life preserving protective reflexes—the bill specifically defines subject levels of anesthesia and exclusions.

reimbursement/insurance program administered by the states, each with the authority (and many with the apparent desire) to set its own standards. Medicare itself has very few requirements for physical environment; in fact, it has two:

1. The ASC must provide a safe and sanitary environment, appropriate to the types of surgery conducted with a separate waiting room and recovery area.
2. The ASC must meet the provisions of the Life Safety Code of the National Fire Protection Association (NFPA–1985 edition). This document includes fire protection, emergency power, medical gas system, construction, and exiting standards for facility design and development.

One may notice that there is no mention of room numbers or sizes, no extra wide corridors, no separation of clean areas from soiled; in fact, none of the spatial characteristics that most people equate with ASCs. That is because it is each state itself, not Medicare, that creates and enforces the entire category of detailed room and process-oriented health care standards. Specific details and the scope of requirements for spatial provision varies widely from state to state, except that they share several common themes:

- Separation of soiled (less clean) areas from clean (more clean) areas;
- Movement of materials from less clean areas, through areas where they are processed to become more clean, then into more clean areas;
- Preservation of patient privacy, both physical and informational;
- Procedure rooms sized to accommodate the maximum need, with appropriate support spaces;
- Fire safety preparedness standards more restrictive than typically applied to medical offices and less restrictive than typically applied to acute care facilities;
- Functional "zoning" of space to provide waiting areas with public toilet access, reception and business areas with private interview space, patient preparation areas including clothing change, staff lounge and changing areas, the surgical suite itself (procedure rooms and ancillary support), recovery areas including stages I and II and lounge, and medical gas/building service areas.

It is also true that the specific details of construction and fire safety standards vary substantially from state to state. They again, however, demonstrate consistency through two basic categories of application:

1. Standards that serve to ensure orderly cessation of procedures in process at the onset of an internal emergency situation. These requirements usually encompass provision of essential emergency power, emergency lighting, smoke and fire compartmentalization, and alarm systems.
2. Standards that serve to ensure a safe and orderly exiting/evacuation of a facility as made necessary by occurrence of an emergency situation. These requirements usually dictate the number and arrangement of exits, the width of exit passageways, exit signs, emergency lighting, alarm systems, smoke and fire compartmentalization, and fire fighting equipment.

Occasionally, a state's standards will require the ability to function in support of a significant emergency external to the facility itself, such as an earthquake or tornado. In California, a free-standing multispecialty ASC may be designated as an "essential facility" and consequently is required to include structural upgrades to withstand significant earthquakes and emergency power for extended full-capacity operation without utility company support.

Despite the variation in specific requirements, the considerations along the way to ensuring regulatory conformance are consistent and categorized by levels of jurisdiction:

- *Mandatory Local Jurisdictions*: Building Codes, Zoning Ordinances, and Fire Safety Standards—applicable to all medical facilities from practice suites to acute care hospitals. These standards address the basic planning and construction of buildings for public occupancy. In most cases, local approval is signified by the occupancy permit for the facility. Facilities that achieve only local approval and none higher (see below) typically cannot negotiate/qualify for third-party facility fee reimbursement.
- *Mandatory State Health and State Fire Marshal Jurisdictions*: Certificates of Need (permission to build) where applicable and licensing standards—applicable to outpatient surgery and acute care facilities. These standards address the spatial details and requirements for licensed facilities including operational characteristics, functional and fire safety planning, and acceptable building construction systems. State approval is usually signified by the granting of a license for the specific type of health care function, such as Ambulatory Surgery. Facilities that achieve licensure are in a relatively good position to negotiate third-party facility fee reimbursement.
- *Optional Federal Jurisdiction*: Medicare certification standards—applicable only to facilities desiring Medicare part "B" (facility fee) reimbursement. These standards are very minimal, as outlined above, leaving the detailed requirements for Medicare Certification to individual states. To date there is no direct federal approval of ASCs.
- *Optional State Health and State Fire Marshal Jurisdictions*: Medicare certification standards—applicable only to facilities desiring Medicare part "B" (facility fee) reimbursement. These standards focus on three areas:
  1. Rules of participation, or what types of facilities can and cannot qualify;
  2. Facility planning, construction, and operation. Many states simply apply their rules for licensure in addition to Medicare's specific regulatory standards. Other states consider Medicare Certifiable facilities as a separate classification, frequently with less restrictive physical environment standards;
  3. Survey and approval process, including plan approval (if available) and site surveys on an initial and periodic follow-up basis.

The first step for developing an ASC anywhere in the United States is simply to define the desired sources of facility fee reimbursement. From that point, establish a list of authorities having jurisdiction and identify their particular standards and regulations in effect:

No Facility Fee (professional fees only)
- If procedures are under local anesthesia only and limited to those traditionally done in an office setting, Local Jurisdiction will direct.
- If procedures are of higher acuity than traditionally done in an office setting or include heavy sedation and/or general anesthesia, contact the State Health Department to determine considerations beyond Local Jurisdiction (if any).

Independent Third-Party Facility Fee Reimbursement
- Local Jurisdiction standards must be met or exceeded.
- Contact each potential third-party payer and identify their minimal standards for facility fee participation. The response may vary from no special facility standards (but minimal reimbursement), to Accreditation, to State Licensure.

Independent Third-Party and Medicare Facility Fee Reimbursement
- As required for independent third-party reimbursement above.

- Contact State Health Department to identify their additional standards for participation. The response may range from the minimal federal requirements outlined above, to State Licensure, to Certificate of Need as well as State Licensure.

Independent Third-Party, Medicare, and State Program Facility Fee Reimbursement

- All standards of all authorities will be applied. Again it is necessary to contact the State Health Department to determine whether a Certificate of Need is necessary and to identify other requirements for licensure as an ASC.

The final word in this primer is one of caution and opportunity. All standards and regulations are subject to interpretation of each authority having jurisdiction, and the most restrictive interpretation from the various authorities will determine what applies. At the same time, this interpretive nature may open the door to "equivalent provision" when literal compliance is not possible or is clearly excessive for the circumstances. Finding a facility in your state, approved with only partial compliance, does not mean you will get the same favorable interpretation, but it does identify the opportunity to investigate possible cost savings for your unique circumstances.

REFERENCES

1. Shore DA. Evaluating accountability mechanisms. Part I. Accreditation. CSAE Forum, February 1990; 74:2.
2. Federal Register: July 23, 1996 (Volume 61, Number 142) Notices, Page 38207.

14. Conclusion

A. JEFFERSON PENFIELD

It is my hope that this book will ease the burdens of surgical practice in gynecology by providing practice guidelines, simplifying techniques, reducing complications, and improving the safety of such frequently performed operations as dilatation and curettage (D&C), first trimester abortion, hysteroscopic procedures, and laparoscopy. The use of local anesthesia and the transferral of many of these procedures to free-standing facilities and office surgeries are innovations that frequently result in improved surgical care for patients. Let me cite some examples.

> A 47-year-old patient, gravida 6 para 6, was previously sterilized. She skipped her last two periods and arrived in the office surgery passing large clots from the vagina. Immediate examination revealed a congested uterus and fresh active bleeding from the cervical os. She had a moderate tachycardia but no significant drop in blood pressure. From her history and examination, I estimated that she had lost at least 500 mL of blood. Consequently, the patient was reassured, counseled, and prepared for an immediate D&C for severe dysfunctional menorrhagia. The examining table then became the operating table as a tray of sterile instruments, always on hand, was brought in. One of the nurses, whom the patient had come to know and trust from previous routine visits, was standing by the head of the table. Within 10 minutes of the patient's arrival in the office, a paracervical block had been administered, the cervix dilated with minimal discomfort, and the curettage accomplished with prompt cessation of bleeding. After a brief interval, the patient walked with assistance to the recovery room, where she rested and was given her postoperative instructions and a prescription for iron tablets. She left within the hour for rest at home that day.
>
> Subsequent histologic examination of her curettings confirmed my initial impression that she was experiencing severe dysfunctional bleeding. Intensive oral iron supplements for 30 days corrected her anemia, and 10 days of progestational therapy each month for 6 months resulted in a regular diminishing monthly flow.
>
> Had this same patient been admitted to the local hospital emergency room, she would have lost approximately another 500 mL of blood before being typed and cross-matched on her way to the operating room. The additional hour's delay would undoubtedly have been accompanied by increasing tachycardia and hypotension, and the hospital anesthesiologist, noting a hematocrit of 28, would have ordered a transfusion before putting the patient to sleep for her D&C. This patient can be handled more efficiently and promptly in the well-equipped office surgery. Most routine D&Cs may be scheduled just as simply and with equal safety in a free-standing surgical unit.
>
> As another example, a young woman was having a miscarriage. Office examination revealed tissue protruding from the cervical os. Immediate uterine evacuation and curettage under paracervical block was carried out in the office surgery. After resting 1 hour, the patient returned in 2 weeks for follow-up examination and contraceptive counseling.

Elective first trimester abortions are appropriately performed in a private office surgery or a free-standing clinic. Local anesthesia is almost always to be preferred over general anesthesia in these cases because it permits normal uterine contractions and thus helps to minimize blood loss.

Laparoscopy can also be performed under local anesthesia in an outpatient or office surgical setting. If the closed technique of abdominal entry is selected, involving the insertion of insufflating needle and/or sharp trocar, then general anesthesia and full laparotomy capability should be available within 10 to 15 minutes in case of major vessel laceration (1, 2).

Aortic and iliac vessel injuries will not occur during abdominal entry by the open technique if the cavity is entered by scalpel incision of the skin and fascia and blunt entry through the peritoneal layer (3). Local anesthesia is adequate for laparoscopy unless the surgeon intends to introduce ancillary instruments through secondary incisions to perform operative procedures such as ovarian biopsies or tubal surgery other than sterilization.

Will American gynecologists follow the lead of other surgical specialists, such as plastic surgeons and ophthalmologists, and turn increasingly to local anesthesia and free-standing facilities?

Some anesthesiologists and some hospital administrators will resist the trend, which they interpret as a rejection of their services and their facilities. Many gynecologists will be slow to modify their long-standing reliance on maximum anesthesia for all surgical cases, arguing that only general anesthesia can abolish all discomfort. Recent graduates of residency programs will be inclined to continue to perform their surgery in the familiar environment of the hospital operating room, where general anesthesia is the norm.

However, the free-standing facility and the office surgery will attract those gynecologists who want to reduce complications, simplify procedures, and minimize risks. In addition, they will appreciate the convenience and ultimate economy of out-of-hospital surgical units. The initial expense of establishing an office surgery or free-standing clinic is offset by the time saved and the ease of patient scheduling as compared with a hospital admission. Quality care may be offered to patients by a skilled physician and a well-trained nursing staff with minimal turnover. In addition to being responsible for the maintenance of surgical instruments, the nurses provide skilled counseling and expert assistance in the operating room. A more personal relationship with the patient is fostered and closer postoperative supervision is possible.

Regarding quality care in outpatient gynecologic surgery, I deeply appreciate the splendid contributions to this text by the guest authors. Dr. Wortman has provided basic instruction in hysteroscopy for the practicing gynecologist, as well as information on pioneering techniques. Dr. Timor-Tritsch and Dr. Monteagudo have convincingly demonstrated the value of on-site transvaginal sonography in an office or outpatient setting. They have also described sonographically guided puncture procedures which require specialized expertise. Dr. Allen has shown how we can harness all of these expanding technologies to best serve our patients by establishing quality control, fulfilling accreditation requirements, and conducting cost-effective outpatient surgical practices.

REFERENCES

1. Penfield, A.J. Needle and Trocar Injuries to Major Blood Vessels. Paper presented at the Second International Congress of Gynecologic Endoscopy, Las Vegas, Nevada. November 22, 1975.
2. Penfield, A.J. Trocar and Needle Injuries. In Laparoscopy (ed. Phillips) Williams & Wilkins, Baltimore, MD. 22:236, 1977.
3. Penfield AJ. How to prevent complications of open laparoscopy. J Reprod Med 1985;30:660–663.

Index

Page numbers followed by "t" or "f" denote tables or figure, respectively.

Abdominal wall
   abscess, open laparoscopy and, 152
   hematoma, open laparoscopy and, 151
Abortion
   complications, 58–64
      antibiotic prophylaxis, 61–63
      cervical disruption, 61, 62f
      cervical incompetence, 63
      endometritis, 63
      late, 63–64
      local vs. general anesthesia, 1
      postoperative depression, 63
      uterine atony and hemorrhage, 58–60
      uterine perforation, 60–61
      uterine synechiae, 63
   first trimester, 41–64, 299
      antibiotic prophylaxis for endometritis, 61–63
      apprehension, 53–55
      complications, 1, 58–64
      counseling, 42–44
      infantile cervix/stenosis of internal cervical os and, 55–56
      informed consent, 43–44
      instruments for, 46, 47f, 48f, 49f
      local anesthesia, 46–47
      manual vacuum aspiration, 51, 52f
      mortality rates, 1
      in obese patient, 55
      obstructing myomata, 56–57, 57f
      operative technique, 46–51, 47f–49f. (*see also* Dilatation and curettage)
      patient education, 43
      pelvic sonography in, 45–46
      postoperative examination, 51–52
      postoperative instructions, 54f
      preoperative examination, 44–45
      preparation, 46
      problems, 53–57
      RU 486, 41–42
      transfer to recovery room, 52–53
      trapped products of conception, 57, 58f
      uterine retroversion and, 55
   incomplete, dilatation and curettage for, 32
   second trimester, 1, 194
Abortion clinics, expansion of services, 21
Abscess
   abdominal wall, open laparoscopy and, 152
   Bartholin duct, incision, drainage, and marsupialization/insertion of Word catheter, 188–190, 189f
   suburethral, 188
   tubo-ovarian, 218, 219f
   vulvar and vaginal, incision and drainage, 188
Accreditation, 245–279
   Accreditation Association for Ambulatory Health Care (AAAHC), 246–279
   Certificate of Accreditation, 250f
   certification vs., 246
   definition, 245–246
   health care accrediting bodies, 246
   Joint Commission on Accreditation of Health Care Organizations (JCAHO), 246
   Medicare ASC certification, 246
   office surgical facility, 25
   organizational chart, 254f
   practice accreditation, 245–246
   reviewing authority's standards, 295–298
Accreditation Association for Ambulatory Health Care (AAAHC), 246–279
   AAAHC standards, 251–279
      administration, 255
      anesthesia services, 274–275
      application of, 248–249
      clinical records, 267–268
      documentation of legality of organization, 252
      documentation of patient satisfaction/dissatisfaction, 256f, 257f
      facilities and environment, 268–274
         design requirements, 271, 272f–273f
         equipment maintenance, 271
         external disaster policy, 270f
         fire prevention, 268–269
         handicapped individuals, 271
         hazardous materials, 271
         internal disaster plan/policy, 269f–270f
         Medicare-related standards, 271
         safety issues, 271
      governance, 252–255
         credentials file, 255
         organizational chart, 254f, 255
         policies and procedures manual, 255
      pathology and medical laboratory services, 278–279
      patient rights, 252, 253f
      pharmaceutical standards, 278
      professional improvement, 268
      quality management and improvement, 258–267
         occurrence screening review worksheet, 258, 260f–262f
         physician peer review, 258, 259f

Accreditation Association for Ambulatory Health Care (AAAHC)—*continued*
  quality improvement program, 258, 263f–265f
  risk management program (*see* Risk management)
  quality of care provided, 256–258
  surgical services, 275–278
    equipment maintenance, 275–276
    Medicare-related standards, 276–278
    transfer and evacuation plan, 275, 276f–277f
    transfer and evacuation plan for situations requiring hospitalization, 275, 276f–277f
  accreditation decision, 251
  accreditation policies and procedures, 248
  Certificate of Accreditation, 250f
  deemed status, 246, 295
  history, 247
  member associations, 247
  programs, 247–248
  survey eligibility criteria, 248
  survey fee, 249
  survey process, 249
  survey site visit, 249
Acidosis, in CO_2 hysteroscopy, 77
Acoustic window, in hysteroscopic myomectomy, 120
Adenomyosis, hysteroscopic endomyometrial resection for, 108
Adhesions
  bowel, 142f
  failed minilaparotomy and, 169
  pelvic, Hulka clip sterilization and, 144
Adnexal mass, in first trimester abortion, 44
Age, outcome of myomectomy, 117
Allen Universal stirrups, 69, 70f
Allergy/allergic reactions
  anesthetic agents, 16
  gold allergy, Hulka clip sterilization, 137–138
Ambulatory service centers (*see* Office surgical facility; Outpatient surgical facilities)
Ambulatory surgery (*see* Office surgical facility; Outpatient surgical facilities)
Americaine (*see* Benzocaine)
American Association of Gynecologic Laparoscopists (AAGL)
  Accreditation Council for Gynecologic Endoscopy (ACGE), 127
  address, 128
  membership survey concerning laparoscopic sterilization methods and complications, 176t
  Operative Endoscopy Guidelines, 128
American Medical Association, Physician Profile Service, 255
American Society of Anesthesiologists, guidelines for sedation and analgesia, 7
Americans with Disabilities Act, compliance with, 271

Amino amide anesthetics, 9
  toxicity, clinical experiment, 15–16
Amino ester anesthetics, 9
  toxicity, clinical experiment, 15–16
Amnesia, midazolam-induced, 6
Amniocentesis, early, transvaginal sonographic puncture, 240
Analgesia
  agents (*see* specific drugs)
  practice guidelines for nonanesthesiologists, 7
Anaphylactic reaction, Hyskon, 79
Anectine (*see* Succinylcholine)
Anesthesia
  AAAHC standards, 274–275
  epidural, 1
  general, 300
    for ambulatory tubal sterilization, 21
    complications, 2
    indications for, 3
    suitability for given operation, 1–2
  intrinsic anesthetic potency, 11
  local. (*see* Local anesthesia)
  local vs. general, 1–8
    patient selection, 3
    selection criteria, 1–3
    suitability for given operation, 1–3
    surgeon selection, 3–4
  selection of type, 1–3
  spinal, 1
Anesthesiologist
  rejection of local anesthesia, 2
  role in hysteroscopic surgery, 99
Antianxiety agents, premedication for local anesthesia, 6
Antibiotic drugs, prophylactic
  in hysteroscopic surgery, 100, 111–112
  postabortal, 61–63
Anxiety
  agents for, 6
  epinephrine-induced, 12
Aortic injury, 300
Apnea, prolonged, 17
Apprehension, in abortion candidate, 53–55
Arrhythmia, cardiac, lidocaine in, 14
Aspiration
  breast cyst, 193–194
  manual vacuum aspiration, first trimester abortion, 51, 52f
Assisted reproductive technology, transvaginal sonographic puncture and catheterization procedures, 231
Atropine
  preoperative, minilaparotomy tubal ligation, 167
  for vasovagal reaction, 17
    in dilatation and curettage, 34
    in office hysteroscopy, 92
AT&T Language Line Services, 258
Autoclave, office surgical facility, 26, 28f
Automated puncture device, transvaginal sonographic puncture procedures, 229, 230f

INDEX

Baby Deaver retractors, 134f
Baby Kocher clamps, 134f
Bartholin duct, cyst/abscess, incision, drainage, and marsupialization/insertion of Word catheter, 188–190, 189f
"Beads-on-a-string" sign
   hydrosalpinx, 218, 219f
   ovary, 211, 212f
Benadryl (*see* Diphenhydramine)
Benzocaine (Americaine), 10t
Bhatt, Rohit, 180
Biopsy
   vaginal
      local anesthesia, 188
      suture ligation of bleeders, 192
   vulvar, local anesthesia, 188
Bladder, laceration, during minilaparotomy, 168–169
Bleeding
   cervical, suture ligation of bleeders, 191
   mesosalpingeal, during minilaparotomy, 169
   postabortal
      management, 58–60
      persistent, dilatation and curettage for, 32
   postmenopausal, dilatation and curettage for, 32
   puerperal, dilatation and curettage for, 32
   uterine (*see* Uterus, abnormal bleeding)
   vaginal, suture ligation of bleeders, 192
Blood pressure, epinephrine-induced increase, propranolol for, 12
Blundell, James, 173
Body water, total, calculation, 110
Body weight, outcome of myomectomy, 117–118
Bowel injury
   during hysteroscopic surgery, 111
   during minilaparotomy, 169
   during open laparoscopy, 139, 142f, 151
Bozzini, 65
Bradycardia (*see* Vasovagal reaction)
Breast cyst, aspiration, 193–194
Briggs, Mary, 179
Bupivacaine (Marcaine), 10t
   clinical considerations, 18
Butorphanol tartrate (Stadol)
   in Hulka clip sterilization, 138
   in minilaparotomy tubal ligation, 159
   preoperative, 187

Carbocaine (*see* Mepivacaine)
Carbon dioxide
   emboli, 77, 93
   pneumoperitoneum, 136–137
   uterine distention medium, 76–77
Carbonic acid, formation, in CO_2 hysteroscopy, 77
Cardiac arrest, 8
   anesthetic induced, 15
Cardiac arrhythmia, lidocaine in, 14
Cardiovascular system, anesthetic toxicity, 14–16
Case report
   chronic progressive unilateral pelvic pain,
      diagnostic laparoscopy under local anesthesia, 134–136
   dilatation and curettage for severe dysfunctional menorrhagia, 299
Catgut suture, 194
Cefonicid, prophylactic, for hysteroscopic surgery, 100
"Ceiling test", nonfunctioning fibers in light cables, 76
Central nervous system, anesthetic toxicity, 14
Certification, 246
   Medicare (*see* Medicare certification)
   office surgical facility, 25
Cervical carcinoma, invasive, hysteroscopy in, 92
Cervical finders, for office hysteroscopy, 70, 70f
Cervical intraepithelial neoplasia, hysteroscopic endomyometrial resection for, 108
Cervical pregnancy
   sonographic diagnostic criteria, 237
   transvaginal methotrexate injection for, 236–238, 237f
Cervical sealing instruments, for office hysteroscopy, 71, 71f
Cervix uteri
   bleeding, suture ligation of bleeders, 191
   conization, 192
   dilatation (*see* Dilatation)
   disruption, during first trimester abortion, 61, 62f
   endocervical resection, 102, 102f
   incompetence, 203, 203f
      postabortal, 63
   infantile, first trimester abortion and, 55–56
   laceration, during dilatation and curettage, 38
   length, in pregnancy, 203, 204f
   loop electrical excision procedure, 192
   nonnegotiable, first trimester abortion and, 55–56
   sonographic evaluation, 202–204, 203f
      in pregnancy, 203f, 203–204, 204f
   sounding, first trimester abortion, 48–49
   stenosis
      in hysteroscopic endomyometrial resection, 102
      internal os, first trimester abortion and, 55–56
Chaturachinda, Kamheang, 181
Childbearing (*see* Fertility)
Chloroprocaine (Nesacaine), 10t
   clinical considerations, 17
   toxicity, clinical experiment, 16
Chlorpromazine (Thorazine), for anesthetic-induced hypertension, 15
Chorionic villi sampling, transvaginal sonographic puncture, 240
Chromosome abnormalities, prenatal diagnosis
   amniocentesis, 240
   transvaginal sonography, 221, 222f, 224
Circulating nurse, role in hysteroscopic surgery, 99
Citanest (*see* Prilocaine)
Cocaine anesthesia, 10t
   historical perspective, 9
Colpotomy, local anesthesia, 193
Communication, AT&T Language Line Services, 258

Conization, cervical, 192
Consent (*see* Informed consent)
Consultation, in hysteroscopy, video documentation for, 80
Contraception, in developing countries, 182
Convulsions
 anesthetic-induced, 14
 syncopal, 8
Corpus luteum
 ectopic pregnancy vs., 215
 sonographic appearance, 211, 212f
Counseling
 abortion, 42–44
 dilatation and curettage, 33
 Hulka clip sterilization under local anesthesia, 137
 local anesthesia, 4–5
 minilaparotomy tubal ligation under local anesthesia, 156, 157
Credentialing
 Accreditation Council for Gynecologic Endoscopy (ACGE), 127
 in hysteroscopic surgery, 99, 127–130
 office-based diagnostic hysteroscopy, 68–69
Cryosurgery, endometrial ablation, 94
Cryptomenorrhea, 190
Cul-de-sac
 abscess, 219f
 fluid collection, ectopic pregnancy, 216
Culdocentesis, transvaginal sonographic puncture, 238–240
Culdoscopy
 local anesthesia, 193
 tubal ligation, 182, 193
Culdotomy, vaginal tubal ligation, 193
Cyst
 Bartholin duct, incision, drainage, and marsupialization/insertion of Word catheter, 188–190, 189f
 breast, fine needle aspiration, 193–194
 ovarian (*see* Ovarian cyst)
 peritoneal inclusion, postoperative, 238
Cystadenoma, ovarian, 213, 214f
Cystourethroscopy, procedure room costs and incidentals, surgical tray list, 292f

David, Charles, 65
Denniston plastic cervical dilators, 48f
Depreciation
 accelerated depreciation methods, 287
 declining balance method, 287
 double declining balance method, 287
 equipment costs in computation of annual fixed costs of office surgical facility, 287
 straight line (time) method, 287
 sum-of-the-years'-digits method, 287, 289f
Depression, postabortal, 63
Dermoid, ovarian, 214f
Desormeaux, 65
Dextran 70 (*see* High molecular weight dextran 70)

Diaphoresis (*see* Vasovagal reactions)
Diazepam (Valium)
 in Hulka clip sterilization, 138
 intravenous, cautionary note, 6
 premedication for local anesthesia, 6
  in seizure disorder, 14
 preoperative, 187
  in dilatation and curettage, 33
  in first trimester abortion, 54
  in minilaparotomy tubal ligation, 167
Dibucaine (Nupercaine), 10t
Dilatation, cervical, 49–50
 for hysteroscopic endomyometrial resection, 100
 for hysteroscopic myomectomy, 118
 for hysteroscopic surgery, 100
Dilatation and curettage, 29–39
 for abnormal uterine bleeding, 30–32, 67
 for abortion, 46–51
  cervical dilatation, 49–50
  instruments, 47f–49f
  local anesthesia, 46–47
  preparation, 46
  sounding the cervix and uterus, 48–49
  standard curettage, 51
  vacuum curettage, 50–51
 advantages and disadvantages, 29
 anesthesia, 34
 cervical laceration, 38
 complications, 37–38
 conclusion, 38–39
 counseling, 33
 curettage, 36, 36f
 dilatation, 35
 for dysmenorrhea, 32–33
 for hematometra, 33
 indications, 30–33, 32t
 premedication, 33–34
 procedure room costs and incidentals, surgical tray list, 292f
 for pyometra, 33
 residual placental tissue, sonographic appearance, 208f
 for severe dysfunctional menorrhagia, 299
 sounding of internal cervical os, 34, 35f
 technique, 33–36, 35f, 36f
 uterine pain during, 29
 uterine perforation, 37f, 37–38
 uterosacral block, 29
 vasovagal reactions during, 38
Dilatation and evacuation, 194
 complications, 1
Dilators, 49
 for office hysteroscopy, 70
Diphenhydramine (Benadryl), for anesthetic-induced allergic reactions, 16
Disaster planning, 269f–270f
Dizziness (*see* Vasovagal reaction)
Documentation
 clinical records, 267–268
 equipment maintenance, 276

legality of organization applying for accreditation, 252
occurrence screening review worksheet, 258, 260f–262f
patient encounters, 282
patient survey questionnaire, 256f
physician peer review, 258, 259f
practice data, 282
surgery satisfaction questionnaire, 257f
video documentation (*see* Video documentation)
Doxycycline
for postabortal infection, 63
prophylactic, for hysteroscopic surgery, 100
Drainage procedures, ultrasound-guided, 238
Drug therapy (*see also specific drugs*)
AAAHC standards, 278
Duranest (*see* Etidocaine)
Dysmenorrhea, dilatation and curettage for, 32–33
Dyspareunia, management, 191

Economic issues
fee estimates, 281f
financial management of practice, 280
insurance claim processing, 289, 290f–294f
office surgical facility, 23
operating room and recovery room pricing analysis, 283–289, 284f–287f
computation of annual fixed costs, 283–284, 284f–286f, 287, 289f
computation of fixed costs per hour, 286f, 287
equipment costs, 284, 285f–286f, 287
fee comparison, 287f, 289
memorandum for insurance carriers, 288f, 289
occupancy costs, 283–284, 284f–285f
personnel costs, 283, 284f
reimbursement, 283–294
insurance claim processing, 289, 290f–294f
Edema, anesthetic-induced, 16
Education (*see* Medical education; Patient education)
Electrocoagulation, laparoscopic sterilization
bipolar tubal coagulation, 150, 175f, 175–176
unipolar tubal coagulation, 174–175
Electrodes, for myomectomy, 121
Electrosurgery, endometrial ablation, 94–95
Electrosurgical unit
for endomyometrial resection, 98
for myomectomy, 121
Embolus(i), in CO_2 hysteroscopy, 77, 93
Embryo, growth and development, 220
Encephalopathy, hyponatremic, 109–110
clinical features, 109t
management, 110
Endometrial ablation, 94–95
Endometrioma, ovarian, 213, 214f
Endometriosis, rectal/rectovaginal, 136
Endometritis, postabortal, 63
antibiotic prophylaxis, 61–63
Endometrium
sonographic anatomy, 206

thickness, sonohysterographic determination, 209–210, 210f
transcervical resection, 95
Endomyometrial resection, 95, 96–108
antibiotic prophylaxis, 100
cervical stenosis and, management, 102, 102f
clinical applications, 108
complications
delayed, 113
immediate, 113t
diagnostic hysteroscopy in, 102
dilatation, 100
equipment, 97–98
electrosurgical generators, 98
fluid collection system, 97–98
fluid infusion system, 97
illumination system, 98
resectoscopes, 98
video system, 98
establishing maximum allowable fluid absorption limit, 100
fluid flow, 101–102
in hysteroscopic myomectomy, 119–120
patient education, 97
patient selection, 96–97
diagnostic hysteroscopy, 96
history, 96
laboratory evaluation, 96
sonogram, 96
postoperative care, 107–108
pregnancy after, 112
procedure, 100–102
resectoscope introduction, 101–102
results, 112–113, 113t
surgical team, 98–99
anesthesiologist, 99
circulating nurse, 99
scrub nurse, 99
surgeon, 98–99
technique, 103–107
anterolateral triangles, 106, 106f
cardinal strips, 104, 104f
electrosurgical fulguration, 106–107
excision of tubal ostium, 106–107, 107f
four-leaf clover appearance
panoramic hysteroscopy, 105f
ultrasonography, 105f
posterolateral triangles, 106, 106f
power setting, 103
resection of anterior cardinal strip, 101f, 103
resection of posterior cardinal strip, 103f
ridge tissue, 106, 107f
specimen collection for histologic analysis, 107, 108f
vasopressin injection, 100–101
video documentation, equipment, 98
Epidural anesthesia, 1
Epinephrine
addition to lidocaine, 12, 17, 18

Epinephrine—*continued*
    for anesthetic-induced allergic reactions, 16
    clinical considerations, 12
Equipment (*see* Instrumentation)
Etidocaine (Duranest), 10t
    clinical considerations, 18

Fallopian tube(s)
    Hulka clip application (*see* Hulka clip sterilization)
    ligation (*see* Sterilization, female)
    transvaginal sonography, 215–218
        ectopic pregnancy, 215f, 215–217, 216f
        inflammatory process, 217–218, 218f, 219f
Falope ring (Yoon band), 150, 175f, 177
Fentanyl citrate (Sublimaze), in Hulka clip sterilization, 138
Fertility
    hysteroscopic surgery and, 117
    postabortal, 64
Fetus
    heartbeat, 220, 221f
    nuchal translucency, transvaginal sonography, 221, 222f, 224
Fibrillation, cardiac, anesthetic induced, 15
Fibroids, uterine (*see* Myoma)
Filshie clip sterilization, 175f, 177–178
Financial management (*see* Economic issues)
Fine needle aspiration, breast cyst, 193–194
Fire prevention, 268–269
Fluid overload
    Hyskon-induced, 79
    in hysteroscopic surgery, 108–110
Flumazenil, for respiratory depression, in office hysteroscopy, 93
Foley catheter, tamponade, for hemorrhage during hysteroscopic surgery, 112
Fongsri, Arunee, 180, 181
Free-standing surgical centers, 21
    accreditation, 25
Friedrich, Ernst, 4
Frozen pelvis, 199
Furosemide, for postoperative hyponatremia, 109

Gentamicin, prophylactic, for hysteroscopic surgery, 100
Gimpelson tenaculum, 71, 71f
Giri, Kanti, 180
Glycine (*see also* Hysteroscopy, low viscosity fluids)
    excess absorption, 108–109
    maximum allowable fluid absorption limit ($MAFA_{limit}$), 100
Gold allergy, Hulka clip sterilization, 137–138
Gonadotropin-releasing hormone (GnRH) agonist, preoperative
    hysteroscopic endomyometrial resection, 97
    hysteroscopic myomectomy, 118

Halogen light, for hysteroscopy, 76
Hasson, Harrith, 131
Hasson cannula, 131, 132f, 143f
Hazardous materials, 271
Hegar dilators, 49, 100
Hematoma
    abdominal wall, open laparoscopy and, 151
    parametrial, cervical disruption during first trimester abortion, 61, 62f
Hematometra
    dilatation and curettage for, 33
    dilatation and drainage for, 112
    in imperforate hymen, 190
    postoperative, hysteroscopic surgery, 112
Hemorrhage
    during hysteroscopic surgery, 112
    postoperative, hysteroscopic surgery, 112
    subchorionic, early pregnancy, transvaginal sonography, 221, 222f
    uterine
        dilatation and curettage for, 30–32
        hysteroscopy in, 91
        postabortal
            local vs. general anesthesia, 1
            prevention and management, 58–60
High molecular weight dextran 70 (Hyskon), uterine distention medium, 78–79
History taking
    in hysteroscopic endomyometrial resection, 96
    in office hysteroscopy, 82
    surgical procedures, documentation for Medicare certification, 277
Hives, anesthetic-induced, 16
Hopkins rod-lens system, endoscope, 74, 74f
Hulka clip sterilization, 137–150, 176
    clip application, 144–145, 145f, 146f
    closure, 146f, 147, 147f
    contraindication, 137
    counseling, 137
    follow-up questionnaire, 149f
    gold allergy and, 137–138
    patient preparation, 138
    patient selection, 137–138
    pneumoperitoneum for, 143
    postoperative instructions, 148f
    premedication, 138
    technique, 139f–147f, 139–147
Hulka tenaculum-sound, 134f
Human chorionic gonadotropin (hCG), β-subunit, after puncture and injection of ectopic pregnancy, 238
Hyaluronidase (Wydase), in local anesthesia, 13
Hydrosalpinx, 218, 219f
Hymen
    dilatation, 191
    imperforate, incision, 190
    tight/rigid, incision, 191
Hypertension
    anesthetic induced, 12, 15
    epinephrine use in, 12
Hyponatremia
    dilutional, in hysteroscopic surgery, 100
    in hysteroscopic surgery, 99, 108–110

management, 109–110
severe, 109
Hypotension (*see also* Vasovagal reaction)
  diazepam-induced, 6
Hypoxia, pulse oximetry, 26
Hyskon (*see* High molecular weight dextran 70)
Hysterectomy
  disadvantages, 67
  for intractable postabortal hemorrhage, 60
  suture ligation of vaginal cuff bleeders, 192
Hysteroscopic surgery, 93–124. (*see also specific procedures*)
  advantages, 67
  antibiotic prophylaxis, 100, 111–112
  complications, 108–112
    bowel injury, 111
    fluid overload, hypoosmolarity, and hyponatremia, 108–110
    hematometra, 112
    hemorrhage, 112
    infection, 111–112
    pregnancy, 112
    prevention, 99
    uterine perforation, 110–111
    uterine rupture, 111
  credentialing (*see* Credentialing)
  dilatation, 100
  endometrial ablation, 94–95
  endometrial resection, 95
  endomyometrial resection, 95, 96–108
  maximum allowable fluid absorption limit (MAFA$_{limit}$), 100
  myomectomy, 95–96, 113–125
  stratification of procedures, 130
  vasopressin injection, 100–101
Hysteroscopy, 65–130
  carbon dioxide
    advantages, 76–77
    carbon dioxide emboli, 77, 93
    CO$_2$ insufflation, 77
    disadvantages, 77
    equipment, 86f
    lack of flow, 91
    lack of pressure, 90
    operating room preparation, 86
    patient positioning, 87
    preoperative checklist, 77, 87
    "red out," 91
    trouble-shooting problems, 90–91
  complications and management, 92–93
    carbon dioxide emboli, 93
    complications secondary to inadequate sedation/analgesia, 92
    respiratory depression/arrest, 93
    uterine perforation, 92–93
    vasovagal reaction, 92
  contraindications, 91–92
  credentialing, 68–69, 127–130
    American Association of Gynecologic Laparoscopists Operative Endoscopy Guidelines, 128
    guidelines for attaining privileges in gynecologic operative endoscopy, 128–130
    learning phases, 127
    process, 127–128
  diagnostic
    advantages, 67
    analgesia, 85–86
    anteverted uterus, 88f
    black spot, 88f, 89
    concept of aiming diagnostic scope, 89, 89f
    failure to enter uterine cavity, 89, 91
    in hysteroscopic endomyometrial resection, 96, 102
    informed consent, 83, 84f
    intravenous sedation, 85–86
    office-based (*see* Hysteroscopy, office-based)
    operating room preparation, 86
    paracervical block, 85, 87
    patient positioning, 87
    patient preparation, 84–85
    preoperative checklists, 87
    procedure, 87–90
    trouble-shooting problems, 90–91
    uterine myomata, 114–115
  education. (*see also* Credentialing)
    physician training, 80, 81
    staff training, 81
  historical perspective, 65–66
  instrumentation, 69–80
    cervical finders, 70, 70f
    cervical sealing instruments, 71, 71f
    dilators, 70–71
    emergency kit, 79f, 79–80
    light cables, 75–76
    light source, 76
    pulse oximeter, 79
    speculum, 69
    telescopes, 71–75
    tenaculum, 70
    uterine distention equipment, 76–79
  introduction to, 66–67
  low viscosity fluids, 77–78, 90
    advantages, 77–78
    disadvantages, 78
    endomyometrial resection, 97–98
    equipment, 87f
    flow of fluid, 91, 101–102
    fluid collection system, 97–98, 104f
    infusion system for, 97
    maximum allowable fluid absorption limit (MAFA$_{limit}$), 100
    operating room preparation, 86
    preoperative checklist, 87
    trouble-shooting problems, 91
  office-based, 67–93
    benefits, 68
    complications and management, 92–93
    credentialing, 68–69
    environment, 82

Hysteroscopy—*continued*
   essentials, 69–82
   examination table, 69
   informed consent, 83, 84f
   instrumentation (*see* Hysteroscopy, instrumentation)
   introduction, 67–68
   patient preparation, 82–84
   protocols, 81–82
   staff training, 81
  operative (*see* Hysteroscopic surgery)
  patient education, 83
  patient preparation, 82–84
   history and physical examination, 82
   informed consent, 83, 84f
   laboratory evaluation, 82–83
   patient education, 83
  postoperative instructions, 83t
  procedure room costs and incidentals, surgical tray list, 292f
  respiratory depression/arrest, 79, 93
  stratification of procedures, 130
  telescopes, 71–75
   accommodation of sheaths, 75
   angle of tilt, 71–72, 73f
   angle of view, 73, 74f
   diameter, 73–74
   flexible fiber optic endoscopes, 73f, 75
   Hopkins rod-lens optical system, 74, 74f
   rigid endoscopes, 72f
   semirigid endoscope, 72f
   semirigid fiber optic endoscopes, 75
  uterine distention, 76–79
   carbon dioxide, 76–77
   high molecular weight dextran 70 (Hyskon), 78–79
   low viscosity fluids (LVFs), 77–78
  vasovagal reaction, 92
  video documentation, 80–81
   medicolegal considerations, 81
   patient education, 80
   physician comfort, 80
   physician communication, 80
   physician training, 80

Iliac vessel injury, 300
Imperforate hymen, incision, 190
Incision
  abdominal, postoperative infection, 152
  for Hulka clip sterilization, 139, 142f
  suprapubic minilaparotomy, 155, 162–163
   wound hematoma, 170
   wound infection, 170
India, laparoscopic sterilization services, 180
Infantile cervix
  first trimester abortion and, 55–56
  intrauterine device insertion/removal, 192
Infection
  incisional, 170
  postabortal, 63

  postoperative
   abdominal incision for open laparoscopy, 152
   hysteroscopic surgery, 111–112
Informed consent
  abortion, first trimester, 43–44
  diagnostic hysteroscopy, 83, 84f
  minilaparotomy tubal ligation under local anesthesia, 156, 157f
  transvaginal sonographic puncture procedures, 230–231
Instrumentation
  diagnostic hysteroscopy, 69–80
  dilators, 49
  emergency oropharyngeal suction equipment, 27f
  equipment costs in computation of annual fixed costs of office surgical facility, 284, 285f–286f, 287
   depreciation, 287
  first trimester abortion, 46, 47f, 48f, 49f
   manual vacuum aspiration, 52f
  hysteroscopic endomyometrial resection, 97–98
  hysteroscopy, 69–80
  maintenance, 271, 275–276
  minilaparotomy, 160f, 160t, 161f
  open laparoscopy, 133t, 134f
  sonohysterography, 208
  sterilization, in office surgical facility, 26, 28f
Insufflator
  hysteroscopic, 77
  laparoscopic, 77
Insurance claim processing, 289, 290f–294f
  HCFA 1500 claim form, 289, 290f
  UB-92 claim form, 289, 291f
  variable costs related to surgical procedures, 289, 292f–294f
International Program for Abortion Services (IPAS), 51
Intrauterine device
  insertion/removal, anesthesia for, 192
  sonographic appearance, 207f
Intrinsic anesthetic potency, 11

Jackson-Pratt drain, dilatation and drainage for hematometra, 112
Johns Hopkins Program for International Education in Gynecology and Obstetrics (JHPIEGO), 180
Joint Commission on Accreditation of Health Care Organizations (JCAHO), 246
  deemed status, 246, 295

Kleppinger, Richard, 176

Labia minora, redundant tissue, excision of, 190
Laboratory evaluation
  AAAHC standards for pathology and medical laboratory services, 278–279
  in hysteroscopic endomyometrial resection, 96
  for office hysteroscopy, 82–83

Laceration
  bladder, during minilaparotomy, 168–169
  bowel
    during minilaparotomy, 169
    during open laparoscopy, 139, 142f, 151
  cervical
    during dilatation and curettage, 38
    during first trimester abortion, 61, 62f
  vaginal, suture ligation of bleeders, 192
Lactated Ringer solution (*see* Hysteroscopy, low viscosity fluids)
Laminaria tent
  in hysteroscopic myomectomy, 118
  in hysteroscopic surgery, 100
  for nonnegotiable cervix, 56, 56f
Laparoscopy, 131–153
  anesthesia, 300
  closed, 131
    risks, 7
  diagnostic, 131, 133–137
    chronic pelvic pain, 134–136
    local anesthesia, 133–134
    pain mapping, 136–137
  microlaparoscopy, 137
  open, 131–132
    abdominal wall hematoma and, 151–152
    bowel injury during, 151
    bowel laceration, 139, 142f
    complications, 150–152
    Hulka clip application under local anesthesia (*see* Hulka clip sterilization)
    instrumentation, 133t, 134f
    outpatient sterilization, 179
    postoperative infection of abdominal incision, 152
    risks, 7
    uterine perforation during, 150–151
  statistics, 131
  sterilization, 131, 174–178, 175f
    bipolar tubal coagulation, 150, 175f, 175–176
    complications (*see* Laparoscopy, open, complications)
    failure rate, 150
    Falope ring (Yoon band), 150
    Hulka clip application under local anesthesia, 137–150
    outpatient, free-standing female sterilization services in United States, 179–180
    tubal thermocautery, 182–183
    unipolar tubal coagulation, 174–175
  stratification of procedures, 130
  in uterine perforation, during abortion, 60–61
Laparotomy, suprapubic minilaparotomy (*see* Minilaparotomy)
Laprocator, 180
Laser surgery
  endometrial ablation, 94
  lower genital tract, procedure room costs and incidentals, surgical tray list, 292f
Lee, Shaio-Yu, 179

Leiomyoma, submucous, 123f
Leuprolide acetate, preoperative
  hysteroscopic endomyometrial resection, 97
  hysteroscopic myomectomy, 118
Lidocaine (Xylocaine), 10t
  for abortion, first trimester, 46–47
  advantages, 12–13
  allergic reactions, 16
  cardiac muscle effect, 14
  chemical structure, 12f
  clinical considerations, 11–12, 17–18
  for diagnostic hysteroscopy, 85, 87
  for dilatation and curettage, 34
  epinephrine plus, 12, 17, 18
  fatalities from, 15
  historical perspective, 9
  for Hulka clip sterilization, 138, 139f, 140f
  for minilaparotomy, 161–162, 164f, 165f
  paracervical block, 17, 34
  safe dosage, 13
  in ventricular arrhythmia, 14
Light cables, for hysteroscopy, 75–76
Light source
  in endomyometrial resection, 98
  in hysteroscopy, 76
  in outpatient operating room, 187
Lipscomb, Gary, 4
Liquid nitrogen, endometrial ablation, 94
Liquid silicone, catalyzed, tubal injection, 183
Local anesthesia
  AAAHC standards, 274–275
  abortion
    first trimester, 46–47
    second trimester, 194
  agents, 9–18
    allergic reactions, 16
    choice of, 17–18, 187
    clinical considerations, 11–13
    conclusions, 17–18
    intrinsic anesthetic potency, 11
    representative agents in common clinical use, 10t
    safe dosage levels, 13–17
    toxic reactions (*see* Local anesthesia, toxic reactions)
    vasovagal reactions, 16–17
  allergic reactions, 16
  Bartholin duct cyst/abscess incision, drainage, and marsupialization/insertion of Word catheter, 188–190, 189f
  benefits, 2, 5
  breast cyst aspiration, 193–194
  cervical conization, 192
  clinical applications, 3
  complications (*see also* Local anesthesia, toxic reactions), 2
  counseling the patient, 4–5
  culdoscopy and colpotomy, 193
  definition, 9
  diagnostic hysteroscopy, 85
  diagnostic laparoscopy, 133–137

Local anesthesia—*continued*
  dilatation and curettage, 34
  dilatation and evacuation, 194
  fatalities from, 15
  gynecologic procedures (*see also specific procedures*), 187–194
  historical perspective, 9
  Hulka clip application via single-incision open laparoscopy, 137–150
  intrauterine device insertion and removal, 192–193
  loop electrical excision procedure, 192
  masking abnormal postoperative pain, 13
  medical (resident) education, 4
  minilaparotomy tubal ligation, 155–171
    prerequisites, 156–159
  outpatient facilities (*see* Office surgical facility; Outpatient surgical facilities)
  paracervical block, 17
  patient selection, 3
  personnel and equipment needs, 7
  pharmacodynamics, 9, 11
  plastic surgery of vulva, vagina, or perineum, 190–191
  practice guidelines for nonanesthesiologists, 7
  premedication, 6–7, 187
  preoperative workup, instructions and scheduling, 5
  psychological benefits, 5
  recovery period, 7
  rejection of, 300
    factors affecting, 2–3
  removal of skin lesions between umbilicus and knee, 194
  resuscitation backup, 8
  staff selection, 4
  surgeon selection, 3–4
  suture ligation of cervical or vaginal bleeders, 191–192
  toxic reactions, 13–16
    amino amides vs. amino esters, clinical experiment, 15–16
    cardiovascular effects, 14–16
    central nervous system effects, 14
    sequence of events, 13–14
  uterosacral block, 29, 30f, 31f
  vasovagal reactions, 16–17
  vulvar and vaginal abscess incision and drainage, 188
  vulvar and vaginal biopsies, 188
Loop electrical excision procedure, 192
Lungren, Samuel Smith, 173

Mannitol (*see also* Hysteroscopy, low viscosity fluids)
  in hysteroscopic surgery, 109
Marcaine (*see* Bupivacaine)
Marsupialization, Bartholin duct cyst, 188–190, 189f
Martin, Purvis, 23
Massage, uterine, postevacuation, 52, 60
Medical education
  in hysteroscopy
    learning phases, 127
  patient care staff, 81
  physician training, 81, 98–99
  video documentation, 80
  in transvaginal sonography, 202
Medicare certification, 246
  anesthesia services, 276–278
  deemed status, 295
  facilities and environment standards, 271, 272–273f, 296
Medicare Peer Review Organization, 277
Medicolegal issues
  female sterilization, 183–184
  in hysteroscopy, video documentation, 81
  informed consent (*see* Informed consent)
  Patient Bill of Rights, 253f
Menometrorrhagia, dysfunctional, dilatation and curettage for, 31–32
Menorrhagia, 94
  severe dysfunctional, dilatation and curettage for, 299
Menstrual cycle, sonographic dating, 206, 207f
Menstruation, derangements, 93–94
Mentally incompetent individuals, sterilization, 184
Meperidine hydrochloride (Demerol)
  in culdoscopy, 193
  in Hulka clip sterilization, 138
Mepivacaine (Carbocaine), 10t
  clinical considerations, 12
  fatalities from, 15
  safe dosage, 13
Mesosalpinx, bleeding, during minilaparotomy, 169
Metal halide light source, for hysteroscopy, 76
Methotrexate, transvaginal injection
  for cervical pregnancy, 236–238, 237f
  for cornual pregnancy, 236
  for tubal pregnancy, 235f, 235–236
Methylcyanoacrylate, tubal injection, 183
Methylergonovine maleate (Methergine), postoperative, first trimester abortion, 53, 58–59
Metrorrhagia, 94
Microlaparoscopy, 137
Midazolam (Versed)
  premedication for local anesthesia, 6
  preoperative
    in diagnostic hysteroscopy, 85
    in dilatation and curettage, 33
  respiratory depression, 93
Mifepristone (RU 486), 41–42
Minilaparotomy, 155–171, 178–179
  bladder laceration during, 168–169
  bowel laceration during, 169
  closure, 167
  complications, 155, 167–170
  failed procedure, 169–170
  incision, 155, 162–163
    wound hematoma, 170
    wound infection, 170
  instrumentation, 160f, 160t, 161f

local anesthesia, 155–159
  anesthetic injection, 161–162, 164f, 165f
  prerequisites, 156–159
mesosalpingeal bleeding during, 169
nurse-counselor's role, 156, 158, 159
operating room environment, 158
operating room personnel, 159
patient positioning, 160
premedication, 159
in premenstrual patient, 5
prerequisites, 156–159
  adequate patient motivation, 158
  gentle handling of instruments and tissues, 159
  informed consent, 156, 157f
  preoperative counseling, 156, 158
  preoperative pelvic examination, 158
technique, 160–167, 163f–166f
uterine perforation during, 168
vasovagal reaction, 161, 167
wound hematoma, 170
wound infection, 170
Misoprostol, pregnancy termination with RU 486, 41
Monitoring
  guidelines for sedation and analgesia, 7
  pulse oximetry (*see* Pulse oximetry)
Morbidity and mortality
  abortion, 1
  local anesthetic toxicity, fatalities from, 15
Morrison's pouch, 216, 217f
Mortality rates (*see* Morbidity and mortality)
Myoma
  clinical presentation, 113
  diagnostic hysteroscopy, 114–115
  evaluation protocol, 114–115
    second opinion, 116
  in first trimester abortion, 44
  obstructing, in first trimester abortion, 56–57, 57f
  sonohysterography, 114, 209f
  submucous, 94
    attachment by anatomic site, 117
    cavity-filling, 123f, 124
    classification, 116
    degree of intramural extension, 116–117
    size and volume, 117
  surgical removal (*see* Myomectomy)
  transvaginal sonography, 114
Myomectomy, 95–96, 113–125
  dilatation, 118
  laminaria tents in, 118
  laparoscopy in, 118–119
  medical pretreatment, 118
  myoma coring technique, 96, 124, 124f
    electrodes for, 121
  myoma resection technique, 96, 122f, 123–124
    electrodes for, 121
  myoma shaving technique, 95, 121, 122f, 123
  operating room setup, 120–121
    electrosurgical unit, 121
    operative hysteroscope, 120–121
    specialized electrodes, 121
    ultrasound, 120

patient presentation, 113–116
  intractable uterine bleeding, 114–115
  recurrent pregnancy loss, 116
  second opinion for known fibroids, 116
patient selection, 116–118
  classification of attachment by anatomic site, 117
  degree of intramural extension, 116–117
  desire for future childbearing, 117
  multiple myomata, 117
  myoma size and volume, 117
  patient age, 117
  patient weight, 117–118
planning the operation, 118–120
  simultaneous endomyometrial resection, 119–120
  sonographer's role, 120
  sonographic guidance, 119, 119f, 120
  techniques, 121–124
    power settings, 121
  thermal destruction, 95
  transvaginal sonography in, 114, 120
  two-stage procedure, 119
  vaporizing electrodes, 121
  vasopressin in, 118
Myometritis, postoperative, hysteroscopic surgery, 111, 112

Naloxone hydrochloride (Narcan), for respiratory depression, in office hysteroscopy, 93
Narcotic analgesics, midazolam plus, respiratory depression, 93
National Fire Protection Association, Inc., *Life Safety Code*, 268, 271
Needles
  for injection of anesthetic, 187
  for injection of myoma, 121
  for injection of vasopressin, 118
Neodynium (Nd):YAG laser
  endometrial ablation, 94, 95
  myolysis, 95
Nepal, laparoscopic sterilization services, 180
Nesacaine (*see* Chloroprocaine)
Nietze, Maximillian, 65
Nitrogen, liquid, endometrial ablation, 94
Nitrous oxide, pneumoperitoneum, 136–137
No-load flow rate, resectoscope, 98
Novocain (*see* Procaine)
Nupercaine (*see* Dibucaine)
Nurse anesthetist, role in hysteroscopic surgery, 99
Nurse-counselor, role in minilaparotomy under local anesthesia, 156, 158, 159

Obesity
  bladder laceration during minilaparotomy, 168
  first trimester abortion and, 55
Oblepias, Virgilio, 180, 181
Office surgical facility
  accreditation (*see also* Accreditation), 25, 245–279
  advantages, 22
  certification, 25

Office surgical facility—*continued*
  cost of, 23
  emergency medications, 27f
  emergency oropharyngeal suction equipment, 27f
  facility regulations and standards, 295–298
    construction and fire safety standards, 296
    federal jurisdiction, optional, 297
    jurisdiction of reviewing authorities, 297
    local jurisdiction, 297
    Medicare requirements for physical environment, 296
    sources of facility fee reimbursement and, 297–298
    spatial provision, 296
    state health and state fire marshal jurisdictions
      mandatory, 297
      optional, 297
  fees (*see* Economic issues)
  floor plan, 24f, 272f–273f
  government regulations, 22
  instrument sterilization, 26, 28f
  monitoring devices, 26
  operating room, 23, 25f, 187
  prerequisites, 22
  reimbursement (*see* Economic issues)
  resuscitation backup, 26, 27–28
  risk management (*see also* Risk management), 279–283
  safeguards, 25–28
  safety, 245
  ultrasound use (*see* Ultrasonography)
Operating table, 187
  for suprapubic minilaparotomy, 162f
Oropharyngeal suction equipment, for office surgical facility, 27f
Outpatient surgical facilities, 21–28
  accreditation (*see* Accreditation)
  choice of anesthetic, 187
  facility regulations and standards, 295–298
  female sterilization (*see also* Sterilization, female)
    free-standing female sterilization services in United States, 179–180
    special considerations, 183
  gynecologic procedures (*see also specific procedures*), 187–194
  instrumentation, 187
  lighting, 187
  Medicare certification, 246, 295–296
  minilaparotomy tubal ligation programs, 178
  premedication, 187–188
Ovarian cancer
  screening, office-based ultrasound, 201–202, 215
  sonographic appearance, 213, 214f
Ovarian cyst, 45f
  sonographic appearance, 213, 213f
  transvaginal sonographic puncture and drainage, 231–232, 232f
Ovary
  cystadenoma, 213, 214f
  cystic teratoma, 213, 214f
  dermoid, 214f
  endometrioma, 213, 214f
  menstrual cycle changes, 210
  normal, sonographic appearance, 210, 211f
  polycystic, sonographic appearance, 211, 212f
  in salpingitis, 218, 218f
  transvaginal sonography, 210–215
    "beads(pearls)-on-a-string" appearance, 211, 212f
    corpus luteum, 211, 212f
    menopausal/postmenopausal, 210
    neoplastic pathology, 213, 214f
    normal ovaries, 210, 211f
    polycystic appearance, 211, 212f
Oxygen therapy
  portable oxygen tank, 26f
  for respiratory depression, in office hysteroscopy, 93
Oxytocic agents, in first trimester abortion, 58–60
Oxytocin (Pitocin), postoperative, first trimester abortion, 52, 58–60

Pain
  abnormal, postoperative, 13
  pelvic (*see* Pelvic pain)
  referred, in CO_2 hysteroscopy, 77
  uterine, during cervical dilatation, 29
    patient counseling, 33
Pain mapping, diagnostic laparoscopy under local anesthesia, 136–137
Pantaleoni, 65
Pap smear surveillance, quality improvement study, 263f–265f
Para-aminobenzoic acid (PABA) esters, 9
Paracervical block
  diagnostic hysteroscopy, 85, 87
  dilatation and curettage, 34, 46–47
    advantage of, 35
  first trimester abortion, 46–47
    advantage of, 52, 57
  intrauterine device insertion/removal, 192
  lidocaine, 17
Pathology services, AAAHC standards for pathology and medical laboratory services, 278–279
Patient, rejection of local anesthesia, 2, 5
Patient Bill of Rights, 253f
Patient education
  abortion, first trimester, 43
  hysteroscopic endomyometrial resection, 97
  hysteroscopy, 83
    video documentation, 80
  local anesthesia, 4–5
Peer review, 258
  occurrence screening review worksheet, 258, 260f–262f
  physician peer review roster, 259f
Pelvic examination
  bimanual, incorporation of transvaginal sonography, 200–201
  postoperative, first trimester abortion, 51–52

preoperative
    first trimester abortion, 44–45
    minilaparotomy tubal ligation, 158
Pelvic pain
    chronic, diagnostic laparoscopy under local anesthesia, 134–136
    mapping, diagnostic laparoscopy under local anesthesia, 136–137
    postabortal, 61
Perforation, uterine (see Uterus, perforation)
Perineorrhaphy, reverse, 191
Perineum, plastic syrgery, 190
Peritoneal inclusion cyst, postoperative, transvaginal sonographic puncture and drainage, 238, 239f
Phenergan (see Promethazine hydrochloride)
Phenol mucilage, tubal injection, 183
Philippines, laparoscopic sterilization services, 180, 181
Physical Environment Checklist for Ambulatory Surgical Centers, 271
Physical examination
    for office hysteroscopy, 82
    surgical procedures, documentation for Medicare certification, 277–278
Pitocin (see Oxytocin)
Placenta previa, transvaginal sonography, 204, 205f
Placental polyp, sonographic appearance, 206, 208f
Planned Parenthood, minilaparotomy tubal ligation services, 178–179
Plastic surgery
    excision of redundant tissue of labia minora, 190
    excision of vaginal septum, 191
    incision of imperforate hymen, 190
    incision of tight/rigid hymen, 191
    reverse perineorrhaphy, 191
    vulva, vagina, or perineum, 190–191
Pneumoperitoneum
    gas for, 136–137, 143
    for Hulka clip sterilization, 143
Polyglycollate suture, 188, 194
Polyp
    placental, 206, 208f
    uterine, sonohysterography, 210f
Pontocaine (see Tetracaine)
Postmenopausal period
    ovarian cysts, 232
    sonographic evaluation of ovary, 210
Potassium chloride, transvaginal injection, for ectopic pregnancy, 235
Pratt dilators, 49, 100
Pre-Term Clinic, outpatient, free-standing female sterilization services in United States, 179
Pregnancy
    after endomyometrial resection, 112
    after sterilization, 184
    cervical
        sonographic diagnostic criteria, 237
        transvaginal methotrexate injection for, 236–238, 237f
        cervical sonographic anatomy, 203f, 203–204, 204f
    cornual, transvaginal potassium chloride/methotrexate injection for, 236
    early, transvaginal sonography, 219–224, 220f–222f
    ectopic
        after bipolar tubal coagulation, 176
        clinical features, 45–46
        culdocentesis, 238–240
        sonography in, 45–46
        transvaginal potassium chloride/methotrexate injection for, 235f, 235–236
        transvaginal sonographic puncture techniques for, 234–238
        transvaginal sonography, 215f, 215–217, 216f
        type I (live, unruptured tube), 215, 215f
        type II, 217
        type III (ruptured, bleeding), 216, 216f
    multifetal
        reduction, 233–234, 234f
        sonographic detection, 220, 221f
    tubal (see Pregnancy, ectopic)
Pregnancy loss, recurrent, hysteroscopic surgery for, 116
Pregnancy reduction, ultrasound-guided, 233–234, 234f
Premenstrual period, minilaparotomy during, 5
Prilocaine (Citanest), 10t
Procaine (Novocain), 10t
    historical perspective, 9
Promethazine hydrochloride (Phenergan)
    in Hulka clip sterilization, 138
    in minilaparotomy tubal ligation, 159
    premedication for local anesthesia, 6, 187
    for vasovagal reaction, 17
Propranolol, for epinephrine-induced blood pressure increase, 12
Psychological issues
    local anesthesia, 5
    postabortal depression, 63
Pulse oximetry, 26
    monitoring, AAAHC standards, 274–275
    in office hysteroscopy, 79
Puncture procedures, 229–241
    amniocentesis, 240
    automated puncture device, 229, 230f
    chorionic villi sampling, 240
    culdocentesis, 238–240
    drainage procedures, 238, 239f
    ectopic pregnancy management, 234–238
        cervical pregnancy, 236–238, 237f
        cornual pregnancy, 236
        salpingocentesis, 235f, 235–236
    free-hand approach, 229
    informed consent, 230–231
    multifetal pregnancy reduction, 233–234, 234f
    ovarian cyst puncture and drainage, 231–232, 232f
    in reproductive endocrinology, 231
    ultrasound slice thickness, 229
Pyometra, dilatation and curettage for, 33

Quality assurance, 258
  pap smear surveillance, 263f–265f
  quality care control report, 266f
Quinacrine, in tubal sterilization, 183

Reimbursement (*see* Economic issues)
Resectoscope
  for endomyometrial resection, 98
  no-load flow rate, 98
Respiratory arrest, in hysteroscopy, 79, 93
Respiratory depression, in hysteroscopy, 79, 93
Resuscitation
  backup for local anesthesia, 8
  office surgical facility, 27–28
Reverse perineorrhaphy, 191
Risk management, 279–283
  AAAHC standards, 258–259, 266f, 267
  audit the practice documentation, 282
  components, 279–283
  develop standard procedures, 280
  document all patient encounters, 282
  financial management, 280, 281f
  goals, 279
  identify key processes and procedures, 279, 280
  infection control practices, 280
  patient profile determination, 280
  quality care control report, 266f–267f
  review and revise procedures, 282–283
  staff development, 280
Room air, pneumoperitoneum, 136–137, 143
RU 486 (mifepristone), 41–42

Safety issues, office surgical facility, 245, 271
Saline
  hypertonic, correction of serum sodium, 110
  uterine distention medium (*see* Hysteroscopy, low viscosity fluids)
Saline infusion sonography (SIS) (*see* Sonohysterography)
Salpingitis, transvaginal sonography, 217–218, 218f, 219f
  acute phase, 217–218, 218f, 219f
  chronic phase, 218, 219f
Salpingocentesis, transvaginal potassium chloride/methotrexate injection, 235f, 235–236
Sargis tenaculum-sound, 134f
Schnepper, Fred, 179
Schroeder, C., 66
Screening studies, ovarian cancer, office-based ultrasound, 201–202
Scrub nurse, role in hysteroscopic surgery, 99
Sedation
  intravenous
    areas of concern, 85–86
    for diagnostic hysteroscopy, 85
  practice guidelines for nonanesthesiologists, 7
Silicone, catalyzed liquid silicone, tubal injection, 183
Skin lesions, removal, local anesthesia, 194
"Sliding organ sign," 199

Society of Reproductive Surgeons, Guidelines for Attaining Privileges in Gynecologic Operative Endoscopy, 128–130
Sodium, serum
  correction, 110
  postoperative, hysteroscopic surgery, 109
Sodium chloride solution, correction of serum sodium, 110
Sonography (*see* Transvaginal sonography; Ultrasonography)
Sonohysterography (saline infusion sonography [SIS]), 206, 208–210, 209f, 210f
  clinical applications, 209–210
  in hysteroscopic myomectomy, 120
  instrumentation, 208
  technique, 209
  uterine myomata, 114, 115f, 209f
  uterine polyps, 210f
Sorbitol
  excess absorption, 108–109
  uterine distention medium (*see* Hysteroscopy, low viscosity fluids)
Sounding
  cervical os, 34, 35f
    first trimester abortion, 48–49
  uterus
    first trimester abortion, 48–49
    retroflexed, 55
Speculum(a), for office hysteroscopy, 69
Spinal anesthesia, 1
Stadol (*see* Butorphanol tartrate)
Staff personnel
  anesthesia selection, 4
  training for hysteroscopy, 81
Stark, David, 4
Stenosis, cervical
  in hysteroscopic endomyometrial resection, 102
  internal os, 56
Sterilization, instruments, in office surgical facility, 26, 28f
Sterilization, female, 173–185
  culdoscopic tubal ligation, 182, 193
  federal funding, U.S. Department of Health, Education, and Welfare regulations, 184
  general anesthesia, 21
  historical aspects, 173–174
  laparoscopic methods, 131, 174–178
    bipolar tubal coagulation, 150, 175f, 175–176
    Falope ring (Yoon band), 150, 175f, 177
    Filshie clip application, 175f, 177–178
    Hulka clip application (*see also* Hulka clip sterilization), 137–150, 175f, 176
    membership survey of American Association of Gynecological Laparoscopists, 176t
  outpatient, free-standing female sterilization services in United States, 179–180
  Pomeroy ligation, 175f
  programs in developing nations, 180–182
  tubal thermocautery, 182–183
  unipolar tubal coagulation, 174–175

legal status, 183–184
mentally incompetent individuals, 184
minilaparotomy tubal ligation (*see also* Minilaparotomy), 155–171, 178–179
outpatient facilities, 21
pioneers, 173–174
popularity of tubal ligation, 174
predictions for future, 184–185
pregnancy rates after, 184
transcervical methods, 183
vaginal tubal ligation, 182, 193
Sterilization, male, 173
Stirrups, for office hysteroscopy, 69, 70f
Succinylcholine (Anectine), for anesthetic-induced convulsions, 14
Suprapubic minilaparotomy (*see* Minilaparotomy)
Surgeon
    rejection of local anesthesia, 2
    training and responsibilities in hysteroscopic surgery, 99
Syncope (*see also* Vasovagal reaction)
    convulsions, 8
    diazepam-induced, 6
Synechiae, uterine, postabortal, 63

Tachycardia, epinephrine-induced, 12
Tamoxifen therapy, endometrial thickness, sonohysterographic determination, 209–210, 210f
Tamponade, for hemorrhage during hysteroscopic surgery, 112
Telescopes, for hysteroscopy, 71–75
Tenaculum
    for abortion, first trimester, 47f
    for office hysteroscopy, 70
Teratoma, cystic, ovarian, 213, 214f
Tetracaine (Pontocaine), 10t
Thailand, laparoscopic sterilization services
    Bangkok, 181
    Chiang Mai, 180, 181
Thermocautery, tubal sterilization, 182–183
Thorazine (*see* Chlorpromazine)
Training (*see* Medical education)
Tranquilizer, premedication for local anesthesia, 6
Transvaginal sonography
    "beads-on-a-string" sign
        hydrosalpinx, 218, 219f
        ovary, 211, 212f
    clinical applications, 199
    dynamic use of, 199
    early pregnancy, 219–224, 220f–222f
        chorionic sac, 219–220
        fetal heartbeat, 220, 221f
        multifetal pregnancies, 220, 221f
        prenatal diagnosis of chromosome aneuploidy, 221, 222f, 224
        vaginal bleeding, 220–221, 222f
    ectopic pregnancy, 215f, 215–217, 216f
    in hysteroscopic endomyometrial resection, 96
    in hysteroscopic myomectomy, 114, 120
    incorporation into bimanual pelvic examination, 200–201
    office use, 197–224
        advantages, 199–200
        availability of equipment, 200
        cervical evaluation, 202–204, 203f
        clinical applications, 199
        early pregnancy, 219–224, 220f–222f
        ease of operation, 200
        fallopian tube evaluation, 215–218
        incorporation into bimanual pelvic examination, 200–201
        ovarian cancer screening, 201–202
        ovarian evaluation, 210–215
        statistics, 198, 198f
        uterine evaluation, 204, 206–210
    ovarian neoplasia, 213, 214f
    in pain mapping, 136
    picture quality, 198
    placenta previa, 204, 205f
    puncture procedures (*see also* Puncture procedures), 229–241
    salpingitis, 217–218, 218f, 219f
        acute phase, 217–218, 218f, 219f
        chronic phase, 218, 219f
    "sliding organ sign," 199
    sonohysterography, 206, 208–210, 209f, 210f
    training, 202
    uterine myomata, 114
Tubo-ovarian abscess, 218, 219f
Tubo-ovarian complex, 218, 218f
Tumor(s), ovarian, transvaginal sonography, 213, 214f
Tyson, Judy, 51

Ultrasonography
    abdominal, in hysteroscopic myomectomy, 119, 119f
    acoustic window, 120
    in hysteroscopic endomyometrial resection, four-leaf clover appearance, 105f
    in hysteroscopic myomectomy, 96, 120
    multifetal pregnancy reduction, 233–234, 234f
    office-based vs. "formal" imaging study, 201
    office use, 197–224
        advantages, 199–200
        cervical evaluation, 202–204
        clinical applications, 199, 202–224
        dynamic use, 199
        early pregnancy detection, 219–222, 224
        equipment setup, 223f
        fallopian tube evaluation, 215–218
        incorporation into bimanual pelvic examination, 200–201
        ovarian cancer screening, 201–202
        ovarian evaluation, 210–215
        picture quality, 198
        statistics, 198, 198f
        training, 202
        uterine evaluation, 204, 206–210

Ultrasonography—*continued*
  preoperative evaluation, first trimester abortion, 45–46
  puncture procedures (*see also* Puncture procedures), 229–241
Urocatcher drape, 97–98, 104f
Urticaria, anesthetic induced, 16
U.S. Department of Health, Education, and Welfare, regulations governing female sterilization, 184
Uterine aspirator, for abortion, first trimester, 49f
Uterine atony, postabortal, 52
  persistent, 59
  prevention and management, 58–60
Uterosacral block, 29, 30f, 31f
  abortion, first trimester, 47
  dilatation and curettage, 34
Uterus
  abnormal bleeding
    dilatation and curettage for, 30–32
    evaluation protocol, 114–115
    hemorrhage (*see* Hemorrhage, uterine)
    hysteroscopic surgery for (*see* Hysteroscopic surgery)
    hysteroscopy in, 67, 114–115
    intractable, 114–115
    laboratory evaluation, 82–83
    menstrual abnormalities, 93–94
    postmenopausal, 94
    quest for treatment, 94
    sonohysterography in, 114, 115f
    transvaginal sonography in, 114
  anteverted
    hysteroscopic examination, 88f
    transvaginal sonography, 204, 206f
  dextrorotation, failed minilaparotomy and, 169
  distention media, 76–79
    carbon dioxide, 76–77
    high molecular weight dextran 70, 78–79
    low viscosity fluids, 77–78
  massage, postevacuation, 52
  myomata (*see* Myoma)
  perforation
    during abortion, 60–61
    during dilatation and curettage, 37f, 37–38, 60–61
    during hysteroscopic surgery, 110–111
      "cold" injury, 110
      "hot" injury, 110–111
    hysteroscopy in, 91
    during minilaparotomy, 168
    during office hysteroscopy, 92–93
    during open laparoscopy, 150–151
  retroflexed, sounding, 55
  retroverted
    first trimester abortion and, 55
    pelvic examination, 44
    transvaginal sonography, 206
  rupture, during hysteroscopic surgery, 111
  sensory innervation, 29, 30f

sounding, first trimester abortion, 48–49
synechiae, postabortal, 63
transvaginal sonography, 204, 206–210
unicornuate, 44
  sounding, 48

Vacurettes, for abortion, first trimester, 48f
Vacuum curettage, for abortion, 50–51
Vagina
  abscess, incision and drainage, 188
  biopsy, 188
  bleeding
    early pregnancy, transvaginal sonography, 220–221, 222f
    suture ligation of bleeders, 192
  plastic surgery, 190
  septum, excision, 191
Valium (*see* Diazepam)
Vaporizing electrodes, for myomectomy, 121
VaporTrode, myoma destruction, 95
Vasoconstrictor agents, in local anesthesia, 12
  hypertensive reaction, 15
Vasopressin
  in cervical conization, 192
  in hysteroscopic myomectomy, 118
  intracervical, in hysteroscopic endomyometrial resection, 100–101
Vasovagal episode(s), 8
Vasovagal reaction, 167
  anesthetic agents, 16–17
  during dilatation and curettage, 38
  during intrauterine device insertion/removal, 193
  during minilaparotomy, 161, 167
  during office hysteroscopy, 92
Ventricular arrhythmia, lidocaine in, 14
Versed (*see* Midazolam)
Video, manual vacuum aspiration, 51
Video documentation
  in endomyometrial resection, 98
  in hysteroscopy, 80–81
    light source, 76
Volonelgesia, 4
Vulva
  abscess, incision and drainage, 188
  biopsy, 188
  plastic surgery, 190

Word catheter, 190
Wound hematoma, minilaparotomy, 170
Wound infection, minilaparotomy, 170
Wydase (*see* Hyaluronidase)
Wynter, H.H., 193

Xenon light source, for hysteroscopy, 76
Xylocaine (*see* Lidocaine)

Yoon, Im Bae, 177
Yoon band (Falope ring), 150, 175f, 177

Augment Your Resources with These Titles:

Procedures in Women's Health
Roger P. Smith, MD, Frank W. Ling, MD, and Douglas W. Laube, MD, MEd

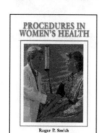

In this practical source you'll find descriptions of common procedures that can be easily done in your office, with nearly 300 photos and drawings that offer the strong visual perspective you need to perform primary care procedures successfully. The material is organized by body region with chapters that cover...

- ophthalmology
- orthopaedics
- ear, nose and throat
- neurology
- colon and rectal procedures
- dermatology
- and urology.

Each chapter takes you through the proper use of instruments, followed by a description of normal and abnormal findings you're likely to encounter, and the text's consistent format helps you find the information you need in a flash.
1997/about 400 pages
#0-683-18219-6

Atlas of Pelvic Surgery Third Edition
Clifford R. Wheeless, Jr., MD

Excellent illustrations and the expert commentary of Dr. Clifford Wheeless bring you a unique perspective on pelvic surgery. This step-by-step guide is organized by organ system for easy reference, and extensive material is included on new operative procedures such as laparoscopy.
1996/544 pages/475 illustrations/#0-683-08956-0

Gynecologic Endoscopy Principles in Practice
Michael J. Sammarco, MD, Thomas G. Stovall, MD, and John F. Steege, MD

Now one text brings together the basics on gynecologic endoscopy, providing a foundation of knowledge and skill that will benefit your patients and your practice. *Gynecologic Endoscopy* is the only text to offer all these benefits:

- integration of skills learned on tissue models with actual cases
- an emphasis on safety, with details on avoiding and managing complications
- outstanding illustrations clearly depicting techniques
- a comprehensive catalog of instruments—unique to this volume!

1996/256 pages/200 illustrations/#0-683-07509-8

Try Them for 30 Days
Preview these titles for a full month. If you're not completely satisfied, return them to us within 30 days with no further obligation (US and Canada only). There's never any risk to you.

From the US:
Phone orders accepted 24 hours a day, 7 days a week
Call: 1-800-638-0672
Fax: 1-800-447-8438

From Canada:
Call: 1-800-665-1148
Fax: 1-800-665-0103

International customers please call:
In the UK and Europe 44-(171) 385-2357
In Southeast Asia 852-2610-2339
All other countries 1-410-528-4223

INTERNET:
E-mail: custserv@wwilkins.com
Home page: http://www.wwilkins.com

Williams & Wilkins
A Waverly Company
351 West Camden Street
Baltimore, Maryland 21201-2436